THIRD EDITION

Effective Patient Education

A Guide to Increased Compliance

DONNA R. FALVO, RN, PhD, CRC

JONES AND BARTLETT PUBLISHERS

Sudbury, Massachusetts

BOSTON   TORONTO   LONDON   SINGAPORE

World Headquarters

Jones and Bartlett Publishers
40 Tall Pine Drive
Sudbury, MA 01776
978-443-5000
info@jbpub.com
www.jbpub.com

Jones and Bartlett Publishers
Canada
6339 Ormindale Way
Mississauga, ON L5V 1J2
CANADA

Jones and Bartlett Publishers
International
Barb House, Barb Mews
London W6 7PA
UK

Jones and Bartlett's books and products are available through most bookstores and online booksellers. To contact Jones and Bartlett Publishers directly, call 800-832-0034, fax 978-443-8000, or visit our website at www.jbpub.com.

Substantial discounts on bulk quantities of Jones and Bartlett's publications are available to corporations, professional associations, and other qualified organizations. For details and specific discount information, contact the special sales department at Jones and Bartlett via the above contact information or send an email to specialsales@jbpub.com.

ISBN-13: 978-0-7637-3157-1
ISBN-10: 0-7637-3157-9

The authors, editor, and publisher have made every effort to provide accurate information. However, they are not responsible for errors, omissions, or for any outcomes related to the use of the contents of this book and take no responsibility for the use of the products and procedures described. Treatments and side effects described in this book may not be applicable to all people; likewise, some people may require a dose or experience a side effect that is not described herein. Drugs and medical devices are discussed that may have limited availability controlled by the Food and Drug Administration (FDA) for use only in a research study or clinical trial. Research, clinical practice, and government regulations often change the accepted standard in this field. When consideration is being given to use of any drug in the clinical setting, the health care provider or reader is responsible for determining FDA status of the drug, reading the package insert, and reviewing prescribing information for the most up-to-date recommendations on dose, precautions, and contraindications, and determining the appropriate usage for the product. This is especially important in the case of drugs that are new or seldom used.

Library of Congress Cataloging-in-Publication Data
Falvo, Donna R.
  Effective patient education : a guide to increased compliance / Donna
Falvo.— 3rd ed.
    p. ; cm.
Includes bibliographical references and index.
  ISBN 0-7637-3157-9
  1. Patient education. 2. Patient compliance.
  [DNLM: 1. Patient Education. 2. Patient Compliance. W 85 F197e
2004] I. Title.
  R727.4.F35 2004
  615.5'071—dc22
6048   2003017072

Production Credits
Acquisitions Editor: Kevin Sullivan
Production Manager: Amy Rose
Associate Production Editor: Karen C. Ferreira
Editorial Assistant: Amy Sibley
Marketing Manager: Joy Stark-Vancs
Marketing Associate: Elizabeth Waterfall
Manufacturing and Inventory Coordinator: Amy Bacus
Cover Design: Kristin E. Ohlin
Composition: Northeast Compositors
Printing and Binding: Malloy, Inc.
Cover Printing: Malloy, Inc.

Printed in the United States of America
11 10 09 08 07   10 9 8 7 6 5 4 3

*This Book is Dedicated
to the Memory of
Christina
and
Armida*

Contents

Preface

With the emphasis on patient education as a patient right and health professional's responsibility, it seems that patients would easily learn how to treat and control disease adequately, as well as how to prevent many diseases. Given the abundance of accessible patient education information, not to mention the level of medical sophistication and technological advances available, it is shocking that large numbers of individuals continue to be incapacitated or debilitated by, or succumb to, conditions that could be controlled or treated effectively, or that they continue to develop preventable diseases.

Of course, anyone who has been a patient or who has worked with patients knows that recommendations given by health professionals are not always followed. Knowing what to do and how to do it does not guarantee patients' willingness or ability to follow health advice. Patients enter the health care system with preexisting beliefs and attitudes, fears and anxieties, previous experiences, and individual life and family circumstances, all of which impact on their willingness and ability to follow health recommendations.

In order to conduct effective patient education, health professionals must be aware of individual patient variables that influence the degree to which they follow health advice, and then use this information to communicate health recommendations in accordance with individual patient need. There is no cookbook approach that works for every patient. Effective patient education is a way of communicating health information that fosters a partnership between patient and health professional. It facilitates open sharing of information so that mutually agreed upon goals can be established. This partnership can exist only in an atmosphere of mutual trust and respect in which patients and health professionals cooperate to identify barriers to patient compliance and overcome them.

This book will help health professionals develop skills and knowledge necessary to conduct effective patient education in a time and resource efficient way. It emphasizes a team approach to patient education, recognizing that, in the complexity of health care today, many health professionals are involved in patient care. The book is, therefore, written for nurses, physicians, physical therapists, dietitians, pharmacists, or other health professionals with responsibility to educate patients to enhance or maintain their health and well being. Case studies are used throughout the book. Although the cases are based on actual situations, the names and details of the cases have been altered in order to protect

nt and health professional anonymity. These fictitious names were chosen to make
cases more alive for the reader, while underscoring the diversity of patients in most
ealth care practices.

The goal of effective patient education is to help patients make informed choices and
to provide guidance and support, so that they have the best opportunity to achieve their
maximum health potential. Effective patient education need not be costly in either time
or resources. Rather, it can increase quality of care by increasing the chances that patients
will be able to carry out health practices that will enhance their general health status.

ABOUT THE AUTHOR

Donna Falvo is a registered nurse, licensed psychologist, and certified rehabilitation counselor. She has been a staff nurse, nursing instructor, counselor, and professor of family and
community medicine, as well as professor of rehabilitation counseling. The author of
numerous articles on patient education and patient compliance, she was named a Mary
Switzer Scholar in 1986 and was elected to Sigma Xi National Scientific Research Society
in 1995. She served for 4 years as chair of the Society of Teachers of Family Medicine's
Group on Patient Education and served on the Steering Committee for the National
Patient Education Conference sponsored by the Academy of Family Practice and Society
of Teachers of Family Medicine. In addition, Dr. Falvo has been an invited speaker at a
number of national patient education conferences sponsored by organizations such as the
American Hospital Association and the American Physical Therapy Association. She has
also been invited to conduct workshops and speak at patient education conferences sponsored by various universities and private corporations. She was elected president of the
American Rehabilitation Counseling Association in 1998. Dr. Falvo serves on the editorial board of the *Rehabilitation Counseling Bulletin* and is also author of the book *Medical and
Psychosocial Aspects of Chronic Illness and Disability.* She currently lives in Chapel Hill, North
Carolina, where she works as a consultant.

Patient Compliance:
A Brief Overview

1

DEFINING PATIENT COMPLIANCE

It was once expected that patients, with minimum information and few questions, should and would follow advice given by their health professionals. Times have changed. With social changes in all segments of society, it is now generally accepted that patients should be fully informed about health-related matters and should be involved in and accept more responsibility for their health and health care. The importance of seeking patients' active cooperation and involvement in decisions about their health is now widely recognized. Patients have access to more information than ever before and have more responsibility in directing and managing their own care. The expectation is that with increased information, patients will follow treatment recommendations; however, this does not always seem to be the case. Despite increased access to information, and increased responsibility for their own care, studies indicate that a large number of patients still fail to follow recommendations given by the health professional (Blessing-Moore 1996, Butler et al. 1996, Vivian and Wilcox 2000).

At a time when there is increasing information available to patients and increased focus on patient autonomy, patient's rights, and consumerism, it is ironic that patient compliance continues to be a problem and that a term such as "patient compliance," with its authoritarian and coercive connotations, is still found in health-related literature.

In the 60 or more years since the concept of *patient compliance* was first recognized (Koltun and Stone 1986), and over the last 35 years intensely studied, there has been considerable controversy over use of the term. The term *compliance* has long been criticized as denoting a power differential between patient and health professional. The term, for many, implies yielding or obedience to authority. In an attempt to diminish the paternalistic and authoritarian nature of the term *compliance*, terms such as *treatment adherence, therapeutic alliance, collaboration,* or *concordance* have been coined as substitutes to describe the extent to which patients follow the advice and recommendations provided by health professionals. Semantics, however, sometimes become cumbersome, distracting from the problem they are used to describe. No matter what the problem is called, a problem still exists.

Despite information available to patients, and despite advances in knowledge and sophistication of technology for the prevention, diagnosis, treatment, or cure of disease, patients continue to succumb to diseases that could have been prevented or effectively treated. Although treatment failure or iatrogenic causes account for some patient morbidity and even mortality, in a wide number of instances the cause is that patients simply did not adhere to recommendations given to them.

Assuming that the patient's condition has been accurately diagnosed and the appropriate treatment prescribed, the only way that recommended preventative measures or therapeutic regimens can be effective is if patients correctly follow recommendations and advice given by the health professional. Compliance, or more to the point, noncompliance, continues to be a problem that needs to be identified, studied, and understood. The problem of noncompliance extends to all health professions. There is a wide and diverse body of literature in the area of patient compliance that spans most health professions, including medicine, dentistry, nursing, physical therapy, and social sciences to list a few (Trostle 1997).

Although specific words used to describe a phenomenon significantly influence how a phenomenon is understood, semantics may not be as important as the philosophical context in which they are used. For simplicity's sake, the word *compliance* is used in this book because the term continues to be used frequently in the literature (Lutfey and Wishnet 1999) to convey the extent to which patients follow recommendations given by their health professional (Lutfey and Wishnet, 1999). In the case of this book, it is *not* used to imply a power differentiation between patient and health professional, or to suggest that patients should follow recommendations blindly. The underlying assumption of this book is that compliance is a reflection of good communication and fit of ideas about treatment between patient and health professional. Compliance is the end product of a relationship that is built on respect, active participation, and partnership between patient and health professional, not coercion or manipulation on the part of either.

IMPORTANCE OF COMPLIANCE

Compliance to health recommendations has been the focus of research for a number of years because of its importance to the health and well being of patients, the health care system, and society as a whole. The health benefit of properly treated and controlled disease is obvious. Many disease conditions, complications of disease, as well as disability and death can be forestalled or prevented through patients' control of their health behaviors and through appropriate adherence to therapeutic regimes (Johnson and Bootman 1995, Liberman and Rotarius 1999, Hernandez 1995, Nicolucci et al. 1996). Compliance with treatment recommendations can also have an impact on general public health, especially in the treatment or eradication of infectious disease, such as tuberculosis or HIV (Freeman et al. 1996, Johnston and Mann 2000). Failure to follow health recommendations impacts society in other ways as well. Noncompliance, which results in increased morbidity, mortality, disability, or increased use of health care services, causes decreased productivity through lost work days and drives up insurance and other health care costs (Feldman 1982).

Noncompliance is a pervasive problem with implications not only for the health of patients but also for the effective use of resources. Patients who seek medical attention but do not follow medical advice overutilize health services. The role and importance of patient compliance in treatment of acute conditions is one example. Acute conditions, such as infections, can often be cured with short courses of medication or treatment. Patient failure to adhere to recommended treatment, however, can result in progression of the condition or development of complications that require increased medical care and treatment with consequences of increased morbidity and, in some instances, mortality (Birkhead et al. 1989). Likewise, medications purchased but never taken are wasted. Patients who miss appointments misuse the time of the health professional and perhaps waste a time slot that could have been used by another patient. Patient compliance plays an important role in disease prevention as well. For example, the health risks brought about by tobacco use, excessive consumption of alcohol, sedentary life style, and poor dietary practices are well known. Engaging in healthy life-style behaviors can significantly decrease the risk of developing a number of diseases such as cancer, heart disease, stroke, or other serious illnesses (Burke and Dunbar-Jacob 1995, Evangelista and Dracup 2000). When failure to follow recommendations results in development of chronic disease, there are ramifications for the patient, the health care system, and society.

Compliance with treatment recommendations in the control of chronic diseases such as diabetes, heart disease, and hypertension has been shown to decrease morbidity rates and permanent disability, enabling patients to continue to live active and productive lives (Evangelista and Dracup 2000).

Although considerable time and expense have been used to develop highly effective and relatively safe treatments for a number of diseases, patients continue to be incapacitated or debilitated by, or die from, conditions for which effective treatments are available (Morrison et al. 2000). Likewise, although health risks for a number of serious diseases are known, millions of people continue to engage in unhealthy behaviors that predispose them to a number of diseases. A variety of factors can contribute to this phenomenon, however a major factor is that often patients simply fail to follow recommendations they have been given by their health professional.

Ensuring the success of treatment becomes increasingly important as health care costs rise. Health outcomes from treatment rely to a large extent on the degree of patient compliance (Horowitz and Horowitz 1993, Haynes et al. 2001). Noncompliance not only jeopardizes patients' health but has economic consequences for the health care system. The health costs of noncompliance can be high. The estimated cost of noncompliance in the United States has been estimated to be 100 billion dollars per year (Breen and Thornhill 1998). There is significant cost to the individual personally, and the health system in general, when, due to noncompliance, acute conditions that could have been cured develop into chronic conditions, when chronic conditions that could have been controlled develop into debilitating illness, or when disease develops that could have been prevented.

As health care costs rise, there is an increasing tendency to lower costs by decreasing inpatient stays. Consequently, patients are expected to assume more responsibility for their own care in the home setting. Patients' failure to follow recommendations in the outpatient setting can result in complications that require increased medical attention or readmission to the inpatient facility. Diagnostic procedures or additional treatments may be needed, which increase not only cost but also perhaps risks to the patient's continued health. Noncompliance can also interfere with the ability to determine treatment efficacy for various diseases. Measurement of effectiveness of a new treatment is based on the assumption that patients have accurately complied with the treatment protocol. If patients have not accurately followed treatment recommendations, it is difficult to determine the extent to which treatment is effective. Compliance with outpatient therapy is important to reduce the patient's risk of developing additional complications, as well as to reduce costs.

In an era when efficacious therapies exist, or are rapidly being developed, the health and economic consequences of such high rates of noncompliance are alarming. The consequences of noncompliance seem apparent, but the effects may not be fully appreciated.

High rates of noncompliance can have a profound impact on both the health of the individual and the health care system. As medical care becomes more sophisticated and effective in its ability to treat and prevent disease, patient compliance becomes more crucial. Noncompliance is costly: it wastes medical expertise and health care resources as well as being harmful to patients. Highly advanced medical procedures and treatments are of limited use in improving health status if patients neglect to follow recommendations provided to them.

Noncompliance produces substantial adverse effects on quality and cost of care directly, by disrupting or negating potential benefits of therapies or preventive measures prescribed, and indirectly, by exposing patients to unnecessary diagnostic procedures and additional treatments that may otherwise not have been needed. In addition, noncompliance may interfere with the patient's cure, causing serious complications from a disease that has not been adequately controlled.

EXTENT OF NONCOMPLIANCE

The extent to which patients follow recommendations of health professionals has been studied from a variety of perspectives. The rate of noncompliance with prescribed therapeutic regimens has been found to be alarmingly high. Over three decades ago, in one of the first studies about the extent of noncompliance, Davis reported a range of noncompliance from 15% to 93% (Davis 1968a). A number of other classic studies of compliance reinforced Davis' findings. In a review of 50 studies, Blackwell (1973) found 25 to 50% of all patients noncompliant, whereas Sackett and Haynes in a comprehensive review of 256 articles reported compliance rates from 40% to 80% (Sackett and Haynes 1976). Although compliance behavior can take many forms, more recent studies of rates of noncompliance continue to show that patients are noncompliant with health recommendations at least 50% of the time (Haynes 1999). Despite differences in compliance rates reported, there appears to be general consensus that a high percentage of patients still fail to follow health and treatment recommendations of health professionals.

Such findings suggest that a substantial proportion of individuals seeking medical treatment fail to receive maximum therapeutic benefits because of nonadherence to recommendations. The consequences of noncompliance are far reaching.

FORMS OF PATIENT NONCOMPLIANCE

Patient noncompliance can take many forms; these include failure to keep appointments; take medication as directed; follow recommended dietary, exercise, or other life-style changes or restrictions; follow other aspects of treatment; and follow recommended preventative health practices. Noncompliance in any of these areas can have varying effects, depending on the seriousness of the condition and the degree of noncompliance. Specific examples of types of patient noncompliance and their potential effects will help illustrate the scope of the problem.

Appointment Keeping

Patients' failure to keep an appointment can have serious consequences for the individual patient, but it is also an inefficient use of time by the health professionals, who have set aside a specified period to work with that patient. The missed appointment may be for a regular checkup, follow-up of a previously treated medical problem, diagnostic procedure, or referral to a specialist for evaluation.

Patients who fail to keep an appointment for a regular checkup run the risk of allowing early stages of disease to go undetected; a medical problem that could have been solved rather simply could become a major problem because of the lack of early intervention. Such was the case of Mrs. Lappas, a 50-year-old postmenopausal woman, who failed to keep her appointment for a routine Pap smear. She had decided that during a time of economic strain, such an examination was not worth the money. Some time later, when she began having abnormal vaginal bleeding, she consulted her physician. At that time, she was diagnosed as having cervical cancer that had become far advanced, requiring extensive surgical intervention and yielding a rather poor prognosis for her longevity. Earlier detection of the disease could have had an impact not only on how the disease was treated but also on the patient's prognosis as well.

Appointments for follow-up of a previously treated condition can also be a source of noncompliance. A study of psychiatric patients demonstrated consequences of noncompliance with follow-up appointments (Nelson et al. 2000). The study examined whether patients discharged from an inpatient psychiatric facility would have lower rehospitalization rates if they kept their follow-up appointments after discharge. Results showed that patients who failed to keep their outpatient follow-up appointments after discharge from the inpatient facility were twice as likely to be rehospitalized in the same year as those patients who had kept at least one follow-up appointment. When annual rates for readmission were examined, it was discovered that patients who kept follow-up appointments after discharge from the psychiatric facility had a 1 in 10 chance of being rehospitalized compared to those patients who had been discharged but who were not compliant with follow-up appointments. The readmission rate for these patients was one in four.

Other potential consequences of a missed follow-up appointment can be illustrated in the case of Mr. Jones, who was found to have hypertension. His physician prescribed an antihypertensive medication and told him his blood pressure should be closely monitored. The physician asked Mr. Jones to come for a follow-up appointment every month to assess the effectiveness of the medication. Mr. Jones experienced no symptoms and consequently saw no reason to return for follow-up visits. Six months after the initial visit, having gone to no follow-up visits, Mr. Jones experienced a stroke.

Referral appointments with specialists may also be missed; such failure can postpone diagnosis and treatment of specific disease entities. Such was the case of Mr. Ling. During a routine examination by his dentist, a growth was found in Mr. Ling's mouth. The dentist, concerned about the growth, immediately referred him for evaluation by an ear, nose, and throat specialist. The dentist informed Mr. Ling of the importance of having the growth evaluated. Being a busy man, however, Mr. Ling continued to postpone consultation. When, a year later, Mr. Ling began to have difficulty breathing and swallowing, he consulted his regular physician, who found the growth had grown considerably. On further evaluation, the growth was found to be cancerous.

Not all missed appointments have the consequences described in the examples above, however patients' failure to keep appointments can affect health care delivery, not only in terms of time and money but also in delays of treatment.

Medication Noncompliance

Noncompliance with prescribed medication regimens can also take several forms and can result in a number of serious consequences. Numerous examples of consequences of medication noncompliance can be found in the literature. Poor adherence to antihypertensive medications has been found to lead to unnecessary complications and early death (Chin and Goldman 1997). Psychiatric patients with schizophrenia who were noncompliant with medications have been found to have an increased risk of rehospitalization, homelessness, and symptom exacerbation (Olfson et al. 2000). Noncompliance with medication for treatment of asthma has been found to be linked to asthma deaths (Birkhead et al. 1989).

Such noncompliance with medication may consist of never having the prescriptions filled. Some patients may alter the prescribed dose—taking either too much or too little of the medication or varying the time interval at which the medication is taken. Other patients may neglect to follow the full course of treatment, stopping the medication as soon as their symptoms subside. Such forms of noncompliance can have deleterious effects. The following example illustrates these points.

Mrs. Cellini was pregnant with her third child. During her prenatal checkup it was discovered that she had a urinary tract infection. She was given a prescription for treatment. The family had limited income, and because her daughter also had needed medication, Mrs. Cellini reasoned that her first priority was her daughter's medication. Consequently Mrs. Cellini's urinary tract infection progressed to pyelonephritis, necessitating hospitalization.

Underutilization of a drug may deprive patients of anticipated therapeutic benefits, possibly resulting in worsening of the condition being treated. Patients who discontinue use of a mediation after symptoms subside but before the condition is fully cured may run the risk of recurrence of the condition because the shorter course of therapy was not enough to eradicate it. This may necessitate additional visits to the health professional and may have deleterious effects on the patient. In addition, the health professional who is unaware of the patients noncompliance and who sees the condition neither improved nor controlled may prescribe higher doses of the drug or additional drugs, exposing the patient to an increased possibility of adverse side effects if he or she decides to take all the prescribed drugs at different intervals. In other circumstances, if drugs are not used up, patients may store them, potentiating inappropriate use of the medications by themselves or others at a later time.

The seriousness of lack of compliance with a prescribed medication regimen can vary from one situation to another. In those cases in which medication is a continual, ongoing part of controlling the disease itself, such as in hypertension or diabetes, failure to comply can have life-threatening consequences. Virginia, an 18-year-old insulin-dependent diabetic, was repeatedly treated at the local hospital emergency room for hyperglycemia. Her physician, attributing the problem to inadequate amounts of insulin, continued to alter the dosage accordingly. Eventually, she was brought into the emergency room in a diabetic coma. Upon more careful questioning of family members the nurse discovered that Virginia had frequently neglected to take her insulin in the prescribed amounts. All along the problem had not been the amount of insulin prescribed but Virginia's failure to take it accurately.

In other cases when medication is intended to prevent a medical problem from becoming a more serious threat to health, noncompliance can also have serious consequences. Julie, a four-year-old girl, was brought to the neighborhood health clinic by her mother because of cold, fever, and sore throat. She was diagnosed as having strep throat and was placed on a regimen of penicillin. The nurse explained to Julie's mother that the medication was not only to help Julie's sore throat but also to prevent the infection from involving other parts of the body as well. Before the course of treatment was over, the family went to visit Julie's grandparents for the weekend and forgot to take along the medication. Upon returning from the visit, the parents never resumed Julie's mediation regimen; she seemed so much better, and she had missed several days of the medication anyway. Julie later developed rheumatic fever.

Less serious medication noncompliance may still have an impact on the health care system itself by causing patients with recurring symptoms to be readmitted to the hospital or to return to outpatient clinics for treatment conditions that could have been cured with proper compliance the first time. The health care provider is thus diverted from caring for other individuals who may have more serious needs for health care.

Medications are not without side effects. Patients who err on the side of excess run the risk of drug interactions, drug toxicity, and a variety of other impairments related to side effects from misuse or overuse of prescribed, therapeutic medications.

Dietary and Other Life-Style Changes

Dietary and other behavioral or life-style changes are frequently required in the management of various conditions. Life-style changes may be recommended to prevent disease from occurring, such as smoking cessation for prevention of heart and lung disease or cancer. In other instances, dietary or life-style changes constitute a major portion of treatment of disease, such as patients on hemodialysis for end-stage renal disease who are asked to adhere to a strict regimen of fluid and diet restrictions or individuals with diabetes who are taught to regulate and monitor food intake, exercise, and other self-care behaviors.

Dietary and other life-style changes require significant discipline and motivation on the part of the patient. Recommendations associated with life-style changes can be some of the most difficult recommendations for patients to follow but can also have some of the most severe consequences if the patient fails to comply (Brown 1990, Morgan 2000). Take the example of Ms. Burnett. Ms. Burnett, a 20-year-old single woman, was pregnant with her first child. During one of her prenatal visits, the nurse noted that Ms. Burnett's blood pressure was elevated, there was protein in her urine, and she had a substantial weight gain since her last visit. Upon questioning Ms. Burnett, the nurse found that she had been eating large quantities of junk food, including potato chips and other foods high in calories and salt. Ms. Burnett was referred to the dietitian for consultation. In addition, her physician restricted her activity, asking her to elevate her feet as much as possible to reduce swelling when out of bed and to remain in bed as much as possible. Ms. Burnett, however, a student working her way through school, continued working at her part-time job at a fast-food restaurant, where one of the perks was free food. She continued to stand for long periods during work and continued to eat the free food she was provided as part of her job. Eventually, she began having blurred vision and headaches. She consulted her physician and was promptly admitted to the hospital for treatment for preeclampsia.

Failure to Follow Other Aspects of Treatment

Treatment modalities other than keeping appointments, taking medications, and following dietary and other life-style restrictions may also be prescribed. Examples include treatments such as applying heat or cold to areas of the body, wrapping extremities with elastic bandages for sprains or strains, applying warm soaks, changing bandages, and so forth. Nonadherence even to these rather mild, noninvasive forms of treatment can have serious consequences, as is illustrated by the case of Mr. Schmidt. He had circulatory problems in his lower extremities for some time due to arteriosclerosis. Although he had been warned about the danger of attempting his own foot care, he tried to remove a callous from his right foot. As a result he sustained an injury that subsequently became infected. Upon consulting his physician, he was instructed to soak his foot several times a day and to keep it under a heat lamp for 30 minutes three times a day. Mr. Schmidt, a farmer, discounted the importance of the instructions and continued to do farm chores, stating that he didn't have time to sit around three times a day and pamper his foot. Although he used the heat lamp sporadically, he stopped soaking his foot altogether. The wound did not heal; the infection became worse, his foot became gangrenous, and he was eventually admitted to the hospital for amputation.

Preventive Health Practices

The role of prevention in maintaining health has been known for more than 40 years. As early as 1964, the Surgeon General of the United States Public Health Service issued a warning based on an accumulation of evidence that smoking is hazardous to health (Luther 1964). It is now widely accepted that tobacco use is related to heart disease, stroke, emphysema and cancer (Bartecchi et al. 1994,

MacKenzie et al. 1994, He et al. 2001, Aubry et al. 2000). The influence of diet and exercise on people's health and well-being has also been well publicized. The importance of weight control in reducing risk from heart disease (Rao et al. 2001), hypertension (Hooker-Whitman, 2002), osteoarthritis (Hart and Spector 1993), diabetes (Roth and Berger 1960), and recently, cancer (Calle et al. 2003) is widely accepted. The importance of good dental hygiene in preventing tooth loss and gingivitis, which has been linked to other inflammatory processes in the body, is also recognized (Gustafsson et al. 2002).

A variety of health professionals try to teach patients how to prevent disease from occurring and promote good health. Physicians, nurses, dietitians, dentists, and a variety of other health professionals and professional organizations give countless recommendations to patients about how to stay healthy and prevent disease. Programs designed to help people follow preventive health practices have been established with varying degrees of effectiveness.

Nonetheless, countless numbers of patients fail to heed the advise of health professionals and other sources of information on disease prevention. Thousands of people still smoke, still eat foods they know are bad for them, overeat, fail to exercise, or neglect dental care.

Obviously, patients who ignore preventive health advice also run a considerable risk of developing disease and conditions that can result in disability or death. They may also require other therapeutic treatment, another potential area of noncompliance.

Lack of adherence to preventive measures can be illustrated by the case of Mr. Martinez. Approaching middle age, Mr. Martinez had an extensive family history of heart disease. Soon after moving to a new city with his family, he established health care for himself and his family at a nearby Family Practice Clinic. During his first visit to the clinic for treatment of a cold, the nurse noted that he smoked nearly three packs of cigarettes a day, consumed nearly 20 cups of coffee daily, slept a maximum of five hours a night, and generally consumed large amounts of alcohol on a regular basis. The nurse talked with Mr. Martinez about aspects of prevention, giving him a variety of brochures on the subject to take home. The physician outlined an exercise program for Mr. Martinez, referred him to a smoking cessation clinic, and talked with him about ways to cut down on his coffee and alcohol consumption. Throughout the next year, each time Mr. Martinez came to the clinic, the Family Practice staff continued to reinforce the importance of prevention to prevent heart disease as well as a number of other ailments; however, he continued to ignore the advice given, stating that given his family history his days were numbered anyway, so he might as well make the most of life while he could. Almost two years to the day after moving to the city, Mr. Martinez was hospitalized with his first heart attack.

Both the nurse and the physician as well as other members of the clinic staff felt very frustrated. Not only had Mr. Martinez's noncompliance endangered his health, but considerable time and effort had been spent helping Mr. Martinez learn ways to modify his behavior to adhere more closely to prescribed preventive health measures. Now he was being treated for a condition that was partly caused by his own failure to put the recommendations into practice, a behavior that could possibly have prevented his heart attack from occurring.

CAUSES OF PATIENT NONCOMPLIANCE

Patient noncompliance has been attributed to a number of factors; these include factors specific to the patient, the disease or treatment, and the health professional (DiMatteo and DiNicola 1982, Amundson 1985). To increase compliance, it is logical that the health professional should have some understanding of the causes of noncompliance. Health professionals hold a variety of misconceptions, however, about patient noncompliance and its causes, as well as its cures. In many instances, health professionals' lack of understanding of compliance issues can itself be a factor in noncompliance. For example, health professionals frequently have misconceptions about the extent of patient noncompliance. At first glance, it does seem totally irrational that a patient seeking and paying for health advice would choose not to follow it. As cited previously, however, studies indicate that this certainly is true for a large number of patients. Various studies have demonstrated that health professionals grossly underestimate the extent of noncompliance in patients with whom they have been working (Roth and Berger 1960, Charney 1972). If health professionals are unaware of patients' noncompliance, causes for it cannot be identified and thus corrected. This in turn can result in patients' unnecessary exposure to additional treatments and tests, plus the possibility of worsening of the condition itself.

Many health professionals also hold the misconception that noncompliance is common only to outpatient practices. Patient noncompliance can occur in any setting in which recommendations are given. Even hospitalization does not guarantee compliance (Blackwell 1997). In an early study by Roth and Berger (1960), 75 hospitalized patients in a gastrointestinal ward were prescribed liquid antacid. Although general supervision was done by nurses on the ward, actually taking the medication was left up to individual patients. Later, measurement of patient compliance showed that less than 50% of the medication was taken as prescribed.

Health professionals may also have misconceptions about patients who are at risk of noncompliance. It is often assumed that patients who are uneducated or from lower socioeconomic groups are less likely to follow recommendations; research has not shown this to be the case. Variables such as age, gender, race or ethnic background, educational level, marital status, socioeconomic level, and religion have been studied as determinants of patient compliance. Few demographic variables have consistently been shown to be related to patient noncompliance (Turk and Meichenbaum 1991, Lutfey and Wishnet 1999). Although such inconsistent findings may be attributed in part to different research designs, different study populations, and different forms of compliance measurement, the fact that many other researchers have not been able to identify potentially noncompliant patients according to these variables suggests that the variables are not a reliable explanation for noncompliance. Although demographic variables may be a factor in noncompliance for individual patients, they certainly do not appear influential for the patient population as a whole.

Other possible reasons for noncompliance have also been studied; these include features of the disease itself, its diagnosis and severity, and its symptomatology and chronicity. Again, it seems logical that where failure to follow medical advice would be the most harmful, patient compliance would be greatest. Although findings in this area are inconclusive, in many instances this also has not seemed to be the case. Classic early studies found that patients with less-severe medical problems were actually more likely to follow through with medical advice than those with more-severe illness (Davis 1968b).

Some early studies found patients' increased perception of disease severity as being significantly related to the likelihood of their compliance (Becker et al. 1972). Leventhal's classic work (1971), however, suggested that for asymptomatic individuals, low levels of perceived severity were not sufficiently motivating to produce increased compliance, while very high levels of perceived seriousness raised fear and anxiety and were inhibiting, thus decreasing the chances that patients would comply with the treatment regimen. Other studies have shown little consistent correlation between any disease features and how closely patients follow a therapeutic regimen (Haynes 1979). Findings from classic studies suggest that compliance, as related to a disease condition, is based on individual differences rather than factors generalizable to patients as a group.

Compliance originally was viewed as a patient-related phenomenon. Early classic studies looked toward patient-related variables as a way of understanding and predicting patient noncompliance. However, given results from many of the early studies that indicated that sociodemographic and disease features had little consistent correlation with patient compliance, researchers turned to other variables that might be found to explain the phenomenon. When studying features of the therapeutic regimen itself, several features were found to be correlated with compliance. Early studies found that the greater the extent to which patients must alter personal habits, behavior, or other aspects of life style as part of their treatment, the less likely they were to follow recommendations (Donabedian and Rosenfeld 1964, Davis 1967). In addition, researchers found that the less complicated the treatment regime, the higher the rate of compliance (Cohen 1979, Lane 1983). Studies of these variables have been replicated by many researchers in the years since the first studies were conducted. A number of studies over the past two decades have confirmed these findings (Spector 1985, Coutts et al. 1992, Kolton and Piccolo 1998).

REVIEW OF INTERVENTIONS TO INCREASE COMPLIANCE

With growing interest in factors of the therapeutic regime itself as potential determinants of compliance, a number studies related to strategies and interventions specifically designed to enhance the likelihood of increased compliance began to be seen in the literature. Two popular interventions were behavioral techniques and specifically designed apparatuses that would help patients to remember to take their medication (Azrin and Powell 1969, Eshelman and Fitzloff 1976).

Although studies using apparatus often showed an increase in patient compliance, one flaw in the strategy was the assumption that forgetfulness was the major factor that caused noncompliance. Even when forgetfulness was a factor, use of the device still required patients to remember to fill it and to be motivated to use it. It might seem reasonable to assume that if patients could not remember their medications, they may also be unable to remember to use the apparatus designed to increase compliance. Although the apparatus may be helpful to some patients, the method did not appear to be the panacea for all compliance problems.

Other strategies included specific behavioral techniques involving differential reinforcement, extinction, shaping, modeling, and desensitization. These methods were found to have varying degrees of success for some regimens, although there were still not a panacea. To succeed, behavioral approaches require motivation and cooperation by patients themselves. Patients must be willing to follow through with these techniques on their own in the home environment or to see the health professional responsible for instituting the techniques on a regular basis. The more frequent the interaction between patient and health professional, the more likely the technique will be successful in increasing compliance. Use of behavioral techniques, which over time have shown success in many instances, can be costly in terms of the health professional's time. If the patient is motivated enough to carry out the techniques independently, then much of the compliance battle has already been won. Behavioral techniques are less useful when patients who are noncompliant have little motivation to carry out the regimen, let alone the behavioral techniques designed to improve compliance with the regime itself. Before behavioral techniques can be implemented, the patient must also understand clearly what he or she must do. Even if the health professional has explained the procedure, the explanation may have been given in terms the patient does not understand, or the patient may view the procedure as an impossible task.

Another problem with the strict use of behavioral techniques to increase compliance is the accurate identification of the target behavior to be changed. The behavior the health professional considers in need of change may, in fact, not be the behavior that needs to be changed. The case of Ms. Grossman, an obese college student, is an example of such an occurrence. Ms. Grossman had been going to the obesity clinic for several months, without success. A variety of behavioral techniques had been implemented to help her control her eating behavior. She seemed motivated, visiting the clinic regularly and appearing genuinely sincere about carrying out the plans she had been given. After several months, when she still had not lost weight, the nurse at the clinic questioned her more closely about her behavior away from the clinic. Although Ms. Gross-man had complied very well with the recommendations to control her eating at home, her downfall appeared to be her eating behavior in public. She ate a meal at noon daily at the student center, and other food intake occurred at social events on weekends. Painfully shy, Ms. Grossman tended to overeat when in a group. While she was eating, she did not have to engage in conversation. In addition, at social events she hovered at the food table so she did not have to mingle in a group or be forced to sit alone, waiting for someone to approach her to talk. The target behavior originally identified as contributing to her obesity was daily eating behavior. It became more obvious that the behavior that actually contributed more to her obesity was her social behavior. Once the target behavior was correctly identified and work began on helping her improve her social skills, her weight-reduction program became successful.

Although apparatuses and special techniques were used with varying degrees of success in increasing compliance, most studies concluded that compliance dropped when the specific interventions or programs designed to increase compliance were discontinued (McKenney et al. 1973).

Other interventions to increase patient compliance include patient contracting. Stark and colleagues (Stark et al. 1987) introduced behavioral contracting as a method to increase compliance of an 11-year-old girl with cystic fibrosis to her chest physiotherapy treatment. The technique produced positive changes in her compliance, physiologic measures, and family functioning during the contracting period and at 9-week follow-up. Although this application of behavioral contracting appeared to show success for 9 weeks, it is difficult to know the extent to which, over time and without additional interventions, there would be a lapse in the compliance evident in the study itself. Likewise, although behavioral contracting may be helpful to increase compliance for some, the circumstances of other patients may change the effectiveness of this approach.

Other interventions have also been developed in an attempt to increase compliance. Wolosin (1990) studied the effect of appointment scheduling and reminder postcards on women's likelihood of complying with recommendations for mammography screening. One group of women was examined, told about mammography, and instructed to make an appointment for themselves, whereas another group had appointments scheduled for them at the visit, which was followed up with a reminder postcard. The women who had appointments scheduled for them had higher rates of compliance with recommendations for mammography screening than did those who had to make their own appointments. Although this intervention apparently increased patient compliance with recommendations, variability of patient populations and socioeconomic differences in different locations, and other extraneous variables, make generalization of results questionable. In addition, even though compliance was apparently increased, the question of whether such an intervention merely maintains dependence as opposed to helping patients accept responsibility for their own health must be asked.

Information-giving would appear to be an important intervention in increasing compliance. Patients obviously cannot be expected to comply with a treatment plan they do not understand. It would seem reasonable to speculate that the better informed a patient is about his or her condition and treatment, the more compliant the patient will be. Studies, however, have not consistently shown this to be the case (Bartlett 1983, Sands and Holman 1985, Blessing-Moore 1996). In a study of diabetic patients, knowledge about diabetes and its control was increased with an educational program, but compliance with the medical regimen was not (Watts 1980).

Patients may be able to repeat facts without having a true understanding of the material presented. Although some information is especially relevant to patient adherence, such as knowledge of what the therapeutic regimen requires and how and when to do it, acquisition of knowledge is not necessarily followed by appropriate action (Blessing-Moore 1996).

ROLE OF THE HEALTH PROFESSIONAL IN PATIENT COMPLIANCE

One variable that had not yet been studied in detail with relationship to patient compliance was the role health professionals might play in influencing patient behavior. As researchers began to study the health professional–patient relationship in the context of patient compliance, interesting findings began to emerge. Poor communication has been found to be one of the most important factors in determining the extent to which patients comply with treatment (McLane et al. 1995, Kirchner 2000). A positive influence on patient compliance appeared to be strongly related to the health provider's communication and explanation skills (Schmidt 1977). Communication, in this context, appears to go beyond verbal exchange of information, extending to the very relationship between patient and health professional.

The ability of health professionals to demonstrate warmth and concern for the patient (Falvo et al. 1980), to demonstrate empathy (Luborsky et al. 1985), and to generate a trusting, cooperative environment that provides patients with freedom of choice appear to be important components in the relationship between patient and health professional to facilitate compliance (Langer 1999). Helping patients feel comfortable discussing concerns or perceived difficulties with the recommended treatment by demonstrating empathy is built on a relationship of trust (Waeber et al. 2000). This type of relationship helps patients feel that the health professional is listening and understands their feelings, concerns, and limitations without judging them. Health professionals who take time to explain to patients elements of treatment in an informative and nonthreatening manner encourage patient participation and enhance the likelihood of compliance (Miller 1997). Having an open relationship between patient and health professional so that the patient's concerns are accepted and in which the patient and health professional work together to develop a mutually agreeable plan appears to be a major factor in promoting patient compliance.

PATIENT EDUCATION AND PATIENT COMPLIANCE

Educating patients about their condition, treatment, risks, and benefits is an essential part of patient care. It stands to reason that patient education is also a major factor in patient compliance because patients are unable to follow recommendations for which they have no knowledge or understanding. Having knowledge of disease or treatment alone, however, has not been found to be a strong predictor of patient compliance (Bernard-Bonnin et al. 1995).

Perhaps one of the difficulties is equating information acquisition with education. Education in any setting is more complex. In a highly mechanized age when so many materials to enhance learning are available and when so many sources of information are produced, it is not surprising that many people think of patient education simply as information transfer. Although information transfer is a part of the educational process, educational endeavors in any setting usually have goals that include more than giving information that individuals then regurgitate. Educational goals generally consist of procedures that help individuals gain knowledge so that they will be able to incorporate the knowledge into their lives through learning of skills, behavior, or attitudes. Patient education then, in order to be truly effective, must be more than simply repeating directions to patients or handing out printed materials. Effective patient education might be better thought of as a clinical skill that incorporates many of the attributes found to be important in patient compliance. It is a process that involves precise clinical skills on the part of the health professional in terms of data gathering, individualization of instructions, support, evaluation, and follow-up of patients' success in implementing the treatment plan.

COMPLIANCE AS COLLABORATION

There has been a tendency to oversimplify both patient education and patient compliance. There appears to be no cookie-cutter approach that works for all patients with all conditions. Factors in both patient education and patient compliance are much more complex. Effective communication and collaboration between health professional and patient, guided by factual information and experience of the health professional, allows patients to make informed choices about an agreed-upon regimen (Saltzman 1995, Quill and Brody 1996). By providing patients with clear, factual, unbiased information, identifying and acknowledging their concerns and limitations, altering treatment plans as appropriate, and conducting evaluations and follow-up, increased compliance is more likely to result (Bender and Milgrom 1996, Roter et al. 1998, Graziani et al. 1999).

REFERENCES

Amundson, L.H. 1985. Review of patient compliance: I. Magnitude and determinants. *Continuing Education* September:621–630.

Aubry, M.C., Wright, J. L., Myers, J.L. 2000. Smoking and pulmonary and cardiovascular diseases: the pathology of smoking-related lung diseases. *Clinics in Chest Medicine* 21:11–35.

Azrin, N.H., Powell, J. 1969. Behavioral engineering: the use of response priming to improve prescribed self-medication. *Journal of Applied Behavior Analysis* 2:39–42.

Bartecchi, C.E., Mackenzie, T.D., Schrier, R.W. 1994. The human costs of tobacco use. (first of two parts). *New England Journal of Medicine* 330:907–912.

Bartlett, E.E. 1983. Restoring credibility to the field of patient education. *Patient Education Newsletter* 6(6):11.

Becker, M.H., Drachman, R.H., Kirscht, J.P. 1972. Predicting mothers compliance with pediatric medical regimens. *Journal of Pediatrics* 81:843–854.

Bender, B., Milgrom, H. 1996. Compliance with asthma therapy: a case for shared responsibility. *Journal of Asthma* 33:99–202.

Bernard-Bonnin, A.C., Stachenko, S., Bonin, D., Charette, C., Rousseau, E. 1995. Self-management teaching programs and morbidity of pediatric asthma: a meta-analysis. *Journal of Allergy and Clinical Immunology* 95(Part 1):34–41.

Birkhead, G., Attaway, N.J., Strunk, R.C., Townsend, M.C., Teutsch, S. 1989. Investigation of a cluster of deaths of adolescents from asthma: evidence implicating inadequate treatment and poor patient adherence with medications. *Journal of Allergy and Clinical Immunology* 84(Part 1):484–491.

Blackwell, B. (Ed.). 1997. Treatment compliance and the therapeutic alliance. Newark: Hardwood Academic Publishers.

Blackwell, B. 1973. Drug therapy—Patient compliance. *New England Journal of Medicine* 289:249–252.

Blessing-Moore, J. 1996. Does asthma education change behavior? To know is not to do. *Chest* 109:9–19.

Breen, R., Thornhill, J.T. 1998. Noncompliance with medications for psychiatric disorders. *CNS Drugs* 9:457–471.

Brown, S. 1990. Studies of educational interventions and outcomes in diabetic adults: a meta-analysis revisited. *Patient Education and Counseling* 16:189–215.

Burke, L.E., Dunbar-Jacob, J. 1995. Adherence to medication, diet, and activity recommendations: from assessment to maintenance. *Journal of Cardiovascular Nursing* 9:62–79.

Butler, C., Rollnick, S., Stott, N. 1996. The practitioner, the patient and resistance to change: recent ideas on compliance. *Canadian Medical Association Journal*, 154:1357–1362.

Calle, E.E., Rodriquez, C., Walker-Thurmond, K., Thun, M.J. 2003. Overweight, obesity, and mortality from cancer in a prospectively studied cohort of US adults. *New England Journal of Medicine* 348:1625–1638.

Charney, E. 1972. Patient-doctor communication: implications for the clinician. *Pediatric Clinics of North America* 19:263–279.

Chin, J.H., Goldman, L. 1997. Correlates of early hospital admission or death in patients with congestive heart failure. *American Journal of Cardiology* 79:1640–1644.

Cohen, S.J. 1979. New directions in patient compliance. Lexington, MA: Lexington Books.

Coutts, J.A., Gibson, N.A., Paton, J.Y. 1992. Measuring compliance with inhaled medication in asthma. *Archives of Diseases of Childhood* 67:332–222.

Davis, M.S. 1968a. Variations in patient compliance with doctors advice: an empirical analysis of patterns of communication. *American Journal of Public Health* 58:274–288.

Davis, M.S. 1968b. Physiologic, psychological and demographic factors in patient compliance with doctors orders. *Medical Care* 6:115–122.

Davis, M.S. 1967. Predicting non-compliant behavior. *Journal of Health and Social Behavior* 8:265–271.

DiMatteo, M.R., DiNicola, D.D. 1982. Achieving patient compliance: the psychology of the medical practitioner's role. New York: Pergamon Press.

Donabedian, A., Rosenfeld, L.S. 1964. Follow up study of chronically ill patients discharged from the hospital. *Journal Of Chronic Disease* 17:847–862.

Eshelman, F.N., Fitzloff, J. 1976. Effect of packaging on patient compliance with an antihypertensive medication. *Current Therapeutic Research* 20:215–219.

Evangelista, L.S., Dracup, K.A. 2000. A closer look at compliance research in heart failure patients in the last decade. *Progress in Cardiovascular Nursing* 15:97–103.

Falvo, D., Woehlke, P., Deichmann, J. 1980. Relationship of physician behavior to patient compliance. *Patient Counseling and Health Education* 2:185–188.

Feldman, R.H.L. 1982. A guide for enhancing health care compliance in ambulatory care settings. *Journal of Ambulatory Care Management* 5:1–12.

Freeman, R.C., Rodriquez, G., French, J.F. 1996. Compliance with AZT treatment regimen of HIV seropositive injection drug users: a neglected issue. *AIDS Education and Prevention* 8:58–71.

Graziani, C., Rosenthal, M.P., Diamond, J.J. 1999. Diabetic education program use and patients perceived barriers to adherence. *Family Medicine* 31:358–363.

Gustafsson, B.K., Hakansson, J., Klinge, B. 2002. Oral health and cardiovascular disease in Sweden. *Journal of Clinical Periodontal* 29:254–259.

Hart, D.J., Spector, T.D. 1993. The relationship of obesity, fat distribution and osteoarthritis in women in the general population: the Chingford study. *Journal of Rheumatology* 20:331–335.

Haynes, R.B. 1999. Compliance: the state of the science. Conference Proceedings, April 1999, Waltham, MA.

Haynes, R.B. 1979. Determinants of compliance: the disease and the mechanics of treatment. In: Haynes, R.B. et al. (Eds.), Compliance in health care. Baltimore: Johns Hopkins University Press, 49–62.

Haynes R.B., Montague P., Oliver T. 2001. Interventions for helping patients to follow prescriptions for medications (Cochrane Review). In: The Cochrane Library, Issue 2. Oxford: Update Software.

He, J., Ogden, L., Bazzano, L., Vupputuri, S., Loria, C., Whelton, P. 2001. Risk factors for congestive heart failure in US men and women. *Archives of Internal Medicine* 161:996–1002.

Hernandez, C.A. 1995. The experience of living with insulin dependent diabetes: lessons for the diabetic educator. *The Diabetic Educator* 21:33–37.

Hooker-Whitman, J. 2002. Medical complications of obesity. *Clinics in Family Practice* 4:2.

Horowitz, R.I., Horowitz, S. 1993. Adherence to treatment and health outcomes. *Archives in Internal Medicine* 153:1863–1868.

Johnson, J.A., Bootman, J.L. 1995. Drug-related morbidity and mortality: a cost of illness model. *Archives of Internal Medicine*, 155:1949–1956.

Johnston, R.K., Mann, T. 2000. Barriers to antiretroviral adherence in HIV infected women. *AIDS Care* 12:377–386.

Kirchner, J.T. 2000. Patient compliance in filling new prescriptions. *American Family Physician* 62:201–206.

Koltun, A., Stone G.C. 1986. Current trends in patient noncompliance research: focus on diseases, regimes, programs and other provider disciplines. *Journal of Compliance in Health Care* 2:21–32.

Kolton, K.A., Piccolo, P. 1998. Patient compliance: a challenge in practice. *Nurse Practitioner* 13:37–50.

Lane, S.D. 1983. Compliance, satisfaction and physician-patient communication. In: Bostrom, R.N. (Ed.), Communication year book 7. Beverly Hills: Sage, 772–799.

Langer, N. 1999. Culturally competent professionals in therapeutic alliances enhances patient compliance. *Journal Of Health Care For The Poor and Underserved in Nashville* 1:19–26.

Leventhal, H. 1971. Fear appeals and persuasion: the differentiation of a motivational construct. *American Journal of Public Health* 61:1208–1224.

Liberman, A., Rotarius, T. 1999. Behavioral contract management: a prescription for employee and patient compliance. *The Health Care Manager* 18:1–10.

Luborsky, L., McLellan, A.T., Woody, G.E., O'Brien, C.P., Auerbach, A. 1985. Therapist success and its determinants. *Archives of General Psychiatry* 42:602–611.

Lutfey, K.E., Wishnet, W. 1999. Beyond compliance: is adherence improving the prospect of diabetes care. *Diabetes Care* 22:635–639.

Luther, T. 1964. Smoking and health: report of the advisory committee to the surgeon general of the public health service. Public Health Service, Washington, DC: PHS Publication No. 1103.

MacKenzie, T.D., Bartecchi, C.E., Schrier, R.W. 1994. The human costs of tobacco use (second of two parts) *New England Journal of Medicine* 330:975–980.

McLane, C.G., Zyzanski, S.J., Flocke, S.A. 1995. Factors associated with medication noncompliance in rural elderly hypertensive patients. *American Journal of Hypertension* 8:206–209.

McKenney, J.M., Slining, J.M., Henderson, H.R., Devins, D., Barr, M. 1973. The effect of clinical pharmacy services on patients with essential hypertension. *Circulation* 48:1104–1111.

Miller, N.H. 1997. Compliance with treatment in chronic asymptomatic disease. *American Journal of Medicine* 102:43–49.

Morgan, L. 2000. A decade review: methods to improve adherence to the treatment regime among hemodialysis patients. *Nephrology Nursing Journal* 27:299–304.

Morrison, A., Wertheimer, A.I., Berger, M.L. 2000. Interventions to improve antihypertensive drug adherence: a quantitative review of trials. *Formulary* 35:234–255.

Nelson, E.A., Maruish, M.E., Axler, J.L. 2000. Effects of discharge planning and compliance with outpatient appointments on readmission rates. *Psychiatric Services* 51:885–889.

Nicolucci, A., Cavaliere, D., Scorpiglione, N., Carinci, F., Capani, F., Tognoni, G., Benedetti, M.M. 1996. A comprehensive assessment of the avoidability of long-term complications of diabetes. A case-control study. SID-AMD Italian Study Group for the Implementation of the St. Vincent Declaration. *Diabetes Care* 19:927–33.

Olfson, M., Mechanic, D., Hansell, S., Boyer, C.A., Walkup, J., Weiden, P.J. 2000. Predicting medical noncompliance after hospital discharge among patients with schizophrenia. *Psychiatric Service* 51:216–222.

Quill, T.E., Brody, H. 1996. Physician recommendations and patient autonomy: finding a balance between physician power and patient choice. *Annals of Internal Medicine* 125:763–769.

Rao, S.V., Donahue, M., Pi-Sunyer, F.X., Fuster, V. 2001. Obesity as a risk factor in coronary artery disease. *American Heart Journal* 142:1102–1107.

Roter, D.L., Hall, J.A., Merisca, R., Nordstrom, B., Cretin, D., Svarstad, B. 1998. Effectiveness of interventions to improve patient compliance: a meta analysis. *Medical Care* 36:1138–1161.

Roth, H., Berger, D. 1960. Studies on patient cooperation in ulcer treatment: observation of actual as compared to prescribed antacid intake on a hospital ward. *Gastroenterology* 38:630–633.

Sackett, D.L., Haynes, R.B. 1976. Compliance with therapeutic regimens. Baltimore: Johns Hopkins University Press.

Salzman, C. 1995. Medication compliance in the elderly. *Journal of Clinical Psychiatry* 56(suppl 1):18–22.

Sands, D., Holman, E. 1985. Does knowledge enhance patient compliance? *Journal of Gerontological Nursing* 11:23–29.

Schmidt, D.D. 1977. Patient compliance: the effect of the doctor as a therapeutic agent. *Journal of Family Practice* 4:853–856.

Spector, S.L. 1985. Is your asthmatic patient really complying? *Annals of Allergy* 55:552–556.

Stark, L.J., Miller, S.T., Plienes, A.J., Drabman, R.S. 1987. Behavioral contracting to increase chest physiotherapy. A study of a young cystic fibrosis patient. *Behavioral Modification* 11:75–86.

Trostle, J.A. 1997. The history and meaning of patient compliance as an ideology. In: Gochman, D.S. (Ed.), Handbook of health behavior research III: provider determinants. New York: Plenum Press, 109–124.

Turk, D.C., Meichenbaum, D. 1991. Adherence to self care regimens: the patient's perspective. In: Sweet, J., Rozensky, R., Tovian, S. (Eds.), Handbook of clinical psychology in medical settings, Vol. 19. New York: Plenum Press, 249–268.

Vivian, B.G., Wilcox, J.P. 2000. Compliance communication in home health care: a mutually reciprocal process. *Qualitative Health Research* 10:103–116.

Waeber, B., Burnier, M., Brunner, H.R. 2000. How to improve adherence with prescribed treatment in hypertensive patients? *Journal of Cardiovascular Pharmacology* 35(suppl):S23–S26.

Watts, F.N. 1980. Behavioral aspects of the management of diabetes mellitus: education, self-care and metabolic control. *Behavior, Research and Therapy* 18:171–180.

Wolosin, R.J. 1990. Effect of appointment scheduling and reminder postcards on adherence to mammography recommendations. *Journal of Family Practice* 30:542–547.

The Evolution of Patient Education

2

IMPORTANCE OF PATIENT EDUCATION TODAY

To some extent, health professionals have always given patients information about their condition and treatment, as well as information about prevention of disease or complications from illness and injury. The type and amount of information, however, has varied greatly. The culture and atmosphere of health care has changed from one of paternalism, where patients had limited access to information and limited participation in decisions about their care, to one of patient autonomy and active participation in decision making. A natural outgrowth of this change has been increasing interest in patient education and how information can be delivered most effectively and efficiently to patients. Increased interest in patient education can also be attributed to the advent of managed care, in which patients are being discharged from hospitals earlier and asked to assume more responsibility for their own care at home, care that once would have been provided in an inpatient setting. The current health environment, which emphasizes preventing illness, improving outcomes, containing costs, and increasing patient participation in informed decision making and responsibility for their own health, has made the value of patient education evident.

Underlying attitudes and expectations, however, sometimes change more slowly than societal or professional mandates. There was a time when neither patients nor health professionals expected that patients should be fully informed. The widely held belief that patients did not have the training or background to understand the full explanation of their disease or treatment limited the amount and type of information that patients were given. Patients often shared the view of health professionals that they had insufficient training or experience to understand details about their condition and treatment. Consequently, even when health professionals attempted to give explanations, patients were not always receptive to receiving information about their condition, treatment, or preventive practices. Instead, patients frequently chose to remain passive, placing full faith and responsibility for their health and health care with the health professional.

In other instances, there was the belief that full disclosure of information to patients could lead to misinterpretation, causing needless anxiety and perhaps even adverse effects on patient outcome. Turf issues between health professionals frequently arose, in which there was lack of clarity over who was responsible for or who had the authority to give full information to patients about their condition or treatment.

When information was given to patients, it often consisted of what the health professional considered essential rather than information based on the patient's need or desire to know. Information was often presented to patients in a disorganized way, with little attention given to whether patients actually understood. Even less attention was given to whether patients actually carried out the recommendations given. This, in part, was due to health professionals' assumption that because they were in a position of authority, patients would automatically follow their recommendations. If a health professional discovered that the patient did not follow recommendations, rather than investigating reasons for patient noncompliance, more frequently the patient was labeled as "uncooperative" or "difficult." Attention was rarely given to exploring why recommendations were not followed or to questioning what could be done to increase the likelihood that patients would comply.

In the past several decades, of course, the general attitude about and approach to informing patients has changed. The emphasis on patient education as an important and mandated part of health care has increased. It is now expected that health professionals have the responsibility to fully inform patients about their condition and treatment, and to give them information about how they can prevent complications from occurring. Legally and professionally, it is expected that health professionals inform patients about their health and health care so that they may be fully aware of all aspects of their condition and treatment (Lester and Smith 1993). It is expected that patients are to be given full and accurate information that will enable them to make truly informed choices about their health and health care (Kabel 1984).

Many patients today no longer accept a passive role. They become involved in their own health and actively seek information about their condition, care, and treatment. In addition to the health professional, a number of other health-related information sources now exist. It would seem that with more opportunities for patients to gain health information that a more informed and sophisticated patient population would make noncompliance an issue of the past. Unfortunately, this does not seem to be the case. First of all, not all patients have equal access to information. Likewise, although information about a number of health topics are available, information from various sources is sometimes inconsistent and usually not specific to the patient's individual situation. A more important point, explaining why compliance continues to be problematic despite proliferation of information available, is that information alone is insufficient to motivate patients to take appropriate action. Consequently, even though information is available to patients, noncompliance remains a significant problem.

Given recognition that information does not necessarily mean that patients will comply with treatment recommendations, it would seem that interest in patient education would be diminishing; however, patient education efforts continue to expand. Several reasons help to explain this growth:

1. Because of growth in medical advances and technology, more people live longer with chronic diseases to which they once would have succumbed at an earlier age. Consequently, patient education efforts to help an increasing number of patients and their families manage and live with their condition, as well as helping them learn how to prevent complications from occurring, has become imperative.

2. The aging population is growing dramatically. Patient education directed toward helping older adults maintain their maximum level of health and independence is crucial to the health and well being not only of the individual but also to society as a whole. In addition, as individuals age, incidence of chronic disease increases, with the potential of several chronic conditions existing at one time. Helping older adults and their families understand and manage chronic disease, especially in the context of changes brought about by normal aging, adds a complexity that has made patient education a crucial factor in the health care of older adults.

3. As more is known about the role of prevention in the reduction of chronic disease and disability, patient education efforts directed toward helping patients reduce their risk of developing disease or complications of disease and reducing risk of injury, which could result in disability, become paramount.

4. Patients are now being discharged from hospitals earlier and given greater responsibility for managing care and treatment at home. Helping patients and families gain the knowledge and skills necessary for this level of care is an increasing challenge for patient education efforts.

5. Patients' access to patient education information about their condition, care, and treatment is no longer a luxury but rather a mandate. Because of mandates that dictate patients' rights to be fully informed and to participate in and make decisions about their own health and care has made patient education a necessity in outpatient as well as inpatient settings.

6. Even though information does not guarantee compliance, knowing and understanding recommendations increases the chances that patients will be better able to follow the treatment plan. Patients are unable to follow recommendations unless they are given appropriate information and understand the recommendations they have been given. The recognition of cost of noncompliance

in terms of human and financial resources has increased focus on strategies that may help alleviate or at least reduce the patient compliance problem.

With the increased recognition of the need for and importance of patient education, there also has been increased awareness that patient education is more than merely giving information. There has been recognition of the importance of developing an organized, effective, and individualized approach to patient education activities. It has taken a number of years for the concept to evolve.

PATIENT EDUCATION: A HISTORICAL PERSPECTIVE

Early in the era of organized health care, the possibility of patients benefiting from health care was scarcely greater than chance. Iatrogenic complications flourished, and exposure to the health care system was often more detrimental than helpful. The possibility of exposure to infection was great because of inadequate sanitary conditions in health care facilities. Organized health care was viewed as a last resort, and hospitals were considered a final alternative before death.

Consequently, much of the care of the sick was provided by members of the patient's family. Health professionals' efforts were directed toward teaching the family how to care for the patient and how to protect themselves from disease, especially if the patient's illness was thought to be infectious. Most patient education was done by physicians and nurses, who—because of their degree of patient contact—had the opportunity to conduct patient and family education. Nurses, although not always given authority for treatment, frequently carried out patient education in many of their activities, interpreting physicians' instructions for the patient.

As knowledge of disease processes and the mechanism of disease transmission grew, health care also changed. No longer were medical care and hospitalization viewed as last resorts for the hopelessly ill. Knowledge and technological advances made disease prevention a part of medical care. As a result, programs in sanitation, immunization, and maternal and child health became important components of the public health system. The term *health education* was frequently used to define these programs. The concept of health education might be thought of as a forerunner of patient education as we know it today.

After World War II, greater awareness of the rise of chronic disease and the increased longevity of those with long-term disabilities sparked additional interest in educating patients and their families not only about the control of communicable disease through sanitation and immunization but also about their diseases or disabling conditions as well. Health education thus began to expand its focus from disease prevention to include management of chronic conditions.

Although educating people about their health had begun with health education, most of the effort was still directed toward the general public. There was little effort directed specifically toward people who were actively being treated in the health care system. In 1950, the need for education of patients as an organized part of total health care became increasingly evident. The first references in literature to *patient education* can be found in the early 1950s. During this time, Veterans Administration hospitals, committed to total patient care, began to include selected patient education programs (Beauchamp 1974). At the same time, members of the National Tuberculosis Association were also devoting time and attention to teaching patients and their families about the disease and about a chronic disease program that became part of the public health service (Breckon 1982). As the success of these programs grew, more government funds were designated for the implementation of pilot projects, the focus of which was to teach patients about their disease conditions. Programs focusing on diabetes and rheumatic fever, renal dialysis, cancer, and stroke soon became available.

Although programs designed to teach patients with specific disease conditions were more prominent, the terms *patient education* and *health education* continued to be used interchangeably. Patient education as a separate concept was still in its embryonic form. Until this point, major emphasis had been placed on health education in the schools or on health education of the public at large. In 1964, the American Medical Association held the First National Conference on Health Education Goals. Much of the focus remained on community health programs; however, another significant outcome of the conference was development of an objective focused on educating individuals to be better able to assume responsibility for maintaining their personal health. Although much of the emphasis remained on prevention, the concept of direct participation by patients in their own health care and helping them assume more responsibility for their own health was beginning to be recognized as important.

At the same time, interest in the education of specialized target groups of patients who were already in the health care system and who were under the care of a health professional were also developing. Information given to these specialized groups went beyond disease prevention, which had been the focus of health education. Information for special patient groups was now directed toward increasing their understanding of the disease process and treatment as well. The term *patient education* was beginning to be used by health professionals to convey the idea of dissemination of information to patients who had specific disease conditions. *Patient education* and *health education* were beginning to be viewed as two separate, although related, concepts.

A publication from the Department of Health, Education, and Welfare in 1971, entitled "The Need for Patient Education," implied the need for a more specific concept of patient education—one that would not only include teaching patients how to stay healthy but also provide information about their disease conditions and treatment (US Dept HEW 1971). The article pointed out that although patient education was being provided by some individual health professionals and institutions, most health facilities had no specific program to provide patient education. Most patient education was being conducted on an incidental or ad hoc basis.

As a result of the recognition that patient education for the most part was being provided only sporadically, and because of concern that patients were not being given necessary information about their condition and treatment, the health education section of the American Public Health Association formed a Committee of Educational Tasks in Chronic Illness. The committee provided a forum for a more formal approach to patient education. As part of its recommendations, the committee spoke of the use of an educational prescription that would base patient teaching on each patient's individual needs (American Public Health Association 1968). The committee also recommended that the educational prescription be included as part of the patient's record. This was one of the first mentions of patient education as an organized health care activity worthy of documentation.

Continued interest in and development of patient education was brought about by the convergence of many factors. In 1971, in a health message to Congress, President Nixon used the term *health education*. Later, he appointed a committee to explore the feasibility of a public/private health education foundation. Committee members worked together for 2 years, generating much enthusiasm and interest in health education. Among their recommendations was one that had great impact on the future of patient education. Although still using the terms *health education* and *patient education* interchangeably, the committee recommended that hospitals offer health education to families of patients (Weingarten 1974). As a result of the committee's recommendations, a health education focal point was established in what was then the Department of Health, Education, and Welfare.

Another result of the committee's recommendations was the American Hospital Association's 1973 appointment of a special Committee on Health Education. Although the term *patient education* was still not widely used, the concept itself was becoming more established. The American Hospital Association Committee concluded that hospitals, as well as other health care institutions, had an obligation to provide educational programs for patients. These programs were to be established with the goal of "improved quality of patient care, better utilization of outpatient facilities, shorter lengths of stay and reduced health care costs" (American Hospital Association 1974). The Committee's recommendations not only made clear that patient education was more than giving information, by specifying that it should also have clear-cut outlines, but also established an expectation that health professionals were obligated to engage in patient education activities. Experimental patient education programs began to emerge. Many of the first such programs were implemented in an attempt to decrease noncompliance with prescribed medication regimens, thus decreasing subsequent hospital readmissions (Rosenberg 1971). The concept of patient education was beginning to be viewed as having the potential to affect not only the welfare of the patient but also the health care delivery system itself.

At the same time, health education bills began to appear in Congress. Bills introduced in 1974 and 1975 closely followed President Nixon's committee report. As a result, a modified version of bills previously introduced was passed and signed into law by President Ford in 1976. This established the National Consumer Health Information and Health Promotion Act of 1976.

The consumer movement that began in the 1960s was also gaining considerable force. Consumers were becoming more aware of their right to quality products and services as well as their right to be informed about the product or service they were receiving. Health care was beginning to be viewed in the same way. Because of the consumer movement and greater media exposure to issues related to health care, patients were becoming more aware not only of their rights as consumers of health care but also of their influence over the health care system. They became more demanding about being given information on their condition and treatment. Many patients began to insist on being involved in decision making regarding their care and treatment.

Cognizant of the consumer movement, the American Hospital Association published "A Patient's Bill of Rights" in 1975. The document addressed not only patients' rights to considerate and respectful care but also their right to current information on diagnosis, treatment, and prognosis; the right to receive information in understandable terms; and their right to receive information that would enable them to make informed decisions about any recommended treatment or procedure (American Hospital Association 1975). The concept of patient education had further evolved. Not only was patient education seen as an obligation of the health professional with the expectation of specified outcomes, it was viewed as a patient right as well. This patient right came to be protected by the legal process of informed consent.

Patient education was beginning to be acknowledged as a necessary part of quality patient care. Health professionals could now be held legally liable for acts of omission or commission with regard to education for patients and their families. One of the first rulings to substantiate this right came from an Iowa court in 1974. The court ruled that a physician who had failed to advise a patient properly could be tried for negligence (Krosnick 1974).

Although a descendant of health education, patient education had evolved as a concept in its own right—a concept that included more than teaching patients and their families about disease prevention, sanitation, and immunization. Patient education was now considered a part of total, comprehensive, quality patient care; it included teaching patients about their specific disease and treatment as well as about prevention of disease. It had grown into more than a nicety provided to patients for altruistic reasons. It was now recognized as a necessity for quality health care, a patient right, a factor that could increase efficacy of the health care delivery system, and an obligation and legal responsibility of health professionals.

PROFESSIONAL COMMITMENT TO PATIENT EDUCATION

Patient education became an entity in its own right. The responsibility for providing patient education was recognized as fundamental to the provision of quality health care. Although the importance and legitimacy of patient education had been established, another question still remained: Who exactly was responsible for providing patient education? Various groups of health professionals began to consider how patient education fit into their mode of delivery of health care.

Many health professions had traditionally considered communication with patients and their families about disease and treatment a regular part of care. The realization emerged, however, that patient education was often taken for granted and perhaps not always taken as seriously as other aspects of patient care. Physicians, nurses, dietitians, pharmacists, dentists, physical therapists, and other health professionals began to consider their role and responsibility in providing patient education and to outline their formal commitment to it. As a result, a number of professional organizations representing various health professionals began to issue formal statements that delineated their philosophy and role with regard to patient education.

In 1975, the House of Delegates of the American Medical Association adopted a formal statement that addressed patient education as an integral part of high-quality health care (American Medical Association 1975). It was viewed as a way to improve patients' and their families' participation in treatment and as a tool that could aid in the recovery of patients. Although the American Medical Association's statement clearly emphasized the responsibility of physicians in conducting patient education, it acknowledged that the process was also the ongoing professional responsibility of nurses, dietitians, and other members of the health care team. The statement lent further credibility to patient education as a legitimate part of health care. It also emphasized that patient education was not the responsibility of only one health profession but rather was a team effort involving all health professionals who came in contact with the patient. The statement also focused on another point that had only been alluded to previously: that patients shared in responsibility for their health. Patients rights were acknowledged, but the statement also indicated that rights go hand in hand with responsibility. Patients were expected to share in responsibility for patient education outcomes.

Nurses have also had a long history of involvement in communicating with patients about health care concerns. Nursings' role in patient teaching can be documented as early as 1900 in an article in the American Journal of Nursing (Moore 1900). "The Standards of Nursing Practice" of the American Nursing Association also reflected nurses' responsibilities in patient education (American Nurses Association 1973). Although most nurses had long accepted and acknowledged their part in educating patients, their role in the process had not been clearly defined, particularly with regard to the degree of independence with which they should function. In 1975, the American Nurses' Association published a statement entitled "The Professional Nurse and Health Education," which outlined nurses' responsibility in patient education (American Nurses Association 1975). The publication stated that:

> as a health care provider, every professional nurse is responsible and accountable to the patient and family for the quality of nursing care the patient receives. The responsibility and accountability includes teaching the patient and family relevant facts about specific health care needs and supporting appropriate modification of behavior.

The same document also outlined specific responsibilities for nurses in the hospital setting, which included:

> assessing patients' knowledge about his illness, rehabilitation and health maintenance . . . including diagnostic preparation and procedures, preoperative and postoperative care, treatment and drugs, and discharge planning and follow up.

The American Nurses Association's statement not only established a formal commitment to patient education but also carried the concept one step further by listing specific areas about which patients were expected to receive information. The statement strengthened the view expressed by the American Medical Association's statement, which had pointed out that patient education may be beneficial to patient recovery. The American Nurses Association's statement brought the idea into even clearer focus by speaking of the appropriate modification of behavior of patients themselves. Positive outcomes were expected from patient education. It was no longer considered merely information giving, but a mechanism for bringing about a degree of behavior change as well.

Other health professionals also published statements on patient education. In 1976 the American Society of Hospital Pharmacists published a document entitled "Statement on Pharmacist Conducted Patient Counseling," which emphasized pharmacists' responsibility to educate patients about their medications (American Society of Hospital Pharmacists 1976). The statement listed specific information that patients should be given about their medication, including the name of the medication; how it should be taken; its expected action, route, dosage, and administration; special directions for administration; and precautions and side effects. Patients would no longer be taking medications they knew little about. They would be given information to help them become knowledgeable about the drugs they were taking.

The American Dietetic Association also specified patient education as a function of the registered dietitian. The position paper published recommended that dietitians counsel individuals and families in nutritional principles, dietary plans, and food selections; communicate appropriate dietary history in medical records; and compile and develop nutritional educational material for patients receiving dietary counseling (American Dietetic Association 1976). Giving patients information verbally was clearly an expectation, but compilation and development of patient education materials to reinforce information given in the counseling session was added to their role in patient education.

An important reinforcement of patient education as a right and expectation of quality health care came with the 1976 edition of *Accreditation Manual for Hospitals,* published by the Joint Commission on Accreditation of Health Care Organizations (1976). The 1976 edition included statements relating to quality of professional services and patient rights. It expanded the scope of patient education to include services to outpatients, such as emergency room patients and patients having outpatient surgery, as well as to inpatients. The Joint Commission stated that the criteria for quality patient care should include patients' demonstrated knowledge of their health status, level of functioning, and self-care requirements after leaving the hospital. According to the manual, the patient also has the right to be informed about any technical procedure to be performed, including what the procedure involved, why it was necessary, and who would perform the procedure. The Joint Commission emphasized health professionals' responsibility to provide information about the patient's medical problem, the nature of the problem, the prognosis, and information about the treatment plan to be implemented. The manual mandated that evidence of appropriate informed consent be part of the medical record and emphasized the need for final progress notes, which were to include specific instructions the patient and their family had been given. The manual specified that criteria for patient education should be established and that evidence should be provided that patients not only had been given information but that they understood it as well. In addition to further solidifying patient education as a part of quality health care, the 1976 manual firmly set the stage for using a more structured approach to patient education both in delivery and in record keeping, as well as for accountability to assure that patients were able to comprehend information they were given. Failure to ensure that patients were adequately informed could now result in repercussions not only for health professionals but for the institutions they served.

Other health professions also acknowledged their commitment to the concept of patient education and its implementation, outlining roles and responsibilities expected from their members, with some even including patient education as part of their professional practice acts. Although specific roles and responsibilities of members in various health professions varied, a general consensus of perception of what patient education should entail emerged. The consensus seemed to be that:

- Patient education is a part of total health care and should be included in inpatient, outpatient, or emergency settings.
- Patient education is the responsibility of every health professional.
- Patients have the right to information about their condition and treatment, procedures, potential side effects or complications of treatment, and prevention and health maintenance.
- Patient education should be based on the needs of the individual patient.
- Patient education should be directed not only toward giving patients information but also assisting them to achieve goals that will benefit their health status.
- Documentation of provision of information to patients should be included in the medical record.
- Patient education should be a planned, organized activity.

Patient education continues to have support from most health professions. Since it's original mandate in 1976 for patient education, the Joint Commission on Accreditation of Health Care Organizations lists education of patients and families as a function critical to patient care (Joint Commission on Accreditation of Healthcare Organizations 1995). The National Committee for Quality Assurance has also incorporated patient education-related performance measures into the Health Plan Employer Data and Information Set for comparison of managed care organizations (National Committee for Quality Assurance 1999).

ARRIVING AT A DEFINITION OF PATIENT EDUCATION

Although the philosophical basis of patient education and the characteristics it encompasses have been recognized and, in general, agreed upon by most health professions, the actual process of patient education and how it should be carried out has often been interpreted more broadly. The terms *patient education* and *patient teaching* have been used synonymously and the term *instruction* used interchangeably with *education*. In some instances, *patient education* has been equated to *patient information*.

The terms *education, instruction, teaching,* and *information* each imply a focus on knowledge. Certainly, to be able to carry out treatment recommendations, patients must have knowledge about what to do. Knowledge alone, however, is not always a predictor of behavior. This fact can be illustrated by a common everyday example of speed limits on highways. Most people have knowledge that there are speed limits on the open road and that going over the speed limit could result in a traffic ticket. Despite this knowledge, people continue to go over the speed limit and continue to receive speeding tickets every day. The same principle can be applied to health recommendations and the extent to which patients carry them out. Patients' knowledge about their condition and even knowledge of recommendations are insufficient to ensure that those recommendations will be followed.

Consequently, effectiveness of patient education must involve more than knowledge alone. Before patient education can be effective, learning must take place. Ultimately, learning involves more than the ability to regurgitate facts. A comprehensive definition of patient education, then, must encompass more than presenting information to a passive patient.

Over the years, in the literature, several descriptions of patient education as a broader context have been suggested. Examples are:

a process requiring assessment of the total patient needs, including an understanding of social, psychological, educational, socioeconomic, vocational, and cultural characteristics of the patient (Verstraete and Meier 1973).

activities planned to encourage patients with acute or chronic conditions to participate actively and appropriately in their treatment and rehabilitation (Wolle 1974).

the process of influencing patient behavior and producing the changes in knowledge, attitudes and skills necessary to maintain or improve health (American Academy of Family Physicians 2000).

These descriptions imply that patient education is an active, individualized process directed toward not only knowledge but also toward adaptation and behavior change that will produce positive health outcomes. To be effective, this individualized process necessitates communication between patients and health professionals in which patients' needs, experiences, attitudes, preferences, and other factors that impact their health and health care are identified. Patients' perceptions of themselves, their lives, and their problems can have significant impact on the effectiveness of patient education. Because patients' emotional responses are concomitant of their physical condition, the impact these responses play in the patient education process also cannot be ignored.

DEVELOPING PATIENT EDUCATION AS A CLINICAL SKILL

Just as health professionals learn and practice skills needed to perform technical procedures effectively, so must they learn and practice skills in patient education before those interventions can be effective. Even though patient education may be recognized as an important aspect of quality patient care, it is often taken for granted as a skill health professionals develop automatically. The complexity of the patient education process is often overlooked.

Most health professional receive no formal training in how to most effectively conduct patient education. As a result, even with best intentions, patient education is often conducted haphazardly, inefficiently, and ineffectively. Although the vast majority of patients in both inpatient and outpatient settings require, and presumably receive, some information related to their health, condition, or treatment, it is an interesting paradox that so little time and attention traditionally have been devoted to patient education in the curricula of many schools of health professionals. In the past decade, an increasing number of training programs are including at least some aspects of patient education in the curricula. Such training in the basic curriculum can increase both the quality and quantity of patient education. For those health professionals currently in practice who have not had the benefit of such training, continuing education programs and self-education through the literature can assist in gaining the skills needed to conduct patient education effectively.

Part of learning about patient education is also developing an understanding of its importance in the delivery of quality patient care. Every interaction with a patient is an opportunity to conduct some type of patient education. Health professionals must recognize that just as a variety of health professionals are involved in patient care, so are a variety of health professionals involved in patient education. For the benefit of the patient and for delivery of the highest quality of patient education, it therefore behooves health professionals to work together in a coordinated effort to delivery the most effective patient education possible. Each health professional has a responsibility to conduct patient education when the opportunity arises.

In addition to specific skills related to patient education, health professionals must also have sufficient knowledge about the content of information to be taught. If health professionals are not secure in their knowledge of a specific topical area, there is potential for giving inadequate, not to mention inaccurate, information or, in some instances, no information at all. Of course, sufficient knowledge in an area does not guarantee effective patient education. It does, however, increase the probability, especially if the health professional possesses good communication skills as well.

Effective patient education skills, then, consist of more than information giving. To conduct patient education effectively, health professionals must build trust and rapport with the patient and be facilitators of learning and problem solving. They must have the ability to help patients clarify issues and reach decisions regarding their treatment. Health professionals must have the ability to communicate recommendations in a clear way that patients can understand and be able to develop a plan that is compatible with the patient's own priorities and life style. Lastly, they must be able to develop a plan for follow-up and evaluation of the outcome of the patient education intervention.

Ultimately, patients control the extent to which they follow the recommendations they are given. The role of health professionals is to enable patients to act on their own behalf by providing them with information, thereby helping them to identify appropriate alternatives when needed. The health professional's role includes offering acceptance, support, and guidance so that patients have the highest opportunity to integrate information and recommendations to best meet their own goals. This means health professionals must also have an understanding of how patients respond to illness as well as to health.

In addition to good assessment, communication, social, and organizational skills needed in patient education, development of effective patient education skills requires establishing an appropriate philosophical and conceptual base. Without such a base, expectations of what patient education is and what it can accomplish can result in disappointment and disillusion for health professionals as well as patients.

The effectiveness of patient education depends as much on the emotional atmosphere as on the content being taught. Patient education is most effective when health professionals take a helping approach rather than a dogmatic one. Whether patients follow recommendations depends not only on their understanding of what they are to do but also, and probably to a greater degree, on their judgment and feelings about the meaning those recommendations have for them and their lives.

GROWTH AND CHALLENGES FOR PATIENT EDUCATION

Patient education has gained more credibility and acceptance, but the concept continues to evolve. As patient education develops as an integral part of patient care, new challenges arise that must be confronted and resolved if the concept is to meet its full potential.

Many of the challenges facing patient education emanate from the health care system itself. Cost containment, staff shortages, the need for evidence-based practices, and demonstrated effectiveness create increasing pressure on patient education to prove its value in patient care.

A number of issues facing patient education need to be addressed and resolved. Can patient education improve health status, decrease the incidence of complications of disease, or reduce hospitalizations? To what extent does patient education increase patient satisfaction? Is patient education for the sole purpose of helping patients make informed choices sufficient reason to justify expenditure of resources, especially when patient choices may not always be in agreement with what health professionals believe are in the patients' best interest? Does patient education reduce the chance of litigation, and, if so, is this alone an appropriate reason to support patient education? How can patient education be conducted effectively when inadequate staffing exists? Will inadequate staffing and heavy workload result in decreased quality and quantity of patient education?

Are some methods of patient teaching more effective than others? Are technology-based methods such as computer-assisted instruction or audio-visual aids effective in enhancing desired patient education outcomes, or are they an expense that may not be cost effective? How can patient teaching best be adapted to meet needs of a variety of patients, regardless of age, education, cultural background, or medical condition?

How and when should patient education be reimbursed? What type of patient education should be considered for reimbursement? Is prevention teaching as valuable as patient education for chronic illness? Should all health professionals who conduct patient education be reimbursed for their services, or should only health professionals who meet standards that demonstrate competence in patient education skills be eligible for reimbursement? If standards for competence in patient education skills should be established, by whom should these standards be set? How should competence be measured?

Many of the above issues require policy decisions that should be based on data gained by systematic and well-planned research that address these issues. Other issues require careful philosophical and ethical considerations. How each of these issues are addressed will determine the extent to which patient education gains increased credibility and support as a priority in patient care. How these challenges are resolved will depend to a great extent on leadership of health professionals who believe in and are committed to effective patient education as a means to improved health and health care of all patients.

Is having a coordinator of patient education necessary to promote an organized program of patient education that benefits all patients? If so, how should the coordinator of patient education position be funded? Is having patient education programs directed to specific disease entities adequate to meet patient education needs of patients? How can coordinated efforts to meet the patient education needs of all patients be managed?

How can patient education training be included in curriculum of basic preparation programs of health professionals, and what is the best way to provide continuing education so that health professionals already in the field have the opportunity to learn or to enhance their patient education skills? What mechanism should be used to measure competence in patient education skills?

Patient education is not simply a matter of repeating directions to patients or handing out printed materials. It is a process involving the health professional's precise clinical skills in terms of data gathering, individualization of instructions, prompting and support, and evaluation and follow-up of the patient's success in implementing the treatment plan. Patient's errors in interpreting instructions given by health professionals are common. These errors can occur if health professionals fail to carefully instruct patients in specific details of treatment, encourage questions, assess patient reactions, and determine the extent to which patients understand and agree with the recommendations given. To reduce patient errors and thus increase patient compliance with recommendations, health professionals must monitor patient follow-through with instructions they have been given.

The question then remains: How can health professionals fit such a complex process as patient education into their already harried schedules? The answer is in learning how to conduct patient teaching efficiently and effectively. The process of patient education, if incorporated into daily interactions as an organized, structured part of each patient encounter can actually save health professionals time in terms of increased patient compliance and, therefore, the possibility of fewer unnecessary return visits and fewer unnecessary phone calls, and it can decrease other manifestations of patients' failing to understand and/or follow recommendations. In those instances when patients require additional patient teaching, the benefits of patients who are better able and willing to follow treatment plans can well make up for the extra time spent in patient teaching. Using teaching aids such as brochures, films, or pamphlets can supplement and reinforce patient teaching but should never be used to replace the interpersonal interaction. Not only do teaching aids involve considerable expenditure of resources, they can also result in disillusionment for patients as well as staff with regard to the benefits of patient education. When patients feel the health professional understands their concerns, has explained their condition and treatment in terms they understand, has been willing to individualize the treatment plan to the patient's needs, and provides patient education in a personalized, warm, and understanding manner, a positive effect on patient compliance can result (Green 1987). Patient education is a patient right as well as a responsibility of the health professional. If it is to be conducted, then it should be done effectively to gain the greatest benefit for patient and health professional alike.

REFERENCES

American Academy of Family Physicians. 2000. Recommended core educational guidelines for family practice residents: patient education. Reprint No. 284. Kansas City, MO: American Academy of Family Physicians.

American Dietetic Association. 1976. Position paper on recommended salaries and employment practices for members of the American Dietetic Association. Chicago, IL: American Dietetic Association.

American Hospital Association. 1974. The role of hospitals and other health care institutions in personal and community health education. Chicago, IL: American Hospital Association.

American Hospital Association. 1975. A patient's bill of rights. Chicago, IL: American Hospital Association.

American Medical Association. 1975. Statement of patient education. Chicago, IL: American Medical Association.

American Nurses Association. 1973. Standards of nursing practice. Kansas City, MO: American Nurses Association.

American Nurses Association. 1975. The professional nurse and health education. Kansas City, MO: American Nurses Association.

American Public Health Association. 1968. A model for planning patient education: an essential component of health care. New York, NY: American Public Health Association.

American Society of Hospital Pharmacists. 1976. Statement on pharmacist conducted patient counseling. Bethesda, MD: American Society of Hospital Pharmacists.

Beauchamp, G.E. 1974. Patient education and the hospital program. Veterans Administration Technical Bulletin, No. 88. Washington, DC: US Government Printing Office.

Breckon, D.J. 1982. Hospital health education: a guide to program development. Gaithersburg, MD: Aspen Publishers, Inc.

Green, L.W. 1987. How physicians can improve patient's participation and maintenance in self care. *Western Journal of Medicine* 147:346–349.

Joint Commission on Accreditation of Healthcare Organizations. 1976. Accreditation manual for hospitals. Chicago, IL: Joint Commission on Accreditation of Healthcare Organizations.

Joint Commission on Accreditation of Healthcare Organizations. 1995. Comprehensive accreditation manual for hospitals, Vol. 1 and 2. Oakbrook Terrace, IL: Joint Commission on Accreditation of Healthcare Organizations.

Kabel, J. 1984. Diabetes self-care. Potential liability of the treating physician. *Legal Medicine* 5:253–293.

Krosnick, A. 1974. Failure to educate patients may lead to charge of physician negligence. *Diabetes Outlook* 9:4.

Lester, G.W., Smith, S.G. 1993. Listening and talking to patients. A remedy for malpractice suits? *Western Journal of Medicine* 158:268–272.

Moore, E.J. 1900. Visiting nursing. *American Journal of Nursing* 1:17–21.

National Committee for Quality Assurance. 1999. HEDIS 2000. Washington, DC: National Committee for Quality Assurance.

Rosenberg, S.G. 1971. Patient education leads to better care for heart patients. Technical Reports. Reprinted from *HSMHA Health Reports* 86:793–802.

US Department of Health, Education, and Welfare. 1971. The need for patient education. *American Journal of Public Health* 61:7.

Verstraete, D., Meier, M. 1973. Patient education in a health sciences center. *Minnesota Medicine* 56(Suppl 2):31–35.

Weingarten, V. 1974. Report of the findings and recommendations of the president's committee on health education. *Health Education Monograph* 1:11–19.

Wolle, J.M. 1974. Patient education. *Journal of American College Health Association* 22:231.

Psychosocial Factors in Patient Education and Patient Compliance

3

PSYCHOSOCIAL FACTORS IN PATIENT EDUCATION

Patients with medical problems sometimes behave in ways that imperil their health. Some who have not yet developed symptoms of disease neglect measures that might prevent disease from occurring. The fact that patients would purposely behave in a way that would make their condition worse, or cause a disease process to occur, seems totally irrational. It is widely recognized, however, that many patients neglect to take medications as prescribed, resist restriction of activities as recommended, and neglect to follow preventive measures.

If one of the goals of patient education is to produce behavior change that helps patients to improve or maintain their health status, then poor compliance with recommendations may be viewed as a failure in patient education. Such behavior can be frustrating and puzzling for the conscientious health professional devoted to increasing positive health outcomes through patient education. Why would patients deliberately act in ways deleterious to their health despite having received information indicating that they should behave otherwise? Why, for example, would patients with emphysema continue to smoke regardless of knowledge of the consequences of their behavior? Why do some patients neglect self-care even though they know they will be incapacitated by their condition if it is left untreated?

There is, of course, no single answer. All patients, as individuals, have different reactions, experiences, and motives that direct their behavior. Illness, or threat of illness, elicits many responses from individuals and their families. At times, responses are helpful; other responses deter patients from following the prescribed therapeutic regimen. In addition to patients' knowledge, many factors have an impact on their ability and willingness to carry out recommendations. Psychosocial factors such as patients' reactions; beliefs and attitudes; systems of support, such as their family or other social group; and financial circumstances all have a profound impact on patient education and its ultimate effectiveness. Failure to comply with recommendations can often be attributed to these factors.

Health professionals are frequently uneasy dealing with psychosocial factors, however. Some may be unaware of signs that could alert them to factors with an impact on the effectiveness of patient education. Others may be reluctant to act on psychosocial factors when they are identified. Some may believe that considering psychosocial factors is impractical because of time constraints.

If patient education is to be effective, psychosocial factors cannot be avoided. Giving patients information about their condition or treatment without considering factors that may facilitate or hinder their following recommendations is not only an inefficient use of time, it also leads to poor outcomes for patient education. If, for example, the patient does not believe in taking medication, but medication is a necessary part of treatment, ignoring the problem while continuing to teach the patient about the medication is useless. Explaining the importance of treatment and how to take the medication does little good unless the health professional also considers the patient's feelings and takes that factor into consideration.

In other instances, health professionals may avoid psychosocial factors because they seem overwhelming. Psychosocial factors may be avoided because of the health professional's own feelings of inadequacy in handling the problems presented. Again, dealing only with knowledge aspects of patient education is a futile effort. Without a firm understanding of the other factors that have an impact on the effectiveness of patient education, the health professional's efforts in relaying knowledge alone can end in frustration for both patient and health professional.

Data collection and assessment of psychosocial factors should be part of every patient interaction. Health professionals need only be aware of available data sources. Identification of psychosocial factors need not involve extensive use of time. Likewise, if health professionals put psychosocial data into the right perspective, data need not be overwhelming but rather can be helpful in working more effectively with the patient.

Patients frequently drop hints about factors that might influence their degree of compliance with the prescribed regimen. By listening to these hints and exploring them further, health professionals may be able to devise a more effective teaching plan. Take, for example, Mrs. Delengato, a 32-year-old woman with a history of rheumatic fever. Mrs. Delengato was being treated for cardiac dysrhythmias with quinidine and Inderal. The patient had received teaching about her heart condition and had been given explicit instructions about the medication and behavioral restrictions. When evaluating teaching effectiveness at a subsequent outpatient visit, however, the physician discovered that Mrs. Delengato frequently neglected to take her medication and continued to smoke one pack of cigarettes a day despite recommendations to stop smoking. During the clinic visit, Mrs. Delengato stated that she had recently experienced tachycardia, weakness, and pressure in her chest. In the course of describing her symptoms, she mentioned that her mother had had the same symptoms. The physician explored the statement further. Mrs. Delengato revealed that her mother had died at age 35 from a myocardial infarction, although she had had no previous history of cardiac problems. As the physician continued to talk with her, the patient revealed that she believed she was also destined to die at an early age. Mrs. Delengato felt that if her mother had had no previous history of heart disease and still died, that with her own history of rheumatic fever and subsequent health problems, there was little hope no matter what she did. Mrs. Delengato, therefore, elected to do what she wanted, feeling the treatment and restrictions were of little consequence. Because of the new information gathered about the patient, the physician established a new approach to teaching in which the patient's fears and beliefs could also be addressed.

Patients' lives are guided by a set of norms and values—expressed or unexpressed. The meaning of illness and the consequences ascribed to following or not following recommendations are based mainly on how patients perceive them. Patients' symptoms are also relative; whereas some may dramatize symptoms, others are passive in response to their symptoms and conditions. Health professionals also have values and norms that direct their lives and guide their practice. It is important to be aware that these values may quite often be different from those held by the patient.

Health professionals should gain an appreciation of patients' life situations so as to identify and understand patients' beliefs, perspectives, and priorities. Only then will health professionals be able to devise effective teaching plans. Conducting patient education based on the values and needs of the health professional, rather than on those of the patient, can result in patients shutting out and rejecting information given. Once this has occurred, it is difficult to reinvolve patients.

Health professionals' knowledge of psychosocial factors can be used to design teaching strategies that take various patient influences into consideration. Health professionals may recognize the need to gather additional data. Discovering additional psychosocial factors may alert health professionals to the need to refer the patient to another health professional or agency for assistance. Or the services of other health professionals may be incorporated to help meet patient needs. Outcomes of education may have to be negotiated between patients and health professionals, with the establishment of new goals and expectations tailored to meet patients' individual needs best.

The greater the health professional's understanding of psychosocial factors, the greater the chance that such information can be incorporated into a more effective teaching interaction. As a result, there is an increased probability that the teaching interaction will have positive health outcomes. To be effective, patient education must use creative techniques in which psychosocial factors are identified and incorporated. Each patient is an individual; consequently, there can be no generalization about specific factors that affect individuals. The health professional must become skillful, confident, and adept in assessing patients' needs and factors that have an impact on the degree to which patients are willing or able to follow recommendations. The first step toward this skill is to have an understanding of various ways patients react to and cope with illness, the threat of illness, or disability. The following two sections provide background knowledge to assist health professionals in attaining this skill.

THE PATIENT AS AN INDIVIDUAL

Each patient is a unique person with a unique personality, an individual method of coping with stress, a variety of past experiences, and a system of beliefs about the world. The better able the health professional is to tailor patient education to the individual patient, the greater the likelihood that patients will be able to follow recommendations given. A variety of factors about individual patients will determine their reactions not only to symptoms and disease but also to patient teaching and recommendations provided. Recognizing individual patient needs and priorities helps health professionals to present information in such a way that it will be meaningful for the particular patient to whom it is being directed.

Symptoms of disease, for instance, may create different reactions in patients at different stages of life. A skin lesion during adolescence may cause concern because of its appearance, whereas the same lesion in an older person may hint at the possibility of cancer. Although the lesions in both instances may be the same, and the information that could be given to the patients about them may be similar, the teaching approach used may be different because each patient has different priorities and concerns.

Part of patient teaching must also consider patients' past experiences and expectations. A pregnant teenager whose mother had no prenatal care and no resulting complications from pregnancy may see little need for regular visits to the physician during her own pregnancy. The patient who is used to receiving antibiotics routinely for sore throats regardless of the cause may have some difficulty understanding why the physician is only giving instructions about gargling with salt water.

Patients also have varying views about health and illness. Some believe that health and illness are predetermined, and consequently they may take on a "what will be, will be" attitude, assuming little responsibility for the consequences of their own health behavior. They may scoff at preventive practices such as stopping smoking if they have known people who have smoked all their lives and yet lived to a ripe old age. Rather than arguing with these perceptions or expectations, health professionals will be more successful in most cases if patients' needs, priorities, expectations, and perceptions are considered and worked into the teaching plan.

One of the most critical factors in patient education is determining patients' attitudes about their condition and its meaning for them. Despite patients' knowledge or skill acquisition, their medical management and teaching may be extremely difficult if they have not accepted their condition or its seriousness; if they view it as a means of controlling others or of punishing themselves or others; or if they have a variety of other detrimental feelings about their condition.

An example of the effect of attitude is illustrated by the case of Mrs. Yablonski, who was seen in the neighborhood health clinic because of severe hypertension. The clinic nurse, aware of the importance of patient education, spent considerable time with Mrs. Yablonski, explaining hypertension, the particular treatment prescribed, how Mrs. Yablonski was to take the medication, and the possible consequences of not taking it properly. Being very conscientious, the nurse evaluated Mrs. Yablonski's knowledge level after patient teaching and was delighted to find that the patient was able to describe her condition and treatment in detail, why the medication was important, and what might happen if her condition was left untreated. There had not been a problem with skill, and no other barriers, such as inability to purchase the medication, were identified. The nurse felt that the teaching session had been extremely effective and felt certain that Mrs. Yablonski would be extremely compliant in following recommendations.

The patient was seen at the clinic weekly for blood pressure checks, but each week her blood pressure remained elevated. The physician at the clinic continued to add antihypertensive medications to her treatment regimen, until at last it was decided that Mrs. Yablonski should be referred to a nephrologist for further evaluation. Mrs. Yablonski had been at the referral center for about a week when the nephrologist called her physician, saying that all her tests had been negative and that her blood pressure was currently being controlled on one medication. Upon questioning Mrs. Yablonski closely, the nephrologist had found that she had not taken any of the medication prescribed by her physician. When Mrs. Yablonski returned to her regular physician, he questioned her, puzzled as to why she would deliberately not take her medication when she had understood the possible consequences of stroke and even death from her lack of compliance with the regimen. Mrs. Yablonski replied that she viewed her hypertension as deserved punishment for indiscretions she had committed in the past and therefore was accepting the consequences as "payment" for her previous behavior.

The patient's severe guilt would warrant counseling and therapy that were beyond the scope of patient education. Had either the physician or nurse been aware of the patient's attitudes about her condition earlier, however, Mrs. Yablonski's exposure to a potentially dangerous situation might have been alleviated earlier through referral, and a needless expenditure of time, effort, and money could have been saved. Had the physician or nurse developed a relationship with Mrs. Yablonski that enabled her to share her feelings with one of them, the situation also might have been avoided. By referring Mrs. Yablonski to the appropriate health professional for the help she needed, the patient education intervention might have had a more successful outcome.

In this instance, the patient's attitudes, not her level of knowledge, were the determinant of the degree to which she followed the physician's recommendations. Had her attitudes been identified, counseling and support could have been recommended to assist Mrs. Yablonski in dealing with her guilt and thus could have helped to make further educational efforts more effective.

Social Influences

We are all part of a social group, whether it consists of family, friends, culture, or a religious group. Each group establishes its own norms or values to which individuals within the group are expected to subscribe and adhere. Deviation from these values or norms can be the source of ridicule from the group or, in some cases, even expulsion. Groups provide a sense of self and give individuals a framework within which to interpret various aspects of life and ways of responding to a variety of events. Values of health and health care, the meaning of illness, and which treatments are deemed acceptable or unacceptable are learned within the social group.

Patients and health professionals frequently come from different social groups and therefore may have different values, beliefs, and assumptions. Those differences may emerge not only with regard to reactions and interpretations of various life events but also with regard to health and health care in general. If health professionals make the assumption that everyone subscribes to the same values they do, or if differences in values are not identified between health professionals and patients, there is a basis for misunderstanding as well as a barrier to communication.

The influence of social groups is extremely relevant to patient education. Without an understanding of the influence of these groups, health professionals can spend much effort conducting patient education that is irrelevant, or at times offensive, to patients who have values different from their own. Patients will not only be unwilling to follow health advice that conflicts with their own beliefs or values but may also be alienated from consulting with the health professional in the future. Consider the case of Mrs. Taylor.

Mrs. Taylor had just delivered her fifth child. The postpartum unit of the hospital had established a regular patient education session for all patients who had delivered. Part of the regular teaching was on contraception. The nurse proceeded to teach Mrs. Taylor about contraception according to the teaching protocol. She observed that Mrs. Taylor appeared to be more withdrawn as the teaching went on. The nurse interpreted this to mean that she was tired and concluded the session, asking Mrs. Taylor if she had any questions about the information. She also mentioned that she would come back at a later time to continue the teaching session. Mrs. Taylor replied that she had no questions and that it would not be necessary for the nurse to return. Puzzled, the nurse left the room, charting that Mrs. Taylor was uncooperative and resistant to patient education. Had the nurse taken some time before the teaching session began to gather some information about Mrs. Taylor as an individual, she would have learned that the woman was a devout Roman Catholic who was very much opposed to birth control. Not only had the nurse not considered the patient's needs when conducting the educational intervention, she had created a barrier to further teaching as well. The nurse's time was wasted, and the opportunity for future teaching was lost.

Other instances of the influence of social groups may be illustrated by various patients' use of folk remedies or folk healers. Folk remedies endure in various areas of the United States because they are well known, trusted, accessible, and inexpensive. Advice about folk remedies passed down through generations by trusted individuals is often perceived as more helpful than prescribed medical treatments. Recommendations may be distrusted when given by a health professional the patient does not know, someone with whom he or she has insufficient rapport. In other instances, prescribed treatments may be expensive and/or distasteful and may not give the immediate results the patient expects.

In some cultures, folk healers are still intermingled with modern medicine. It does little good to try to discredit folk remedies or the advice of folk healers that has been given to the patient. The folk healer may be a trusted part of the patient's health care system. Efforts to discredit such healers or the advice given by other trusted members of the patient's social group may only alienate the patient, who may distrust the health professional in the first place. It may be far better to identify the folk remedies tried by the patient or recommended by the folk healer and add medical technology to them rather than demanding that the patient abandon them altogether. At times, the consequences of folk practices may be somewhat difficult to deal with, especially if they can cause harm. Such a situation is illustrated in the case of Mr. Romaro.

Mr. Romaro, a patient of Filipino-American background, was seen at the Family Practice Center for epigastric pain. After a number of diagnostic tests, the physician diagnosed the patient as having an ulcer and immediately prescribed a regimen of medication and a restricted diet. Mr. Romaro was referred to the dietitian for diet counseling, during which the diet and its purpose were explained. Sometime later, the patient returned to the clinic with severe worsening of symptoms. On evaluation, the physician indicated that surgery might be necessary and admitted the patient to the hospital for further observation. The dietitian who had done the original diet teaching visited the patient in the hospital. In the course of the conversation about the extent to which the patient had followed the prescribed diet and treatment regimen at home, Mr. Romaro revealed that he had not taken the medication and had disputed the dietitian's advice to avoid spices in his food. In the Filipino culture, spices were actually considered to have healing properties. Obtaining a variety of spices from his grandmother, the patient had proceeded to spice his food liberally. When his condition became worse instead of better, he attributed the worsening to the prescribed treatment and discontinued it.

Such situations are indeed difficult to work with. In this case, the patient's beliefs and folk remedies were the cause of potential harm. Had the dietitian recognized these beliefs in the initial teaching interaction, they could at least have been considered. The situation might have been different had the dietitian been alert to the possibility of culture differences rather than conducting teaching in a standardized manner. The dietitian might have taken the time to ask Mr. Romaro about his beliefs and perceptions. The dietitian might have said: "I know very little about the Filipino culture. I find sometimes even when Americans are born in this country, the traditions of our heritage, of our grandparents and great grandparents, are still important to our own life style. Are there any special things that we've talked about with regard to your diet that are contrary to any of your cultural or personal beliefs?" Additional information about multicultural issues can be found in Chapter 7.

To discount the beliefs completely would only have been a barrier to establishing trust in the future. To correct erroneous beliefs or to criticize advice given the patient by well-meaning friends or relatives may also destroy trust and rapport. In such instances, it is far better for health professionals to identify the beliefs and health practices of patients, and to work within the patient's framework to build a stronger relationship for the future.

In the United States, being slender is considered an attractive attribute. The saying, "You can never be too thin or too rich," is taken quite seriously by many. It is quite easy for the health professionals to assume that all patients view obesity as undesirable, not only in terms of appearance but also in terms of health. Not all cultures hold similar views, however. In many cultures, eating occupies a central role in life. Overweight may actually be viewed as attractive, with obesity a sign of health. In other cultures, food may be equated with love and affection.

In these instances, talking with patients about weight control and its importance may disavow their own perceptions and beliefs and set the stage for failure. If health professionals view obesity as a health threat, it is far more important in the initial teaching session for the professional to assess what eating means to the individual and to begin working with the patient at that level. If the patients' beliefs about weight appear firmly ingrained, it may be better to begin talking with them about other means of prevention or other aspects of the medical regimen than to attack their basic views. On the other hand, if the patients see eating as a source of comfort and solace or a way of dealing with stress, health professionals may need to gradually help them develop other coping mechanisms before patient education can be effective.

The patient's family or peer group are important social groups that have considerable influence over the patient's ability and willingness to carry out medical recommendations. Even if patients have sufficient knowledge, skill, motivation, and attitude to carry out the treatment regimen, their family or peer group can have a profound impact on the extent to which they actually follow health advice. It would seem, for instance, that a patient who has solicited advice about weight control, been counseled accordingly, and appears to have an understanding of the diet regimen would have an excellent potential for success. Surely the health care professional would have every reason to believe that teaching would be effective. If the family considers obesity attractive and criticizes the patient's efforts to lose weight, however, without additional counseling and support, the patient may fail to reach his or her goal. In many instances, the professional's best educational efforts are undermined if the family does not understand the condition for which the patient is being counseled, or the importance of treatment itself, if medical recommendations conflict with their beliefs.

On the other hand, family and friends can also be a great support and can reinforce the patient's effort to maintain the prescribed regimen. Families who offer support and help to the patient following a treatment regimen are a tremendous aid in helping the patient comply.

The importance of understanding the individual patient and the significance of the influence of the social group, especially family or peers, can be illustrated by the case of Janice, a 19-year-old female who had been an insulin-dependent diabetic since the age of 14. Her diabetes had been fairly well controlled, and Janice appeared to manage her diet and insulin quite well on her own throughout high school. She had adapted well to her condition and appeared to have an excellent understanding of diabetes and the importance of diet and the accurate administration of insulin. She also was basically shy and withdrawn, having few friends and dating very little during high school. When she went to college, she had found it extremely difficult to meet and interact with new people. Much to her delight, during the second semester at college, she met a young man who appeared to be interested in her. They began to see each other on a regular basis and eventually talked of plans to marry.

Upon coming to college, Janice had immediately established herself with the University Health Service and had regular follow-ups for her diabetes. Although her diabetes continued to be well controlled for the first 8 months, at one visit to the Health Service, her blood glucose levels were significantly elevated. The nurse reviewed Janice's activity levels and found them to be no different. Her skill at drawing up the insulin and injecting it was observed, and she performed these procedures correctly. Her understanding of her diet was excellent. All levels of knowledge and skill appeared adequate. Because Janice had apparently accepted her diabetes, there was no reason to suspect that her fluctuating sugar levels were caused by denial or maladaptation to the disease. The physician, puzzled by the changes in her condition, placed Janice in the Health Service infirmary to stabilize her. During visiting hours the nurse observed that a young man had come to visit who appeared quite important to Janice.

After the visitor left, the nurse began talking to Janice about the young man. In the course of conversation, the nurse learned that the man, now Janice's fiancé, believed very strongly that illness was a state of mind and that most illnesses could be overcome by force of will. He felt that, with the proper attitude, Janice could gradually be weaned off insulin and could live a life free of medication. Because of his importance to her and her fear of losing him, Janice periodically skipped her insulin dose or decreased the amount. The nurse, now aware of the problem, arranged to have Janice's fiancé come to the infirmary early the next day for a joint teaching session with Janice. In the session, rather than confronting his beliefs directly, the nurse talked about the role of stress in disease and acknowledged that there were still many things that were unknown about the interaction of body and mind and the development of disease. The nurse continued that although emotions could still influence the course of disease, the mind alone could not always help a process that had already begun. She then began to describe the disease process of diabetes, explaining why insulin was important in its treatment. Janice's fiance had had limited previous understanding of diabetes as a disease process. Neither had he had a firm understanding about the role of insulin and the consequences of nonadherence to the prescribed dosages. He was encouraged to help Janice become emotionally strong and calm to help reduce the chances of her developing complications. He was also helped to understand that taking insulin was a very important part of helping Janice reach this goal.

The beliefs, attitudes, and values of a variety of social groups have a tremendous impact on the patient and must be taken into consideration in planning and implementing patient education. Just as it is important to consider these variables, and especially those related to the patient's social group in terms of culture or ethnic background, it is also important not to overgeneralize about the patient's social group. Even within the United States, there may be differences between groups of the same ethnic origin depending on where in the country members were raised. Likewise, there are differences between persons of various ethnic backgrounds who were raised in the United States and those raised in the country of origin. As with all social groups, each member is still an individual, with a personal makeup and past experiences that make him or her somewhat different from every other member of the group. Each patient must still be considered uniquely individual. The key is to gather data about each individual to determine his or her values, beliefs, or perceptions and to translate those values, beliefs, or perceptions into the process of patient teaching.

Environmental Factors

A variety of factors within patients' environments can influence the effectiveness of patient education. Factors that facilitate or impede patients' following recommendations may include the physical environment, the work environment, their schedules, or the personal life styles they have adopted. Even with sufficient and appropriate knowledge, skill, attitude, and support, unless obstacles within the environment that may interfere with adherence to recommendations are identified, patient education may still be less than effective.

Often where environmental factors contribute to patients' nonadherence to recommendations, failure to follow recommendations may be not so much a function of unwillingness or inability to modify the environment appropriately as a lack of knowledge of how changes could be made so that the recommendations could be followed. In these instances, part of patient education must be directed toward helping patients devise a plan whereby recommendations can be followed despite environmental limitations.

Such was the case of Ms. Knoll, an elderly patient who lived alone in the same farmhouse where she had been born. Because of symptoms she had been experiencing, she sought advice from the physician practicing in a small town several miles from where she lived. After examining Ms. Knoll, the physician ordered a variety of tests, one of which necessitated the collection of a 24-hour urine specimen that would have to be refrigerated. The physician carefully explained the tests to Ms. Knoll, how she should prepare for them, and why they were being ordered.

In concluding patient teaching, the physician asked Ms. Knoll if she felt she would be able to carry out the preparations for the tests, or if she felt there were any problems that would make preparations difficult for her. Ms. Knoll replied that she felt there were several problems. First, transportation was difficult for her because she did not drive and was, therefore, dependent on her niece or neighbors to take her places. Although they had always been very willing to help her, the tests were scheduled at such an early time that she was reluctant to ask them. She continued that she had never had electricity put into her farmhouse and, consequently, had no means of refrigerating the urine specimen even if she was able to collect it.

After the physician was made aware of Ms. Knolls' situation, she began to help her find alternatives and resources that would enable her to have the tests. Because environmental factors were identified early, diagnostic procedures and understanding subsequent treatment were not delayed, and the physician's original efforts at teaching were not wasted.

Patients must often be helped to identify ways they can follow the recommendations given. Telling a person who has had a myocardial infarction to avoid going up and down stairs can be unrealistic for the patient whose bedroom and only bathroom are on the second floor. Patients' ability and willingness to comply with recommendations will be much greater if the health professional identifies environmental restrictions and teaches patients how to modify their environment appropriately.

Other barriers that may affect adherence may arise from patients' work or home environments in terms of lifestyle or responsibilities in their daily lives. For example, it is unrealistic to expect a prenatal patient with symptoms of preeclampsia to maintain full bed rest at home when she has several other preschool children at home as well. To maximize the possibility that she will adhere to advice, the health professional must explore with the patient the possibility for provision of child care during the day while her husband is at work. Likewise, a patient whose occupation involves considerable bending and stooping may not be able to follow advice to avoid bending and stooping altogether. It may be far more profitable, in terms of effectiveness and efficiency, to help the patient establish some limits to bending and stooping and seek ways to minimize the bending and stooping that may be required in some tasks; teaching the patient proper body mechanics for bending and stooping when they must be done may also be helpful.

The Medical Regimen

The medical regimen itself can interfere with patients' ability and/or willingness to comply with the prescribed treatment. For instance, if a number of different treatments or medications are instituted all at once, the patient may have more difficulty carrying out recommendations accurately. The more treatments or medications prescribed, the more adverse the effect on patient compliance (Vollmer 1998). Compliance with the medical regimen also decreases with the length of time it must be carried out (Rosenstock 1988). Although, overall, side effects do not appear to affect patient compliance, from a practical standpoint, it makes sense that a patient experiencing unpleasant side effects from a medication or treatment may be prone to discontinue the regimen (Spiker 1991). In other instances, patients may be unable to take medications in their prescribed form. For example, a patient may have difficulty swallowing pills but be able to take a liquid form of the medication. If the patient's inability to take the medication in pill form is not identified, however, the patient may elect to discontinue the medication without telling the health professional.

In areas of diet, exercise, or other life-style changes, patients may find the regimen too difficult, too time consuming, or too unpleasant to follow. Health professionals can greatly enhance the chances that the regimen will be followed by asking for patients' perceptions about the recommendations and their ability and/or willingness to carry them out.

UNDERSTANDING DIFFERENT PERSONALITY STYLES

No two individuals are the same. The personality of each individual is what makes him or her unique. The combination of traits and characteristics that individuals possess as part of their personality determines to a great extent how they interact with others, how they respond to experiences, and how they make decisions. The outward manifestations of personality in terms of behavior are a reflection of the individual's internal mental state. Individual personality characteristics give individuals some degree of consistency and predictability regarding their behavior.

Although the personality of each individual is unique, there are some personality traits that individuals may share in common. These personality traits make up a type of personality style and in part determine which aspect of illness individuals may find anxiety provoking and the techniques they will employ for coping with their anxiety.

Certain personality traits exhibited by patients can be very frustrating for the health professional unless they are recognized as such and consequently taken into consideration when working with patients. The more health professionals are aware of reactions as they relate to an individual's basic pattern of behaving in a nonillness state, the better they will be able to work with the individual effectively when conducting patient teaching.

Take, for example, Ms. Lee. Although she frequently demanded information, direction, and support from Dr. Franklin, she rarely followed the recommendations given. She appeared to be impulsive and unpredictable, praising Dr. Franklin's teaching efforts on some occasions and devaluing them on others.

Patients such as Ms. Lee can be very demanding and produce feelings of anger and frustration in the health professional who is trying to conduct patient education. This type of behavior may, however, merely be a reflection of the patient's basic personality style and its manifestation as a reaction to illness. Patients may experience conflict in which they desire the health professional to rescue them and at the same time fear that the health professional will desert them.

Luckily, Dr. Franklin took time to look at Ms. Lee's behavior objectively, and, in an attempt to discover techniques that would help him to work more effectively with Ms. Lee, he discovered that by using gentle but firm limit setting, Ms. Lee responded by becoming more cooperative and easier to work with.

Another personality type may be illustrated by the example of Mr. Boyce, who had been diagnosed as having hepatitis. The nurse, Mr. Morgan, became increasingly annoyed when trying to conduct patient teaching with Mr. Boyce, who seemed preoccupied with trivial details, seeking more and more information and at the same time being rigid and indecisive. Mr. Boyce became extremely upset at any variation in routine and became very demanding in his expectations of Mr. Morgan. In discussing his difficulty in working with Mr. Boyce with his colleagues, it became evident to Mr. Morgan that Mr. Boyce was desperately struggling to maintain a sense of control in light of an illness he viewed as threatening. With this insight, Mr. Morgan changed his approach to Mr. Boyce, offering a more methodical approach to patient teaching and engaging Mr. Boyce in fuller participation.

Mr. Williams illustrates yet another example of personality style. He seemed very flamboyant with exaggerated emotions. He had been scheduled for coronary artery bypass surgery. The nurse, Ms. Applebaum, had been assigned to conduct the preoperative teaching. It became very difficult for Ms. Applebaum to conduct the teaching session because Mr. Williams seemed to have little interest in understanding the procedure, stating very dramatically that he just wanted to have the procedure done immediately. Ms. Applebaum talked with Mr. William's family physician in an attempt to gain some insight into Mr. William's reaction that would enable her to conduct patient teaching more effectively. She discovered that Mr. Williams appeared to need much attention and reassurance of his physical prowess. Consequently, when she returned to the teaching situation, she offered reassurance regarding his postoperative course and offered him an opportunity to express his own fears about the procedure and consequences.

Some patients are by nature suspicious and mistrustful. When such individuals become ill, these traits may become exaggerated so that every question, procedure, or recommendation is closely scrutinized and motives of the recommendations questioned. Although such hypervigilance on the part of patients can be annoying to health professionals who during patient teaching are asked to justify everything, by attempting to understand patients' viewpoints, being supportive, and keeping some interpersonal distance, health professionals can maintain objectivity and conduct patient education more effectively.

USING KNOWLEDGE OF PATIENTS' SELF-PERCEPTION TO INDIVIDUALIZE PATIENT TEACHING

There are many dimensions of a patient's personality. The more health professionals know about individual patients and the more this knowledge is used to customize patient teaching to the individual's needs, the more likely the patient education intervention is to be effective. Health professionals can learn much about patients in conversation by listening closely to patients' statements and observing their behavior.

One dimension of personality is self-perception. Self-perception is the patient's view of himself or herself. A number of different factors make up self-perception. One of these factors is identity, or how patients characterize themselves. Whether the patient's self-identity is as a professional, homemaker, neighbor, or a number of other labels patients may use in their own self-description, it is important for health professionals to know what the patient's self-identity is and to utilize this information in patient teaching. If, for example, the patient's self-identity is tied to his or her role as a business executive who is capable of handling considerable responsibility and making decisions, to place this patient in a dependent, passive role during patient teaching would most probably decrease the likelihood of teaching effectiveness and may even serve to alienate the patient.

Another factor involved in self-perception is self-esteem, or how well patients like themselves and feel that others like them. Individuals' degree of self-esteem determines how much confidence they have in themselves and their abilities as well as how capable they believe they are in handling certain situations and performing certain tasks.

Illness alone can lower individuals' self-esteem. When individuals already have low self-esteem, illness may contribute to this further. Individuals with low self-esteem may have little confidence in their ability to learn new material or new skills and may seem overly dependent on others. When health professionals are aware of and sensitive to patients' lack of self-esteem, they can use this information in the patient teaching situation to make the intervention more effective. Take, for example, Mrs. Sanders, a 78-year-old woman who had broken her hip, had surgical repair, and had done well in the postoperative period. The nurse, Ms. Friedman, in preparation for Mrs. Sanders' discharge, came to her room to begin patient teaching about her management at home. Although Mrs. Sanders was alert and seemed capable of understanding the information, she told Ms. Friedman that she must wait until her daughter arrived because she probably would not be able to comprehend the directions anyway. When Mrs. Sanders' daughter came, Ms. Friedman proceeded to give them both the information but found that Mrs. Sanders repeatedly made self-deprecating remarks, such as "I'm just too stupid to understand" and "I never could do anything right."

After the teaching session, Ms. Friedman spoke with Mrs. Sanders' daughter and learned that Mrs. Sanders had always been self-critical and had a poor opinion of herself and her abilities. Ms. Friedman used this information in her next teaching session with Mrs. Sanders, making a special effort to compliment Mrs. Sanders and to reinforce her performance. In so doing, Ms. Friedman was attempting to build Mrs. Sanders' self-esteem and also her self-confidence, both of which would be necessary if she was to participate in her own self-management at home and if the patient teaching intervention was to be effective.

A fundamental aspect of self-perception is the individual's belief about the degree to which he or she has control over events in his or her life. Some people believe that most of what happens to them is determined by outside forces and that they have little control over their own destiny. Such individuals usually have a fatalistic view, which may be demonstrated by statements such as, "I suppose I'll try to follow the recommendations, but no matter what I do, it probably won't do any good anyway. Some things are just meant to be." Other people believe that they have considerable control over their lives and believe that their own actions can at least in part determine their own destiny. Statements such as, "Even though it's hard to stay on a low cholesterol diet, I know if I want to be around to see my grandchildren grow up I'd better stick to the diet," are indicative that the patient believes that his or her actions to at least some degree have a relationship to health consequences.

Whether or not health professionals share the patients' views, ignoring their views or attempting to argue with them about their views makes the patient-teaching interaction less than effective. A better approach is for health professionals to utilize this knowledge to make the teaching interaction more effective. If, for example, an individual believes that he or she has little control over his or her health, rather than making the patient more dependent, or arguing and barraging the patient with statistics regarding risk behavior, the health professional will probably be more effective in identifying some immediate concerns, establishing some short-term goals, and helping the patient experience some control and results from accomplishing the goals.

REACTIONS OF PATIENTS TO ILLNESS

Patients differ remarkably in their perceptions of, and reactions to, what may appear to be similar medical conditions. While some individuals react mildly to a disease or condition that might devastate others, others display considerable emotional and physical discomfort at conditions many people would consider minor. Preventive practices likewise are accepted with varying extremes of response by different patients.

Obviously, a variety of psychosocial factors determine individuals' reactions to illness and, consequently, their reactions to the recommendations and advice given. Each patient has a personal, unique perspective on health, illness, and medical care itself. Before health professionals can conduct meaningful education resulting in positive health outcomes, there must be a clear understanding of patients' perceptions as well as their perception of meanings of health and illness.

Patients' reactions to the fact that they are ill or could be ill involve their attitudes toward illness, how they interpret symptoms of illness, and their attitudes toward health care itself. Health professionals frequently assume that patients seeking health advice are motivated to follow advice in order to get well. If patients believe that no matter what they do they cannot get well, it is unlikely that they will follow a regimen they consider to be of no benefit. In other instances, health professionals may assume that symptoms patients present are the reason they are seeking medical care. This may not always be the case. Recommendations given for conditions that are not of primary concern to the patient have less chance of being followed accurately.

Mrs. Connors sought help from her physician with regard to weight control. She was referred to a dietitian for dietary counseling and regular follow-up visits to monitor her weight loss. Mrs. Connors failed to keep her follow-up appointments. When she was next seen by her family physician several months later for an unrelated problem, it was noted that she had failed to lose any weight. Had the physician and dietitian listened closely to Mrs. Connors' needs, they might have recognized that although weight loss was Mrs. Connors' presenting problem, her concern about her blood pressure actually seemed more pressing. Mrs. Connors' unspoken concern was her blood pressure; she had a friend who had recently suffered a stroke. Consequently, Mrs. Connors had done considerable reading on the subject and discovered that obesity was linked to high blood pressure and stroke. After visiting the physician, however, and finding that her blood pressure was normal, it was no surprise that she did not comply with the physician's or dietitian's recommendations. In Mrs. Connors' view, because her blood pressure was normal despite her obesity, the recommendations for weight loss made little sense.

Health professionals may also assume that patients who are sick are motivated to follow recommendations that will help them to get well. Behaviors associated with patients' sick role, however, may not always be consistent with this philosophy. Parsons (1951) noted that the sick role itself is of a mixed nature, and described the sick role with the following characteristics:

- Individuals are not viewed as being in power to overcome being sick by themselves; some therapeutic process is necessary for patients to recover.
- While patients are ill, they are not expected to function in their normal role or to perform their regular obligations.
- Patients are expected to want to get well.
- Patients are expected to seek help for their illness and to cooperate with health professionals in their attempts to get well.

Thus, although people who are ill are excused from social responsibilities, they are also expected to take some responsibility for their recovery. For many patients, being ill is not a positive role to occupy. For others, however, it may be far preferable to the social role they previously occupied. For some individuals, being sick may be a means of legitimizing dependency as well as increasing the amount of attention they receive. Subsequently, patients may be reluctant to return to their former role and obligations. Their motivation to retain their sick role may be greater than their motivation to get well. Although patients may engage in the socially acceptable behavior of seeking medical advice, they may sabotage the treatment plan by not following recommendations. Some patients may vacillate between their wish to be independent and their wish to remain ill and be taken care of. Because noncooperation with medical advice is also not socially acceptable within the framework of the sick role, noncompliance in such instances may be subtle.

Illness itself may be used for coping with personal problems. Mr. Wilson had recently graduated from college with a degree in secondary education. Shortly after taking his first job in a secondary school, he developed flu symptoms and severe congestion. Consequently, he was advised to stay at home for several days. Although Mr. Wilson sought medical care, received a prescription for medication, and had been advised to rest at home, he continued to appear at school, walking there in bad weather, staying for a few hours, and then returning home. He neglected to pick up his medication at the pharmacy until several days after his visit with the physician, saying that he was too ill at the time to go to the pharmacy. The symptoms became progressively worse; however, Mr. Wilson continued his routine of performing his tasks at school in a perfunctory way and then returning home. He continued to seek medical care for his continuing symptoms. After several visits to the health clinic, the nurse began to note that although Mr. Wilson appeared consistent in keeping his appointments, he did not appear to be following any of the other recommendations that, presumably, would help him recover at a more rapid rate. In talking with Mr. Wilson before the appointment, the nurse questioned him about his job. Through their discussion, the nurse noted that although Mr. Wilson stated that he was happy with his work, he also appeared rather vague and uncomfortable when talking about how he perceived his level of performance. Through further discussion with the physician, the patient later revealed that he was quite unsure of his ability to perform in the classroom setting. Because of his illness, however, expectations about his performance were lowered, both by students and his peers. In addition, Mr. Wilson was actually somewhat martyred by coming to school despite his illness.

Although such motivations for being ill are not always conscious, it behooves health professionals to be aware of such possibilities and the impact on patient education and compliance. Health professionals may not always be able to determine immediately patients' levels of motivation to get well or to remain sick. Through astute observation and deduction, however, patients' levels of motivation may be discovered. Health professionals then have the opportunity to work with patients, discussing their feelings and fears, helping them to determine other ways in which their needs can be met.

Patients' responses to illness may also relate in part to the life circumstances surrounding them. Economic consequences of illness, both acute and chronic, can have an impact on patients' receptivity to patient education and, subsequently, on their compliance with medical advice. Although many occupations include fringe benefits of paid sick days, or even time off with pay in which to seek medical care, other occupations have no such benefits. In the latter instance, days taken off from work because of illness or for follow-up visits to the physician may result in decreased income. Unfortunately, many people in this type of occupation may also be part of a socioeconomic group that can least afford to take days off without pay. In such cases, no matter how complete patient teaching is about the necessity of staying home or of returning for a follow-up visit, the likelihood of compliance with such recommendations is slight. An awareness of these factors by health professionals may help them to modify the teaching plan to maximize the patient's ability to comply with recommendations under the given circumstances. In some instances, it may be sufficient for the patient to call the health professional with a progress report rather than returning for a visit. If the patient cannot remain at home for a week, the provision of rest periods during the working day may be sufficient. If rest or follow-up visits are crucial, the health professional may refer the patient to a community agency where financial assistance for such expenses may be available. It is essential, in any case, that the problem be identified if patient education is to be effective.

Economic consequences of illness may, on the other hand, also cause a reverse reaction by the patient. If patients receive disability benefits as long as they are ill and especially if the opportunity for satisfactory employment is slight, complying with a regimen that may return them to healthy status, and consequently decreasing or eliminating the benefits they receive, will probably not have a high priority.

In terms of preventive health practices, patients frequently do not view the benefits of the prescribed recommendations as being worth the cost. For example, people with limited economic resources who have no perceived illness may find it difficult to follow their physician's recommendations to return for an annual physical. Patients with economic concerns who have been treated for a condition such as strep throat or urinary tract infection, even though the reason for the follow-up has been explained to them, may be reluctant to spend additional money for the follow-up if they are not experiencing symptoms. They may choose to take the chance that the infection has been eradicated, rather than spending extra money for a follow-up visit. The health professional who is aware of these financial concerns may be able to work out alternatives with the patient. In taking patient concerns into consideration, health professionals themselves may weigh the benefit of making recommendations they know the patient will not follow.

Other reactions to disease may depend on the meaning of the illness to the individual. If, for example, the patient perceives health as a reward for a life well lived, then illness may be viewed as punishment for transgressions. In such instances, depending on the patient's degree of guilt, following medical advice may be viewed as interfering with the punishment perceived as being deserved. In other instances, patients may feel guilty because they perceive themselves as being responsible for the illness itself. Especially in instances where certain preventive health practices were advised but not followed, the later development of a disease condition may cause patients to blame themselves for their illness. They thus may be more reluctant to follow recommendations given. In either case, before the health professional can conduct patient education effectively, such feelings must be identified and dealt with.

Illness disrupts the way patients view themselves and the world. Most patients experience a feeling of vulnerability. Illness shatters the magical belief that they are immune from illness, injury, or even death. Illness can produce distortions in thinking. Some patients may react with superstition, grasping at straws through which they can again feel they have control. Patients may lose a sense of security and of cohesiveness. Illness may shatter their sense of identity. They may become frustrated and angry at their sense of helplessness or loss; some become self-absorbed, others more dependent. While some patients may draw on hidden resources of strength and courage, others become more demanding, clinging, or regressed. Some patients may react with rebellion against medical advice. Life may become a maze of inconveniences, hazards, and restrictions. With others, recommendations may be adapted into their regular way of life.

One goal of patient education is to help patients to reorganize, make necessary changes, and maximize their resources. This requires a nonjudgmental attitude on the part of the health professional, along with an effort to understand patients and their reactions. If health professionals are unable to empathize with patients and their reactions, such nonacceptance may well in itself push patients into noncompliance. For example, a newly diagnosed 20-year-old diabetic may continue to have difficulty following a diet despite patient education sessions with the dietitian. The dietitian may have observed that the patient showed little interest in the diet instructions during the teaching session. Rather than criticizing the patient for lack of interest or for failure to follow the diet, the dietitian may hypothesize that such restrictions may be difficult for the patient to follow, or that the patient may be having difficulty accepting the condition in general. The dietitian can demonstrate understanding by taking time to listen to the patient and allowing him or her to vent feelings. Such actions show acceptance of, as well as interest in, the patient as a whole. Such an atmosphere is more conducive to working with patients to institute behavior change than one created by an adversary relationship. The latter may result in rebelliousness or rejection by patients, limiting the chances to achieve the level of compliance desired.

COPING STYLES AND METHODS OF ADAPTATION

Stress is a normal part of life even in healthy individuals. Anxiety is a normal reaction to stress. All individuals have a variety of means by which they cope with anxiety and stress. All individuals have predominant coping styles that are used to reduce anxiety and to restore equilibrium when confronted with a stressful situation. Use of these mechanisms can reduce anxiety, helping people to assume balance and productivity in their lives. Although use of coping styles can be helpful, overuse can have the opposite effect, immobilizing the individual.

These same mechanisms can be used by individuals coping with the stress of illness. How persons have coped with stress in the past will determine to some extent how they will cope with the stress of illness. Many people take their health and body for granted, as well as their continued ability to perform daily activities and social roles. When people are ill—whether the illness is acute or chronic, a result of trauma, or a slow progressive disease—their life style is interrupted, and varying degrees of stress are experienced.

Patients' reactions to illness are not always equivalent to the severity of the disease. What may appear to be a minor illness to one individual may elicit a profound anxiety reaction in another. A variety of psychosocial factors affect patients' reaction to their condition and, consequently, their reaction to the health advice they are given.

Illness changes the self-concept of individuals. Those who prided themselves in being independent may now find themselves dependent on others for their care or for performance of some of the daily activities for which they were responsible. Patients' perception of their degree of loss as a result of their illness, whether they experience loss in terms of function, self-esteem, independence, or finances, is often related to the degree of stress and subsequent anxiety they experience.

Coping styles can help patients adjust to their condition and follow recommendations. Coping styles can also, however, be detrimental to positive patient education outcomes. The health professional who is aware of the use of coping styles and their impact on the effectiveness of patient education, however, can foster their use to produce positive outcomes. In instances where they interfere with positive health outcomes, health professionals can help patients gradually verbalize their concerns, thus helping them begin to deal with their anxiety openly.

Denial

A common coping style against anxiety is denial. Although in some instances denial can be a protective process, it can become dangerous when it prevents the patient from seeking medical care or from following advice that is crucial to recovery or to palliation of a condition. An example of the negative effects of this coping mechanism can be illustrated by the case of Mr. Jacob, who had consulted a physician because of what he considered indigestion. After examination, the physician concluded that Mr. Jacob's symptoms were the result of coronary artery disease. He requested that Mr. Jacob have additional tests to determine the extent of occlusion. The physician told Mr. Jacob that he probably had angina and continued to explain what angina is, as well as giving an explanation about treatment and additional tests to be ordered. Upon leaving the office, Mr. Jacob confided to his wife that he felt physicians were just out to make money and that he had no intention of having any other tests because all he had was indigestion anyway. The anxiety of the diagnosis had been so great for Mr. Jacob that he coped with it by denying that his angina existed.

In such instances as the preceding, the reality of the diagnosis of illness is frequently anxiety provoking for patients. Adhering to the advice given would be admitting that the condition exists. To cope with the anxiety, patients may subconsciously incorporate the defense of denial. By not attending to the information and by not following advice, they are, in essence, denying the existence of their illness. Health professionals should not actively engage in taking these defenses away from the individual. It is, however, important to recognize patient anxiety that may be responsible for the denial of a condition and to assess the degree to which the use of this coping style may cause the patient harm.

Other patients may be ambivalent about knowing more about their condition. They may adopt a "What you don't know won't hurt you" attitude, consequently resisting attempts to give them information about their disease. In such instances, forcing information upon the patient is of little benefit. A more efficient approach at this point is to determine what information is essential for the patient to have, proceeding to deliver it in bits and pieces, and monitoring patient acceptance along the way. Another approach might be to ask the patient interesting questions to stimulate interest.

At the other extreme, some patients cope with anxiety about their illness by wanting to know every detail of their condition and its treatment. The use of this coping style can help reduce anxiety by reducing patients' fear of the unknown and by helping them feel as if they are in control of their condition. This type of reaction can, quite naturally, be beneficial to patient education. Health professionals should not only provide initial information to patients in this situation but also make sure that continuing information is provided about their illness and progress. Obviously, this approach also does not guarantee compliance. If health professionals have been inaccurate in assessment and continue to give patients information without ongoing monitoring, such action could have a negative effect. If, however, health professionals find that provision of additional information does help to reduce the level of anxiety, then it may be more likely that less anxious patients are better able to incorporate information into their daily lives.

Compensatory Style

Individuals may learn to compensate for real or imagined weaknesses by becoming stronger or more proficient in another area. If patients become disabled or lose function in one area, as a matter of coping they may find ways to excel in others. For example, the patient who is unable to maintain her level of physical activity because of emphysema may instead develop writing skills or other means of self-expression, thus increasing self-satisfaction without requiring excessive physical strain. Through education, health professionals can teach patients ways to maximize existing skills or to develop new skills to replace those lost because of their condition.

Although compensatory style is generally highly constructive, it may also be destructive and detrimental. For instance. Ms. Kapur felt unattractive after having a radical mastectomy. She compensated for her perceived unattractiveness by becoming promiscuous. Another example of the detrimental use of compensation is the case of the cardiac patient who is no longer permitted to smoke but compensates by beginning to eat excessively. Information giving alone in these instances has little value. Recognition by health professionals of patients' reactions can, however, be the first step in helping them learn to cope with their feelings about their condition and treatment, and can subsequently increase the potential effectiveness of future patient teaching. In both instances such as those just above, the health professional must be aware that it is the *patient's* perceptions, values, and judgments that are at issue. Whether or not the health professional believes that Ms. Kapur is unattractive or that overeating is as detrimental as smoking is of little consequence. It is the patient's perceptions in this coping style that determine behavior.

Blocking Out Ideas

Another coping style that may be used by patients in adjusting to their condition is putting unpleasant or unacceptable ideas or thoughts out of their minds. For example, patients who are severely anxious because of their symptoms may "forget" them rather than recognizing them for what they are. The patient with periodic chest pain and shortness of breath may later forget having experienced such symptoms; he or she may forget an appointment for an examination or may forget other treatment recommendations. Such a coping style not only takes considerable energy but can also be potentially harmful. Recognition of the patient's excessive use of this coping style can help the health professional mobilize a process to enhance more realistic confrontation of the problems at hand. As with most coping styles, forgetting or blocking out ideas can also be a positive mechanism in adjusting to illness. For example, a burn patient who leaves the hospital may forget the severity of pain experienced as a result of a dressing change, instead focusing on the kindness of the hospital staff and the positive aspects of rehabilitation. This patient has used blocking out of ideas in a productive way in adjusting to his illness. In such instances, facilitation of this coping style can help the patient achieve more positive health outcomes. If the health professional recognizes that a patient appears to be a "chronic forgetter" and that such behaviors are detrimental to his or her care, rather than approaching the patient in an accusatory way, the professional may spend some extra time talking with the patient about his or her feelings concerning the condition and treatment. Through a relationship of trust and mutual respect, the professional using this approach will be better able to help the patient identify and disclose feelings, making a problem-solving approach more likely.

Retreat

Some persons use retreat as a means of coping with their illness. Retreat involves removing oneself emotionally or physically from a situation that is anxiety producing. If the situation is potentially dangerous, then retreating or withdrawing from the situation is, of course, constructive. For example, a recovering alcoholic finding herself in the midst of a party in which there is considerable pressure for her to drink might use this coping style positively by choosing to leave. Less constructive use may occur in cases in which individuals refuse to learn needed behaviors because of fear of failure. Such might be the case of the patient with a new amputation who refuses to try to learn to use the prosthesis. Emotional retreat may also have positive and negative aspects. Some emotional retreat or withdrawal may be a necessary part of helping patients cope with the losses experienced because of their illness. Emotional retreat may also, however, interfere with patients' health care and treatment, as well as their receptiveness to patient education. If the patient remains inattentive to the material presented during the teaching interaction, the health professional may suspect that the patient's behavior is an attempt to cope with the anxiety the information is producing. Through this realization, the health professional is better able to attempt to help the patient cope with the anxiety, thus increasing the probability that the teaching will be effective.

Role Modeling

Using role modeling as a method of coping with illness can also have positive and negative consequences. Positive use of this method of coping is the internalization of desirable attributes of another person into the patient's own behavior or attitudes. Health professionals may foster this type of role modeling for patients to help them adjust to their illness by doing such things as asking a patient with a colostomy who is now leading an active life to visit a hospitalized patient with a new colostomy. Role modeling may have a negative effect, however, if patients are exposed to others with similar conditions who have not adjusted well to their illness. In these instances, the patient may incorporate the negative attitudes expressed by these individuals. In this case, role modeling would be detrimental to the adjustment of the patient. In patient education, knowledge of this method of coping can be facilitated by providing role models that help the patient achieve positive health outcomes. Knowledge of role modeling can also help the health professional identify those instances in which negative effects emerge.

Regression

In regression, a person reverts to an earlier stage of development. It is used to some degree by most persons, whether the illness is acute or chronic, a major or minor illness. Most people, even when only ill with the flu, exhibit more childlike behaviors, such as a short temper, excessive emotionality, or dependency, than they may normally exhibit in their adult roles. Regression, especially in the early phases of illness, may even be necessary to eventual recovery. For instance, patients with a new myocardial infarction, as part of treatment, may need to regress to a more dependent role, giving up some of their responsibility and allowing others to take care of them. In such instances, regression is important to avoid relapse. As recovery begins, however, the health professional may need to encourage the patient to do more independently. Patients who use regression on an ongoing basis establish maladaptive adjustment patterns to their illness that can have a negative impact on their ability to function as well as to follow recommendations. Awareness of regression as a coping style can be of value to the health professional conducting patient education. Through increased understanding of behavior, the health professional can adapt teaching accordingly, anticipating potential problems the patient may have in following health advice.

Ascribing Blame

Some persons may attribute their own unacceptable thoughts or feelings to others or blame others for their own mistakes. For example, a patient who has recently sustained an injury to the spinal cord resulting in paraplegia may herself have unacceptable feelings about persons with a disability. Instead of recognizing her own feelings, however, she may ascribe negative feelings to others regardless of whether or not negative behaviors are actually exhibited. Manifestation of this coping mechanism during teaching may be a statement such as, "You don't think people with spinal cord injury have much worth in the world, do you?" The health professional, unaware of the reason behind the patient's statement, may be bewildered or defensive. The effectiveness of patient education under these circumstances may be hindered. If the health professional is aware of the patient's anxiety and feelings, however, the teaching plan can be better adapted first to cope with the patient's feelings rather than pursuing further communication of information about the patient's condition or treatment. For example, rather than responding to the preceding statement with a comment like, "How can you possibly accuse me of such a thing when I've spent so much time trying to help you?" the health professional may offer a response such as, "No, I don't feel that way, but I'm wondering why you asked. Tell me a little more about your question."

By encouraging patients to talk about their feelings, health professionals demonstrate acceptance as well as gain insight into patients' feelings and behavior. To pursue the teaching plan without first gaining more information about patients' statements sets a precedent for less-than-desirable outcomes. Again, although compliance cannot be guaranteed by this action, the more accepting patients are of their own conditions, and the more they feel the health professional is willing to listen to their concerns, the greater the possibility is that patient teaching will be effective.

Patients may also blame their own noncompliance on others, stating that family members are uncooperative or unsupportive of their treatment. Because this may be true in some instances, health professionals should assess the validity of patients' statements before drawing conclusions. If the health professional finds that the patient's family appears supportive and encourages the patient to follow recommendations, in fact, then the use of this coping mechanism by the patient may be suspected. The health professional can then incorporate into the teaching plan methods by which the patient is gradually helped to cope with anxiety and to accept responsibility for his or her own actions.

Self-Blame

Rather than blaming others for their shortcomings, some patients may blame themselves. If patients are unable to express anger or aggression against another person, the feelings they have may be turned upon themselves. For example, if a patient has a spouse who is impatient or unsupportive, the patient may—instead of becoming angry at the spouse—make statements such as, "I have no patience. I'm so selfish. I expect entirely too much from my spouse." Health professionals who are alert to such cues can help patients recognize and express those feelings, thereby offering the opportunity to discuss problems that may interfere with the patient following recommendations.

Rationalization

Rationalization consists of thinking of socially acceptable reasons for behavior. This coping style enables people to invent excuses for not doing things they know they should have done, as well as helping to soften the disappointment of not reaching goals that perhaps had been set. For example, a person with diabetes may rationalize that he went off his diet because "It won't hurt to cheat every now and then." Appointments for various diagnostic procedures may be missed for reasons such as "They aren't going to find anything wrong, anyway" or "Even if they find that I have cancer, they can't cure it, anyway, so what's the use?" Rationalization can also play a positive part in adjustment to disease, however. It can help the patient who has had to limit activities to a great extent because of a disabling condition to say, "I've really had more time to get to know my family since I've been ill. All the other things I used to do were pretty meaningless, anyway." Health professionals can enhance patient education outcomes by reinforcing the positive use of rationalization. In instances in which rationalization produces negative outcomes, health professionals might direct education efforts toward helping patients discuss their feelings about their condition, gradually helping them accept a more realistic view of the treatment regimen.

Hiding Feelings

At times, persons react to their illness or to those around them by behaving in a way that is opposite to their actual feelings or thoughts. The patient using this coping style may appear to be excessively cheerful and unconcerned about the illness and its implications while actually feeling very frightened and sad. In other cases, patients may be especially charitable to family members or individuals around them when they are really feeling hostile and resentful. Hiding feelings as a coping style can be of value in adjusting to illness if it helps the person maintain behavior that is socially acceptable. It is detrimental to the extreme that it is self-deceptive and prevents the person from recognizing and dealing with actual feelings that, if hidden long enough, may result in additional stress.

Through accurate assessment and understanding of behavior, health professionals can alter teaching plans to the individual. Whether this involves referral to another professional or merely encouraging patients to verbalize their feelings, by recognizing the impact of patients' reactions to their condition, health professionals are in a better position to alter the approach during education to meet patients' needs better.

Redirecting Emotions

A common mechanism for coping, used by most people at one time or another, is the redirection of emotion from the person or situation originally provoking the emotion to an individual or object that seems less threatening. Take the example of Mrs. Garcia.

Mrs. Garcia came into the hospital for a hysterectomy because of fibroids. During the routine preoperative exam, the physician also found a lump in her right breast. Upon biopsy, the lump was found to be malignant and a mastectomy was performed. Mrs. Garcia was angry with the physician for giving her an unfavorable diagnosis and one she had not expected. Rather than venting anger at the physician, however, Mrs. Garcia became very disagreeable and hostile to the nurse who attempted to teach her about self-care at home.

Although redirecting emotions can be valuable in the sense that it allows the individual the release of strong emotions without threat of retaliation from what may be perceived as more powerful sources, those persons at whom the anger is directed are frequently alienated. Because she recognized Mrs. Garcia's behavior as a reaction to stress, rather than becoming angry in return, the nurse attempted to encourage Mrs. Garcia to express her feelings. She discontinued further teaching until the patient was more receptive to the information she planned to give her.

Excess of Activity

Some persons react to illness by engaging in activities that distract them from thinking about their condition or by thinking about things other than the issue at hand. Although this coping style can be positive if used in a constructive way (dwelling on symptoms or implications of disease to the point of inactivity is not therapeutic), its overuse prevents people from dealing realistically with their feelings about their condition and the limitations that may be imposed by it.

Such was the case of Mr. Hester, recently diagnosed as having diabetes. Mr. Hester's insulin was to be regulated on an outpatient basis. He was also to return for regular teaching sessions as an outpatient. At outpatient visits, Mr. Hester always seemed extremely pressed for time. He frequently seemed preoccupied with other commitments during the sessions. Both the physician and the nurse noted that Mr. Hester appeared to be overextending himself. When Mr. Hester had an appointment for patient teaching, he often called saying that he had a pressing commitment that kept him from attending. If he arrived, he seemed preoccupied throughout the visit, saying that it would have to be short because he had numerous other appointments to keep. He failed to read most of the materials about diabetes given to him, saying he had been too busy even to glance through them.

The physician and the nurse questioned Mr. Hester about how he might be able to arrange some of his other activities to allow more time for his scheduled appointments. He replied simply that there was no other way to arrange the schedule of an extremely busy man. Aware of the possibility that Mr. Hester might be considerably anxious about having diabetes and using activity to escape facing his discomfort, the physician and the nurse used each contact with Mr. Hester to express some of these concerns until he gradually became aware of the behavior he was using to avoid dealing with his diabetes.

Diverting Feelings

One of the most positive and constructive of all coping styles can be the diversion of unacceptable feelings or ideas into socially acceptable behaviors. Patients with a chronic illness or traumatic injury, for instance, may have particularly strong feelings of anger or hostility about their diagnosis or the circumstances surrounding their injury. If the energy of their emotions can be diverted into positive activity, however, the result can be quite beneficial. An example of such a diversion may be the case of the patient with Parkinson's disease who has strong feelings about the condition but directs that strong emotion into a positive activity, such as helping to establish support groups for other Parkinson's patients and their families.

Health professionals who notice this method of coping during patient education can facilitate positive outcomes through its use. Patients may be encouraged to participate in educational activities for other patients with their condition. They may be asked to serve as role models for those with similar conditions, discussing common areas of concern and offering suggestions and support.

As with all techniques in patient education, indiscriminate use or misuse of this coping style can be very negative. Before health professionals facilitate its use, they should carefully assess the patient's attitudes and knowledge base to be sure that the patient actually is serving as the positive role model. The health professional must also be alert to signs of overuse of this coping style to the detriment of patients' own conditions.

HELPING PATIENTS COPE

Reactions of patients to disease, illness, or disability are variable. The coping styles discussed are common behaviors learned and used by all individuals to some degree to adjust and adapt to the stress of daily life. In illness, individuals may use the same pattern of coping with stress that has been used in their healthy state, or the patterns may become more pronounced. Such methods of coping, because they are part of everyday life, are normal and desirable. The danger emerges when their use is excessive and prevents the individual from adapting to full potential. In the ease of an individual with illness, overuse of such coping styles can interfere with medical care or treatment.

The role of health professionals conducting patient education is certainly not to attempt to alter patients' coping styles drastically. It is important, however, for health professionals to have an awareness of different patterns of coping so they are better able to understand the behavior of individual patients, anticipate potential barriers to effective patient education, and work toward solutions to overcome barriers or problems. The better able health professionals are to view the situation from the patient's perspective, the less likely they are to avoid or dismiss the challenging patient. By understanding patients' perceptions of health and illness, health professionals are better able to emphasize and be more sensitive to the patients' needs, thus organizing the teaching plan accordingly. By understanding patients' coping styles, health professionals are better able to encourage patients to express their feelings and to encourage and motivate them to follow prescribed regimens.

Allowing patients to express their fears and feelings in a nonjudgmental, empathetic atmosphere, along with developing a sensitive teaching plan based on patients' needs, can go a long way in reducing their anxiety, helping them to adjust to their condition, and maximizing the probability that they will comply with the information given.

Patients' anxieties or other concerns can greatly interfere with the effectiveness of education. Timing of the educational intervention is important, especially to the patient's readiness to learn. Early after diagnosis of serious illness or injury, for example, patients may focus only on the restrictions imposed on them by their illness. They may see few positive aspects to information offered through patient education. Although at this stage patient education may not have an immediate impact, it is important for the health professional to meet with the patient to begin to establish a relationship. This early intervention should be directed toward laying a foundation for effective teaching later. Initially, patients may have little awareness of the implications of their condition. During this time, patients' reactions to their condition may be minimal. If rapport with the health professional can begin to be built at this time, then the relationship will be established and better able to withstand a patient's possible later reaction of anger, frustration, or depression.

As patients eventually begin to recognize the impact of their condition on their life style or on longevity, or when they begin to realize the extent of their perceived loss, they become anxious—not necessarily in proportion to the seriousness of the illness. During this phase, anxiety may block learning. It may be far more productive at this time that health professionals—instead of pushing patients to receive extensive information—help them express their fears. Health professionals should then accept their fears rather than offering superficial reassurance. Such phrases as, "Oh, I'm sure everything will be fine" or "Lots of other people have your condition," are likely to be rejected by patients. Such responses by health professionals can set up barriers to further teaching effectiveness.

To help patients cope with their anxiety, any number of combinations of the coping styles discussed earlier may be used. If coping styles are severely impairing the individual's ability to function or are interfering with medical care, referral to other health professionals for in-depth counseling may be indicated. Such suggestions may be met with resistance if offered by a professional who has not established a trusting relationship with the patient, however. Blind persistence at patient education at this stage is a waste of time for both health professional and patient and may also interfere with the possibility of effective patient teaching later. It may be more important for the health professional to work around the patient's disease by gradually providing realistic information in a supportive manner, giving the information with sensitivity, but also not reinforcing the patient's false beliefs.

Patients who accept their condition and subsequent limitations may become depressed as they acknowledge perceived losses. The health professional conducting patient education should not equate this reaction with a lack of motivation or with an inadequate teaching plan or strategy. It is more productive at this point for the health professional to accept the patient's right to grieve, at the same time establishing short-term teaching goals that continue to move the patient forward. To discontinue efforts toward patient education totally or to provide only sympathy at this point may encourage the patient to assume maladaptive patterns of behavior that are not consistent with independence and positive health outcomes.

By accepting, acknowledging, and helping patients to work through their initial reaction to illness, health professionals also help people adjust to new limitations or special treatment regimens that may be associated with the illness. Effective education is greatly dependent on patients reaching this point.

Although there is no way to diagnose coping styles accurately, health professionals should be aware of their existence and check out possibilities. Rather than a coping style, the patient may be reacting to other environmental factors or to a differing belief system. Only through continued observation and assessment, and additional data gathering, can health professionals gain more insight into patients' behavior. The behaviors of health professionals are important in

| TABLE 3-1 | Facilitative Behaviors for the Health Professional |

1. Recognize that coping styles are defenses patients use to protect themselves from threat, either real or imagined.

2. Recognize that patients' reactions to their condition and recommendations will be determined by a combination of personal characteristics, learning history, and current circumstances.

3. Avoid stereotyped approaches to patients or to the content of information presented. Even patients with the same conditions do not adapt and react in the same way.

4. Set aside assumptions, and perform a careful assessment of the present beliefs, reactions, and circumstances of each patient.

5. Recognize that timing of the teaching intervention is important to the patient's readiness to learn and to work toward established goals. If a good relationship has not previously been established, suggesting that the patient change may lead to rejection of other education efforts.

6. Lay the foundation for effective teaching later with empathetic understanding.

7. Acknowledge and accept patients' fears, frustrations, and other reactions in an understanding way.

8. Give sensitive support that recognizes the stress patients feel.

9. In instances of denial or other coping styles that appear to be having a detrimental effect, gently and gradually confront the patient with reality.

10. Avoid agreeing with patients' statements that do not appear to be an accurate representation of fact: do not reinforce patients' negative beliefs.

11. If the coping style is not interfering with the patient's condition or treatment, leave it alone.

facilitating this process. Facilitative behaviors for the health professional are illustrated in Table 3-1.

ENHANCING PATIENTS' MOTIVATION TO CHANGE

Many variables impact an individual's ability and readiness to follow health care recommendations. The impact of patient noncompliance varies in its magnitude of seriousness. Whereas some acts of noncompliance are trivial, others can have significant impact on patients' health, well-being, and overall quality of life. The purpose of effective patient education is to help patients understand the purpose and importance of recommendations given and to enable them to make informed choices. In addition, effective patient education provides motivation to enable patients to follow the recommendations they have chosen.

Motivation, in this sense, should not be confused with coercion. Rather, motivation in patient education should be directed to understanding how patients' ability to follow recommendations can be facilitated. Motivation should be the result of the partnership formed between patient and health professional. By listening to patients and trying to understand their unique perspective and experience, health professionals begin to establish an atmosphere of collaboration and partnership. Health professionals conducting patient education should present themselves to patients as consultants, never criticizing patients' efforts or criticizing their failure to follow recommendations as expected. Patients may have their own reasons for not following recommendations. By providing empathy and support, as well as feedback and guidance, health professionals help patients to consider changes recommended and enhance their ability to follow them.

Understanding patient resistance, lack of motivation, and noncompliance can help health professionals work more effectively in helping patients achieve health-related goals. One model that may provide insight into more effective ways of providing patients with the assistance needed to help them achieve their goals is the Stages of Change model (Miller et al. 1988, Prochaska et al. 1992, Rollinick et al. 1993, Kushner et al. 1998). The model proposes that there are predictable stages of change. By understanding which stage of change an individual is in, interventions appropriate to that stage can be instituted to motivate the individual to change.

Patients at the first stage, that of precontemplation, are not ready for change. In this stage, patients do not see change as necessary and do not recognize their current behavior as a problem. At this stage, to barrage the patient with information or to attempt to coerce them into action may alienate them or make them even more resistant to change. Patient teaching at this stage is better directed toward getting the patient to start thinking about whether or not change is necessary.

In the second stage of change, contemplation, patients may have begun to think about whether change is necessary but are still ambivalent about making a commitment to change. During this stage, health professionals should again avoid pushing patients into change but rather should encourage further dialogue about patients' questions or concerns related to the change that is being contemplated.

When the patient realizes that change is necessary, he or she has reached the preparation stage. Patient education may be most helpful at this stage when directed toward helping patients outline strategies so that change can be accomplished. Facilitating patients' ability to move toward the goal of making change they have recognized to be important also enhances the effectiveness of patient education.

The action stage of change consists of patients taking active steps to accomplish the change they perceive to be necessary. Helping patients establish an action plan with steps that are manageable and achievable should be the focus of patient education during this stage. Patients may need to be helped to see that by accomplishing short-term goals, long-term change can be accomplished.

Even when change has been accomplished, change must be maintained. Patient education directed toward offering continued support, encouragement, and reinforcement can help patients maintain the changes they have made. Continued feedback about patient progress in maintaining their behavior can, in itself, be reinforcing.

Effective patient education using the Stages of Change model demonstrates respect for patients, their views, and their values. As with most patient education efforts, effective patient education focuses on helping patients make informed decisions based on individual needs and circumstances.

REFERENCES

Kushner, P.R., Levinson, W., Miller, W.R. 1998. Motivational interviewing: what, when and why. *Patient Care* 32(14):55–56,58,64,66,69–72.

Miller, W.R., Sovereign, R.G., Drege, B. 1988. Motivational interviewing with problem drinkers: II. The drinker's check-up as a preventive intervention. *Behavioral Psychotherapy* 16:251–268.

Parsons, T. 1951. The social system. New York: Free Press.

Prochaska, J.O., DiClemente, C.C., Norcross, J.C. 1992. In search of how people change: applications to addictive behaviors. *American Psychologist* 47:1102–1114.

Rollinick, S., Kinnersley, P., Stott, N. 1993. Methods of helping patients with behavior change. *British Medical Journal* 307:188–190.

Rosenstock, I.M. 1988. Enhancing patient compliance with health recommendations. *Journal of Pediatric Health Care* 2:67–72.

Spiker, B. 1991. Methods of assessing and improving patient compliance in clinical trials. In: Cramer, J.A., Spiker, B. (Eds.). Patient compliance in medical practice and clinical trials. New York, NY: Raven Press, 37–56.

Vollmer, S. 1998. Compliance: a physician's problem. *Family Practice Recertification* 20:91–108.

4

Patient Education As a Process in Patient Care

Patient education takes place in a variety of settings, for a variety of reasons, and under a variety of circumstances. It can be conducted in an inpatient or outpatient setting. It can be directed toward helping patients or families understand a disease or learn ways to prevent disease from occurring. It can be directed toward helping patients or families understand how to carry out a therapeutic regimen or toward helping patients understand a procedure they are about to undergo. Patient education can be conducted in a formal classroom setting, with a group, or with an individual. It can be conducted "on the run"—such as while giving a bed bath—or while doing a physical examination.

However patient education is done, and whatever its purposes, health professionals need a framework for delivering patient education information in a conscious and organized way. Health professionals must be aware of opportunities for patient education during patient encounters. Patient education need not be viewed as only a formal process to be done in time set aside for teaching patients with particular conditions rather than an intrinsic part of every encounter. Such a narrow view can waste many opportunities for patient education, as well as fostering the misconception that the total process is far too time consuming to be practical. Broadening the view of the process from being a single intervention to an intrinsic part of each patient encounter offers many opportunities for health professionals to collect data about patients, give patients information, answer questions, reinforce information previously given, check the patients' understanding of the information given, and monitor the effectiveness of past patient education. Each interaction is also an opportunity for health professionals to begin building the trust and rapport that are critical to successful patient education.

Much information can be given and gained from patients during routine procedures, physical exams, or when patients pick up a prescription. Health professionals must be aware of the opportunity and seize upon it, using a conscious and organized effort.

TEACHING AND LEARNING

Rather than being a formal procedure specially scheduled to convey information, patient education is more frequently an exchange between patient and health professional in a health care delivery setting during a regular clinical encounter. Many of the general principles of education can also apply to patient education, however.

One can only be a teacher in the exact sense of the word if there is a learner. Merely giving information to individuals does not mean that teaching has taken place because there is no guarantee that learning has occurred. To be effective, information must be presented in a way that makes it relevant and comprehensible. Information must be delivered when individuals are ready and motivated to learn, and it must be presented in an environment conducive to learning. The teacher, therefore, must be able to identify the information the learner needs, as well as consider the learner's feelings, perceptions, motivation, and readiness to learn.

The relationship between teaching and learning is an interdependent one and part of an interactive process. In this instance, the term *process* can be defined as a systematic set of actions directed toward a goal. The goal of teaching in any educational setting is to transfer information from one individual to another, with the hope that it will be incorporated and put to use by the person to whom the information is being presented. Likewise, the goal of patient education is not merely to enable patients to regurgitate the information back to the health professional; rather, it is to enable patients to incorporate the information into their health behavior to improve their potential for positive health outcomes. To reach this goal, patient education cannot happen by chance; it must be part of a process based on an organized and structured sequence of events between patients and health professionals.

Patient education is no different in these respects from education in any other setting; it is an individualized process. The task of the teacher, in this case the health professional, is to identify the needs of the individual patient, to present information according to those needs, to set goals that are realistic and appropriate for the individual, and to assess the results accurately.

Viewed this way, patient education requires the same problem-solving skills that other clinical interventions demand. Just as the same antibiotic is not ordered for all infections or the same diet therapy given to every person with a particular illness, neither should all patients receive the same type of patient education. A treatment is not prescribed without collecting data to arrive at a diagnosis. Patient management and the treatment prescribed are based on diagnosis and the individual patient's situation. To be effective, patient education requires a similar process. There must be data collection and assessment of the patient and his or her educational needs. These data must then be synthesized to formulate an individual teaching plan; the plan must be implemented and then monitored to evaluate whether, and to what degree, the goal has been reached and to identify alternatives that may be necessary.

It may seem that patient education could, under these criteria, be a time-consuming process. However, conducting patient education without using a structured, organized approach can also be time consuming and ineffective. To conduct patient education effectively, it is not necessary for health professionals to change roles from health professional to teacher. Education can be conducted at many points during encounters with patients. Health professionals must, however, be aware of teachable moments, be able to identify patient needs, and be able to make a conscious and organized effort to conduct education in a way that will be most meaningful to the individual patient.

CATEGORIES OF LEARNING

Patient education is directed toward increasing patients' knowledge about their condition, treatment, or measures of prevention. The goal of patient education, then, is to help patients increase their ability to make decisions about their health and health care, to cope with a specific illness, and to improve their health-related behavior. Health professionals who only think of patient education in terms of factual information may be disappointed when health care outcomes are not what was anticipated. One reason for failure may be the health professional's inability to assess adequately the type of patient teaching needed.

There are three categories of human learning: (1) cognitive, (2) psychomotor, and (3) affective (Bloom 1956). All three categories, or domains, are included at one time or another in patient education. Before beginning teaching, health professionals should identify which (possibly all) of these aspects are to be addressed.

The cognitive domain refers to the actual knowledge and understanding individuals have or are given about a certain subject. For example, a nurse teaching a patient with a colostomy about colostomy irrigation is working within the patient's cognitive domain when including information about underlying anatomy and physiology as well as the purpose of the irrigation.

If the nurse's goal is to enable the patient to do colostomy irrigations at home independently, however, then providing only facts about the colostomy and the procedure is not enough. The patient must also be taught the physical skills needed to implement the procedure. These skills involve the patient's psychomotor domain. Patient teaching would thus be directed toward helping the patient to learn an activity or the physical skills associated with the cognitive information previously received. Reading about or listening to an explanation of colostomy irrigation is not the same as actually doing the irrigation. To include knowledge without teaching the physical skills involved, in this instance, would do little to help achieve the stated goal. On the other hand, teaching the patient the mechanics of a colostomy irrigation without helping him or her to understand its purpose and necessity may also end in less than desirable results. Here, cognitive and psychomotor teaching go hand in hand.

The affective domain is also critical in reaching the desired goal of patient education. The affective domain refers to the patient's attitude. The patient may have the knowledge and skills needed to perform a procedure but be unwilling or unmotivated, because of a reaction to a condition or treatment, to carry it out. If the patient has gained the knowledge and skills needed for colostomy irrigation but views the procedure as distasteful or dirty, the goal of independent performance of the procedure at home will probably still not be reached. Although the affective domain is perhaps more difficult to identify than cognitive or psychomotor aspects of instruction, it can have a profound impact on the success of patient teaching.

A relationship exists between all three categories of human learning. Although cognition involves recall and recognition of information presented, it also refers to comprehension of the material taught. Recall and recognition, or patients' willingness to recite facts, are of little benefit if they are unable to understand the meaning of the facts, how they can be put to use, or why they are important. Before patients or learners can do this, they must first receive the information and be willing to listen to what is being said. Only when patients are ready to receive the information can health professionals actually teach.

Beyond the level of comprehension is patient's ability to apply the knowledge or perform the skill they have learned. Patients with diabetes, for example, may fully understand the diet exchange sheet and be able to recall food items included in the various exchanges. A fuller measure of patients' understanding, however, might be their ability to apply the information in a practical situation, such as being able to choose food for lunch from the hospital cafeteria line. Cognitively, patients must be able to analyze situations and apply the knowledge gained. They must be able to synthesize knowledge to fit new situations and adapt knowledge and behavior accordingly. Patients must also be physically able to perform the behavior learned.

Comprehension and the ability to apply knowledge, or to perform a skill, are only part of the equation in learning, however. The affective domain, or the patient's willingness and motivation to incorporate the learning into life, is crucial for teaching effectiveness. In the preceding example, despite the patients' ability to pick out the appropriate foods in the hospital cafeteria, they must also be willing to continue voluntarily to choose appropriate foods after leaving the hospital, when the direct supervision of the health professional is no longer available.

The goal of patient education is to help individuals gain knowledge and skills that they will be able to incorporate into their behavior. Ideally, effective patient education helps patients organize information they are given so that it is compatible with their own value system and incorporate it into their daily activities. Implementing this type of impact is possibly the greatest challenge in patient education.

MOTIVATION TO LEARN

Identifying the type of knowledge to be transmitted through patient teaching is only one step in the process. Patients must also be motivated to learn the information that is to be presented. Before they can be motivated to learn, they must recognize that they have a need for the information to be presented, and they must be physically and mentally ready to receive it. Assessing patients' motivation to learn is another step in patient education.

Identifying the Need to Know

What motivates people to learn? Before they can be motivated, they must first recognize a need to know. The teaching-learning process usually begins with an individual identifying a need for gaining knowledge or for learning a skill. This need may first be identified by either the teacher or the learner. If the learner has identified the need, then obviously he or she will be more motivated to seek out information and to learn the material once it is presented. If the teacher has identified the need, the job is not only to relay the information in such a way that the learner is able to understand it but also to demonstrate to the learner why this information is important.

Either the patient or the health professional may identify the need for patient education. Patients who ask, "What exactly will the surgery involve?" or "Exactly how do I go about changing my dressings after I go home?" have clearly recognized the need to learn. In these instances, the patient has identified a lack of knowledge or skill he or she perceives as needed. The patient has instigated the teaching-learning process and will more likely be motivated to learn information given in response to his or her questions. Obviously, the more the patient recognizes the need to learn, the more relevant and important he or she feels the information is, the more motivated they will be to learn and incorporate the information presented.

In some instances, it is the health professional who identifies patients' need to know. The nurse who observes a new mother diapering and dressing her baby awkwardly may start patient teaching by explaining principles about carrying and handling a new infant. The physician who, after treating a young woman for persistent urinary tract infections, discovers that she has been wiping her perianal area from back to front after elimination has also identified a patient's need to know. The patient in this example, unaware of the possible relationship between this practice and her chronic urinary tract infections, may be unaware of the information she lacked. Recognizing the patient's need to know, the physician can proceed to explain the importance of wiping from front to back to help prevent further urinary tract infections from occurring.

Initiating patient teaching seems relatively simple and straightforward. Either the patient or the health professional may recognize the need for information; consequently, the process of patient education is begun. The need to learn, however, is not always as easily recognizable as in the examples presented. The need to know can be quite obvious if patients ask direct questions or if the health professional observes obvious cues indicating that education is needed. At other times, however, patients may not ask direct questions because they do not know what to ask or have not realized their need for information. Likewise, health professionals may be unaware of cues given by patients indicating that they lack knowledge in a certain area. In some instances, health professionals may assume or take it for granted that patients have a better understanding of the condition or treatment than they really do. Misunderstandings or misconceptions may exist that health professionals have not recognized. Therefore, no attempt to give further information or to correct misconceptions may be made. If health professionals are not alert to the cues that signal patients' need to learn, very little teaching or learning will take place. An example of a less direct cue that indicates the need for patient education might be the casual remark by a patient at an annual checkup who says, "I guess I'll be going through menopause soon. I hear so many stories about all the symptoms other women experience. It's sure not something I'm looking forward to. I just hope my husband understands that I'll be a different woman." Although perhaps not consciously aware of her question, the patient is nonetheless demonstrating a need for patient education, or at least a further exploration of her information base. If the statement is ignored or if the patient does not become insistent or more direct in her request for information, the opportunity for patient education is lost.

In other instances, there may be incongruence between the patient's and the health professional's view of the patient's need to know. The health professional may perceive the need for patient education when the patient does not. For example, consider the following response by a patient to a pharmacist. After filling a prescription, the pharmacist tried to give the patient further information about the medication, including possible side effects. The patient responded: "Oh, I trust the doctor. Whatever he ordered is fine. After all, he's the doctor; there's no reason why I should have to know all the details." In this instance, the patient obviously had not perceived a need to know. Teaching content is useless unless it is perceived by the learner as useful and as advantageous to learn. In this example, the best approach may have been for the pharmacist to help the patient understand why the information was important, a factor of which the patient may be totally unaware. The pharmacist might also attempt, however, to discover more about the individual patient's feelings. The patient's statement may be related to how he or she views the patient's and physician's roles within the health care system, or it may be related to the patient's difficulty in accepting the condition for which he or she is being treated. Taking an approach that identifies the patient's feelings may do more to facilitate future education than any other approach at this time. If the pharmacist blindly persists in presenting information despite the patient's obvious disinterest in receiving it, there is risk of alienating the patient from receiving further information. In addition, such persistence wastes the pharmacist's time and effort in presenting information the patient perceives as useless.

Individuals who are coerced into receiving information they are not ready to learn or have no interest in learning will probably have decreased comprehension and retention of the material. Thus, chances are slim that information these patients have been given will be incorporated into their health behaviors.

Readiness to Learn

Learning readiness is determined by many factors. Anything that affects physical or psychological comfort can affect an individual's ability and motivation to learn. After the need to know has been identified, patients' readiness to receive information at that particular time must also be assessed. There may be many barriers to patient learning that, if identified and overcome, can facilitate the learning process. Patients who are unreceptive to information at one time may be more receptive to the same information at another time. For example, patients who are experiencing pain or who are in some other way physically uncomfortable are unsuitable candidates for learning about their present condition and causes of the pain. Pain and physical discomfort are a distraction to learning. The same patients may be quite receptive to learning about their condition at a later time, however, when the pain has subsided.

In addition to physical discomfort, patients may have other priorities that supersede information given them in patient teaching, thus affecting their learning readiness. A patient with allergies who has taken a lunch break from work to visit the physician may not be attentive to learning about how to eliminate allergies in the home if he or she is concerned about returning to work on time. The same patient may be far more receptive to the same information when he or she has fewer time constraints.

Patients' reactions to their illness can also influence their learning readiness and motivation to learn. Emotional upheavals are a powerful distraction from learning. Such was the case of Mrs. Peterson, who had consulted her physician because of pain and lesions she had found around her perineal area. After examining her, the physician diagnosed Mrs. Peterson's condition as genital herpes and spent additional time explaining the condition to her. An outside observer might have rated the information given as very comprehensive and the physician as extremely proficient in conducting patient teaching. The physician explained the condition thoroughly and in terms that Mrs. Peterson could understand—if she had been listening. Mrs. Peterson had become so upset by the diagnosis—believing it meant that her husband had been cheating on her—that she had heard nothing more the physician had said. Even though the physician, from all indications, did an excellent job of patient teaching, the patient was not ready to learn. Consequently, little was gained from the time spent teaching.

Patients' levels of anxiety can also determine their readiness to learn and subsequent ability and willingness to carry out a therapeutic regimen. Health professionals once held a common belief that patients could be frightened into compliant behavior. Presenting information vividly so that patients had a clear understanding of the severely detrimental consequences of their behavior if they did not adhere to medical advice was thought to increase the likelihood that they would comply with recommendations. It may be difficult to imagine, for example, that a person with a strong family history of heart disease would persist in smoking three packs of cigarettes a day after being told the probability of mortality for heavy smokers with a strong family history of heart disease. The same might be said for people who are told the horrors of a variety of other diseases that are possible if they continue in their current behavior patterns.

Although realization of the potential health risk and hazard of various behaviors may be sufficient to motivate some people to change their behavior or to adhere more closely to health advice, in many instances, such tactics have the opposite effect. For many individuals, such knowledge merely raises their anxiety to such a level that the information and advice are rejected, having caused too much discomfort for them to deal with.

Studies indicate that scare tactics do little to motivate people to follow health advice, preventive or otherwise. Whereas some anxiety may stimulate learning, severe anxiety is incapacitating and can, in fact, interfere with the learning process (Leventhal 1971, Rudd 1995). Severe anxiety can lead to denial by patients. When the diagnosis or its implications are too anxiety provoking for patients to accept, their reaction may be to block out the information totally. They may rationalize that although the possibility of danger may be present for some individuals, the information is not applicable to them personally—they will beat the odds.

Health professionals who blindly proceed with patient teaching under these circumstances not only conduct a futile exercise but run the risk of losing rapport and trust that could enhance future efforts. A far better approach at this time might be to acknowledge the patient's anxiety and feelings and to demonstrate acceptance of them. Patients may not be consciously aware of their level of anxiety. Health professionals who persist in bringing information to patients that they are not ready to hear only drives them further away. By demonstrating an understanding of the patient as an individual and thus beginning to build a relationship in which the patient may be helped to recognize fears and anxiety, health professionals begin to create an environment conducive to a discussion of fears and, thus, gradually conducive to learning readiness. It is only at this point that patients will actually be able or willing to incorporate the information given.

ASSESSING PATIENT NEEDS

The goal of patient education is to assist patients in obtaining knowledge, skills, or attitude that will help them attain behaviors that will maximize their potential for positive health outcomes. Before patient education can be effective in reaching this goal, however, health professionals must determine what type of information or change is appropriate for the patient and what factors specific to that individual may facilitate or impede learning and behavior change. As a process, patient education involves not only giving patients information but receiving information from patients as well. Health professionals should not be so anxious to inform patients that the patients' needs are ignored. Before giving patients information, health professionals should not forget to collect data from patients that would enhance delivery of information and formation of strategies to help patients achieve designated health behaviors. Making this determination is called behavioral diagnosis.

Behavioral diagnosis has been defined as the systemic identification of health practices that appear to be causally linked to the health problem or problems identified in the epidemiological diagnosis (Bartlett 1982). Just as medical diagnosis enables health professionals to identify the probable cause of the medical problem and determine an appropriate treatment, behavioral diagnosis makes possible the identification of factors that have an influence on health behaviors. In turn, it helps health professionals select optimal strategies to assist patients in altering or improving health status. Specific steps in conducting behavioral diagnosis appear in Table 4-1. Knowledge is only one variable that helps or hinders adherence. Other factors that influence patients' ability to comply with recommendations given by health professionals may be categorized as (1) individual factors, (2) social factors, (3) environmental factors, and (4) the medical regimen (Bartlett 1982).

TABLE 4-1   Steps in Behavioral Diagnosis

1. Distinguish between behavioral and nonbehavioral causes of the problem. That is, does the patient's behavior contribute directly to the problem, or is the problem a result of heredity or other factors beyond the patient's control?

2. List behaviors the patient must exhibit to follow the recommendations. That is, does the patient have to modify diet? Does he or she need transportation for follow-up visits? Must medication be taken on a daily basis?

3. Rank the behaviors listed in order of importance. For example, is it more important for the patient to take medication daily than to change his or her diet? Is having diagnostic tests more important at this point than following other aspects of the regimen?

4. Rate each behavior according to changeability. From assessment of the patient, is the patient more likely to take a medication daily than follow other recommended aspects of treatment, such as increasing exercise? Is the patient willing to cut down on smoking but not stop altogether?

5. Prioritize behaviors in order of importance and changeability. Make those behaviors target goals for patient education. That is, develop specific goals. What behavior is most important and most likely to be changed? What specific expectations for change are there?

Individual needs can refer to the immediate teaching situation as well as to those things that may interfere with patients' carrying out the recommended regimen. In terms of immediate needs, health professionals should assess whether the individual is ready to learn at this particular time or whether there are physical, emotional, mental, or other barriers that would interfere with the person's receptiveness and ability to learn.

Individual needs also include the patient's current level of knowledge. Does the patient have insufficient knowledge to carry out the regimen or lack understanding of its importance, thus decreasing the possibility that the recommendations will be followed? Does the patient have misconceptions about his or her condition or treatment that need to be addressed before teaching or learning can take place?

Individual needs also include patients' attitudes. Health professionals must address patients' attitudes and beliefs about their condition and treatment and, in some cases, about health care in general. Is the patient motivated to carry out the treatment plan? Is he or she fearful about the diagnosis, treatment, or prognosis? Has the patient accepted the condition as well as the need for treatment, or is the person in a phase of denial? How does the patient perceive the severity of the disease? What meaning does the disease or condition have for the individual personally?

Patients' individual skill levels must be assessed by health professionals. Does the patient have the ability to carry out the regimen, or will teaching of new skills or modification of old ones be necessary? Will other family members or special devices be needed to help the patient perform the skills needed to follow the recommendations?

Social factors and their impact on an individual patient's ability or willingness to follow recommendations must be assessed if patient education is to be effective. What social influences may either impede or facilitate learning and the patient's ability to follow the recommendations given? What is the patient's system of social support? How well does it function? Will family, friends, employers, or others with whom the patient has contact support him or her in achieving the educational goals, or will such influence interfere with the patient's following the recommended behavior? Do values of the individual's social, ethnic, or religious group conflict with recommendations or with the patient's ability to carry them out?

Environmental factors may help or hinder patients' ability to learn or to carry out recommended procedures. Does the patient have inadequate housing, inadequate transportation, or a scarcity of other resources that make carrying out the regimen more difficult, even impossible? Does the individual's daily schedule, responsibilities, or work schedule make it impossible to follow advice?

It is also important to assess the basic teaching environment. Is the atmosphere conducive to learning? Is there adequate privacy? Is the patient in a comfortable environment for learning?

In terms of the medical regimen itself, is it too complex for the patient to carry out? Are there side effects that prohibit the patient from continuing treatment? Does the patient have the skills and/or ability to follow the recommendations?

In making a behavioral diagnosis, it is important for health professionals to consider the impact of these factors on patients' ability to learn and carry out the behaviors education is to address. To what extent do factors predispose to the patient's problem? To what extent do the factors enable the patient to engage in the specified behaviors? Do the factors reinforce patient behavior? If so, how— and how much? Health professionals should consider both positive and negative effects these factors may have on patient behavior.

Making an accurate behavioral diagnosis enables health professionals to make an appropriate educational plan for initiating behavior change. Collecting data about patients to make these determinations and then using data in patient education requires sensitivity and skill. As with any clinical skill, a certain amount of knowledge and understanding is required to perform it efficiently and effectively. The more detailed description of the factors to be considered in behavioral diagnosis presented in Chapter 3 provides a knowledge base for the development of skill in patient teaching.

PROBLEM SOLVING IN PATIENT EDUCATION

Identifying the individual, social, environmental, and medical regimen factors through appropriate data collection is the health professional's first step in patient education. The next is to determine, based on the data collected, the approach that is most appropriate and most conducive to learning for the particular patient. This step includes determining the amount and sequence of information to be given, the type of information needed, and the educational interventions best suited to the patient.

The patient's profile and associated strengths or problems influence the health professional's use of words, the depth of information given, its sequence according to the patient's priorities, and the type of teaching intervention used. For example, if a patient who has Parkinson's disease is discouraged about its progressive nature and about the inability to control it, patient teaching about the anatomy and physiology of the condition is probably of little benefit. At this point, teaching might be directed to helping the patient talk about his or her feelings or referral to a Parkinson's disease support group where the person can meet and talk with others who might be sharing similar experiences. In other instances, if the health professional discovers that the patient's main problem is not lack of understanding of the condition or what the treatment involves but merely difficulty in remembering to implement the regimen, teaching may be directed toward designing a method that would help the patient remember the prescribed treatment.

Effective patient education encompasses a deliberate, problem-solving approach. The process of patient education is a series of steps in which data about the patient are gathered and assessed, a plan for education developed and implemented, and evaluation of teaching effectiveness conducted.

Considerable space has already been devoted in this chapter to increasing health professionals' awareness of factors to be considered in patient education. At first glance, it may seem as if effective patient education is a nearly impossible task. If incorporated into total patient care, however, it should really take very little time. Many data are available from everyday interactions with patients. If the health professional has an ongoing relationship with the patient, data have been picked up over time through numerous interactions. Additional time spent explaining recommendations or answering the patient's questions can save time in the long run by eliminating misunderstanding or by correcting knowledge, skill, or attitude deficiencies that would have prevented the patient from accurately following recommendations.

There are obviously many levels of patient education and many circumstances in which it can take place. Although the exact approach may differ according to the setting and the type of patient education given, many general principles remain the same. To be effective, health professionals must have an organized, structured approach to patient interactions so that information about the patient can be gathered and incorporated into the teaching plan. In so doing, health professionals are best able to meet patients' information needs. Data gathering requires awareness of information needed, astute observation, and active listening by health professionals. Systematic assessment enables health professionals to individualize patient teaching, thus maximizing the probability that it will be effective. Data gathering and assessment provide a basis for behavioral diagnosis on which a teaching plan can be developed that is best suited to patients' needs; the plan can then be evaluated to see how effective it was in actually meeting those needs.

Data Collection and Assessment

Although some data collection and assessment may involve formal interaction with the patient, much information—both objective and subjective—can be gained in routine patient interactions. Every patient contact is an opportunity for data collection. Major areas of information needed include the following:

- demographic information about the patient as an individual, including age, marital status, occupation, education, ethnic or cultural background, and the like
- the patient's physical and emotional readiness to learn
- the patient's perceived information needs and priorities
- the patient's current level of knowledge and/or skill
- the patient's attitudes, reactions, and feelings about his or her health status, condition, and treatment, and about health and health care in general
- the patient's system of social support and any other pertinent social or environmental factors that might have an impact on teaching or on the patient's ability to carry out the treatment

Data about patients can be collected from many sources and in many ways. Simple observation can be a great source of information if the health professional is aware of opportunities for it and makes a conscious effort to observe cues from patients.

For example, in an outpatient setting, much information can be gathered simply by glancing into the waiting room. Noting who brought the patient to the clinic, or who is with the patient, may give the health professional some idea about family or other systems of social support. Observation of the patient's general appearance, manner of dress, hairstyle, and general affect can also provide important information. The patient may demonstrate a variety of nonverbal cues, such as facial expressions, posture, or general body movements that can give the health professional much information about the patient's general feelings at the time. For example, some physicians routinely call patients from the waiting room themselves just to make this type of observation. When preparing the patient for examination, the nurse also has the opportunity to observe behavior. Does the patient's expression indicate fear, anxiety, sadness, or anger or does the patient appear calm and relaxed? While waiting for the physician, does the patient engage in foot tapping, squirming, or other signs of general restlessness? Does the patient seem distraught? Peaceful?

Much information is available to health professionals in the hospital setting as well. By glancing into the patient's room at visiting hours, the health professional may be able to gain information about the patient's social support by observing who visits regularly and what type of interactions take place between patient and visitors. While distributing medications or performing treatments, other general observations can be made about the patient's general affect. Does he or she appear apprehensive or assured? Does the patient appear to be comfortable physically, or are there signs indicating pain or some other type of physical discomfort that might interfere with the teaching process?

Skilled observation can be an extremely valuable assessment tool when combined with other sources of data, such as the patient's chart. A brief review of the chart can provide demographic information and possibly some information about patients' past health history, which may also be a clue to past experiences. These experiences may influence patients' reactions to their condition, their treatment, or the health care they are currently receiving. Notes on the chart by other health professionals may help supply information about the patient's reactions, strengths, or other specific characteristics that can be helpful when individualizing a patient teaching plan.

Perhaps the most valuable sources of information are the patients themselves. Information can be gained from patients both informally—through casual conversation—and formally—through a structured interview. Through casual conversation, astute health professionals may begin to note clues about patients' life styles, whom they feel close to, their general attitude and feelings about their condition and treatment, and their openness to receiving more information.

Through simple verbal interchange, health professionals can also determine anger, anxiety, and sadness from patients' tone of voice as well as from words spoken. Information may be gained about learning capabilities by noting the patients' language structure and level of communication. Such information can be obtained any time there is contact, such as while preparing the patient for an exam, while carrying out a treatment, or while conducting a physical examination. Gathering data in the normal context of patient care requires no extra time; it does, however, provide for more efficient use of time already spent.

A more formal approach to data gathering makes it possible to gather information about the patient that is not available from other sources and to begin to validate perceptions of the patient that have begun to be formulated from data already obtained. This formal approach usually involves talking with the patient with the specific purpose of gaining information. This process can also begin to establish a relationship of trust that can facilitate the teaching process. Formal data gathering should be a prelude to direct patient teaching. If the health professional has not already formulated a view about the patient's knowledge level and learning readiness, this type of interaction provides the opportunity to assess the patient's knowledge, beliefs, and attitudes more completely.

Beginning assessment may be done while building rapport. After initial rapport has been established, the health professional may continue assessment. A beginning approach to further assessment may be a statement such as the following:

> Mrs. Ellis, I wanted to talk to you a little bit about your hypertension today and to answer any specific questions you may have about it. It would help me to know something about the information you already have about your condition. Could you tell me a little bit about your understanding of hypertension?

Such open-ended questions can provide health care professionals with much more data by allowing patients to respond in their own words. Through this approach, health professionals may gain information about patients' understanding of their condition and about their feelings concerning that condition, as well as their questions and priorities. These types of data may be obtained not only by listening to patients' words but also by observing their willingness to talk about their condition and by observing other nonverbal cues made by patients while talking about their condition.

The time needed for this type of formal data gathering depends on patients' needs and the complexity of the condition or regimen for which they are receiving information. Some patient teaching can often be incorporated into this initial data-gathering session. If questions are raised in the explanation of the patient's condition, the health professional need not wait for a formal teaching session to answer them. Questions that at first may seem irrelevant can indicate patients' greatest area of interest. By answering questions promptly and honestly, health professionals not only acquire patients' attention but further enhance patient trust in the health professional as someone genuinely interested. This trust and rapport may be one of the most important factors in effective patient education. One approach to this part of the process is illustrated by the following case.

Mr. Oliver had been hospitalized because of peptic ulcer; subsequently, he had a subtotal gastrectomy. The nurse on the surgical ward noted from reviewing Mr. Oliver's chart that he was Caucasian, 42 years of age, and divorced. From observations, the nurse noted that Mr. Oliver, a certified public accountant, appeared concerned about his business while in the hospital; he had numerous phone conversations with his business associates. He had few visitors other than his 18-year-old daughter, who visited him daily. During his daily care, the nurse discovered that Mr. Oliver engaged in few recreational activities other than sailing on weekends with his daughter, who would be going away to college in the fall. Although pleasant, Mr. Oliver appeared restless, tense, and very anxious to return to work.

After the initial postoperative period, when Mr. Oliver was experiencing relatively little pain, the nurse began more formal data gathering as a prelude to teaching him about the regimen he was to follow at home. The nurse chose a time when Mr. Oliver's roommate in the next bed had gone to x-ray, thus allowing more privacy for the interaction and lessening the chance of distractions. The nurse found Mr. Oliver going over some book work that one of his colleagues had brought to him:

Nurse: Mr. Oliver, I hope I'm not interrupting. I wanted to begin to talk to you about the instructions you are to follow when you go home. Should I come back later?

Mr. Oliver: No, now is fine—anything to get me out of here sooner so I can get back to work.

Nurse: I know that Dr. Lane explained your condition to you before surgery and has talked with you some after surgery, but sometimes when people are ill, they find it difficult to concentrate on everything they're told. So that I don't repeat information you already have, could you tell me a little bit about what you know about your condition?

Mr. Oliver: Well, I know I had an ulcer in the lower end of my stomach, and they had to take out about half of it. I suppose that means I'll only be able to eat half as much now.

Nurse: Although you may have to increase your intake of food gradually, most people who have had the type of surgery you've experienced can eventually increase their food intake to normal capacity.

Mr. Oliver: That's a relief. I really enjoy eating. My daughter and I go out to eat frequently, and when she goes away to college, most of our times together will probably consist of when I drive up there to take her out to dinner. She's really all I have right now. I'd sure hate to have to give up those special times.

Nurse: I see no reason why you should have to. There will be a special diet that you'll need to follow for a while. Have you had a chance to look at the diet sheet that the dietitian left with you?

Mr. Oliver: Yes, but it looked pretty rigid to me. It had a lot of meals during the day—that could be a lot of food. I'll look like a blimp!

Nurse: Actually, although you'll be eating frequently during the day for a while, the food is in relatively small amounts. What is your schedule like during the day? Will it be difficult for you to eat at frequent intervals?

Mr. Oliver: Yes, sometimes I'm on the road traveling between places at those times.

Nurse: Since your stomach has a small capacity, the six small meals a day provide you with adequate nutrition without distending your stomach. Let's talk about ways in which you may still be able to do that even though you are traveling.

In this case, the nurse gained considerable data that can be used to formulate a behavioral diagnosis and thus be incorporated into a plan for patient teaching. The interaction also served to facilitate rapport and trust between patient and health professional.

Looking at specific points in the interaction, several principles of the first step in patient education can be identified. The nurse's first statement, offering to come back at a later time, not only demonstrated that the nurse was sensitive and respectful of the patient's time but also revealed something about Mr. Oliver's readiness to learn and his motivation as well. He was receptive to discussing his treatment at that time, and his motivation to go home appeared great. The nurse may also assess from Mr. Oliver's statements that work is quite important to him. If the importance of following the regimen to prevent complications that could keep him from work again is emphasized, Mr. Oliver's compliance with the prescribed regimen may be greatly enhanced. By asking the patient about his understanding of his condition, the nurse began to gain some information not only about Mr. Oliver's knowledge level but also about his priorities and concerns. The nurse recognized Mr. Oliver's concern about being able to eat only half as much. By responding and by offering reassurance and support, the nurse communicated a sensitivity to his concerns as an individual.

The nurse identified Mr. Oliver's need to know more about his diet as well as offering clarification about the total amount of food intake within the prescribed program. The nurse also identified potential barriers to Mr. Oliver's ability to carry out the recommendations.

The data collected through informal means also provided the nurse with useful information in formulating an effective plan for patient teaching. It became evident that Mr. Oliver's daughter was a strong source of social support. Since the nurse knew that Mr. Oliver's daughter would be leaving in the fall, further assessment of the impact her absence would have on his ability to follow recommendations may be a focus of further sessions. The nurse also learned that Mr. Oliver is divorced, indicating that assessment of eating habits and food planning and preparation may be needed. Does Mr. Oliver eat mainly in restaurants, or does he cook for himself? How involved is his daughter with helping him prepare and plan food eaten on a daily basis?

Through observation, the nurse also recognized that Mr. Oliver appeared quite involved with his work, with few sources of recreation other than those he enjoys with his daughter. The nurse may therefore need to teach Mr. Oliver about methods of stress reduction or about the importance of recreation as a source of relaxation.

Some analysis and synthesis of the data were done by the nurse throughout the interaction. Further processing of the data is done in formulating the problem base and, subsequently, the teaching plan. The problem-solving approach specifies learning needs, potential barriers to learning or to carrying out the regimen, and the patient's strengths. From the information currently available, a preliminary problem base might be as follows:

- learning needs: information regarding specifics of diet, stress-reduction techniques
- potential barriers: work schedule, ability to prepare food on diet
- strengths: social support of daughter, patient's motivation

The case of Mr. Oliver illustrates assessment and formulation of a problem-solving approach in an inpatient facility. Because health professionals have the opportunity to interact with patients over extended periods of time, data may be collected throughout the hospital stay. Although interactions with patients in outpatient facilities are shorter, the same process of data collection, assessment, and behavioral diagnosis can be used. If patients are regular patients at the outpatient facility, health professionals may have opportunities over extended periods of time to develop an extensive data base about patients and their families that can be used in formulating an effective plan for patient teaching.

Data collection, assessment, and behavioral diagnosis are key components of effective patient education. Because the probability that patients will follow recommendations is greater when the plan is developed around their individual needs, the significance of this process cannot be overstated.

Developing a Plan for Patient Teaching

Once data about the patient have been gathered and assessed, the next step is to incorporate the information into a plan. Information gathering requires a systematic, conscious effort, and the information gathered must be incorporated into a systematic plan to meet patients' individual needs best. Steps in creating an educational plan are illustrated in Table 4-2.

The plan for patient education that is developed should incorporate goals or expected outcomes of patient teaching. The approach to patient teaching should reflect patients' individual needs as well as their strengths. Part of effective patient education is to set goals with patients that are realistic and achievable. The purpose of planning teaching in an organized, individualized way is to arrive at this type of reachable goal.

Because patient education takes place under a wide range of circumstances, there is no standard format that applies to all situations. In the example of Mr. Oliver, discussed previously, the individual goals of patient teaching may include helping Mr. Oliver understand his diet and its importance and helping him arrange his schedule so it is reasonable for him to be able to take the six small meals prescribed. Because the nurse also noted that Mr. Oliver appeared somewhat stressed at his job, part of the plan might include teaching him about the part stress can play in his condition as well as techniques of stress reduction. In addition, the nurse noted the importance of his daughter to Mr. Oliver. Therefore, part of the teaching plan may include teaching the daughter about the treatment regimen. With increased understanding, she may be able to provide

TABLE 4-2	Steps in Patient Education

Step 1. Set goals for the educational session

A. What is necessary for the patient to learn?

B. What are the priorities of learning (i.e., medical urgency, logical sequence)?

C. How will success be measured?

Step 2. Assess the patient

A. What is the patient's learning potential (i.e., knowledge, skills, attitudes, ability)?

B. What factors will help or hinder the patient in carrying out the plan?

C. What are the patient's priorities?

Step 3. Implement the plan

A. Select the best method to meet goals that is appropriate to the patient.

B. Consider the dimension of time from the patient's standpoint as well as from a medical standpoint.

C. Plan with the patient; give the patient the opportunity to share responsibility.

D. Mobilize patient resources.

E. Break the plan down into manageable steps according to priority.

Step 4. Assess outcomes

A. To what extent has the patient reached the established goals?

B. If goals have not been reached identify reasons (i.e., was the problem correctly identified and analyzed?). Were solutions appropriate to the problem?

C. Alter plan accordingly.

the support needed for Mr. Oliver to follow the treatment plan, as well as assist him in carrying it out.

Mr. Oliver appeared receptive to the information; therefore, the nurse may not need to spend additional time preparing him to receive information. In another situation with a different patient, someone not as receptive or perhaps someone having more difficulty accepting his or her condition, the situation might be different. A major portion of the teaching plan might be devoted to building trust with the patient, working with him or her to help express feelings about the condition and treatment, and helping the patient toward gradual acceptance of the condition and treatment.

In the case of Mr. Oliver, types of patient teaching focus on the cognitive domain, with some teaching in the psychomotor domain for performance of specific relaxation techniques. Although the affective domain was assessed, it did not appear that significant time needed to be spent in patient teaching in the affective domain because his acceptance of his condition and treatment appeared adequate. In other circumstances with other patients, time spent in each of the domains may vary.

Because Mr. Oliver was hospitalized, teaching interactions could occur throughout the hospital stay. The health professional was able to determine the amount of teaching time needed to reach the stated goals by Mr. Oliver's responses during the teaching interactions. These responses indicated his degree of understanding and acceptance.

In other situations, such as outpatient clinics, teaching interactions may take place at one office visit or over several visits, depending on the receptiveness of the patient, the complexity of the regimen, and the degree of patient understanding. In some instances, patient education may only be directed toward giving patients information about their treatment regimen. The process of assessment and data collection, as well as development of a teaching plan, remains the same regardless of the circumstances surrounding patient education, although the amount, scope, and focus of assessment and data collection might be narrowed in various circumstances.

The purpose of the patient teaching plan is to help health professionals to develop clear, concise descriptions of planned teaching actions. The plan is based on information gathered about the individual patient and should include the following:

- what type of information the patient should be given (cognitive, psychomotor, affective, or a combination of the three)
- when the teaching will be done (at special appointments, during regular patient encounters, etc.)
- where the teaching should be done (in the immediate environment or in another setting)
- how the teaching will be done (through individual teaching sessions; group sessions; supplemental activities, such as films, pamphlets, and the like; or through a combination of several different activities)
- who will do the patient teaching (one individual or a variety of health professionals)

Although an important aspect of the patient teaching plan is to give patients information that will enable them to carry out the plan, another important consideration is the development of strategies to help patients comply with the recommendations given. Some conditions that involve complex information may require several formal teaching sessions and may involve a variety of teaching approaches. Complex teaching situations may require the use of several team members teaching patients about different aspects of their condition or the recommendations they are to follow. Less complex regimens may require a shorter interaction with only one health professional.

The teaching plan also specifies the expected final outcome of patient teaching. The importance of setting realistic goals cannot be overemphasized. No matter how comprehensive the teaching plan is, patient education cannot be effective if the specified goals are impossible for the patient to reach. In some instances, the health professional does better to set small, short-term goals that are more attainable rather than idealistic goals that are not likely to be reached.

Implementation

Implementation involves carrying out the teaching plan that has been developed. Obviously, the most carefully made plan is of no value if it is not carried out. The implementation phase of the process should be consistent among all health professionals involved in patient teaching if the interaction is to involve more than one professional. Although the consistency of having one caregiver may be important in building the relationship and information base between the health professional and patient, such is not always possible, especially when there is rotation of health professionals providing care. In these instances, information consistency is provided through communication between health professionals. If more than one professional is involved in patient teaching, each member of the teaching team must be aware of what the patient has been told, the level of the patient's understanding, and any additional learning needs that have been identified. Such communication prevents redundancy and promotes consistency, thus increasing the probability that patient education will be effective.

Whether implementation of the patient teaching plan involves a one-to-one interaction or whether several health professionals are involved, the implementation phase is another source of data collection and assessment that can determine the need for alteration of the plan. If additional barriers to patient teaching or to the patient's ability to carry out the regimen are identified during the implementation phase, the teaching plan and implementation phase may need to be altered accordingly. To be effective, patient teaching must also be flexible. Information given during a teaching session may need to be altered according to new patient needs identified during the session. In some instances, there may be a need for alteration of the original treatment plan itself. In such cases, patient teaching must obviously be altered to fit the alternative treatment plan.

The case of Ms. Hernandez can be used to illustrate this point. Ms. Hernandez was a new patient seen by a physician in an outpatient clinic for the first time for a urinary tract infection. The physician, through observation and by talking with the patient, assessed Ms. Hernandez as being pleasant, relatively well spoken, well dressed, and apparently receptive to learning more about her condition than simply how to take the medication. The physician also assessed from the original interaction that Ms. Hernandez had not had a urinary tract infection before. The physician therefore proceeded with a teaching plan that included a brief description of urinary tract infection, measures that might prevent reoccurrence, and a description of the regimen to be followed and its importance. Implementation of the teaching plan was as follows:

> *Physician:* Ms. Hernandez, in examining a sample of your urine under the microscope, I've confirmed my diagnosis of urinary tract infection. Urine normally contains no bacteria or germs, but since there were some found in your urine, that indicates that an infection is present. Since you have no other symptoms of fever, or back pain, I believe it's confined to the bladder, which is the storage place for urine.

> *Ms. Hernandez:* Is this the same thing as a kidney infection?

> *Physician:* No, the kidney is located higher up in your lower back. This infection is only in your bladder, which is located in your lower abdomen. It's important to treat the infection in your bladder early, however, so the infection doesn't become chronic and doesn't eventually infect the kidney. There are several different factors that can predispose to urinary tract infection and several ways in which urinary tract infections can consequently be prevented. A common source of infection, especially for women, is the rectum. One way you can prevent contamination of the urinary tract, which can predispose to infection, is to wipe from front to back after eliminating. Another factor that predisposes to bladder infections is allowing long periods of time to elapse without emptying the bladder. Some people go all day at work without urinating. This causes organisms that may have entered the bladder, but would normally have been washed out, to begin to grow; therefore, an infection can become full blown. In addition, if you drink enough fluids, the bladder stays flushed out.

> *Ms. Hernandez:* I already wipe from front to back. I'm not much of a water drinker, but maybe I could start drinking juice or orange drink or something to increase my fluid intake.

> *Physician:* Good. Even four to six glasses of liquid a day is a good start. Now I'd like to explain how to take the medication I'll be giving you to treat the infection. The medicine is called Bactrim DS. It's a double-strength antibacterial agent that will kill the germs that are causing the infection. You'll need to take one pill every 12 hours for 10 days. It's important that the medication is taken at 12-hour intervals so that the level of the medicine in your body remains high enough to kill the germs or bacteria, so try not to miss any doses. After taking the medication for a few days, you may also note that your symptoms disappear. It's important that you continue taking the medication every 12 hours for the full 10 days, otherwise the bacteria may not be killed, and the symptoms may reoccur in a few days.

> I would like to have you return for an appointment at the end of the 10 days so we can test your urine again and make sure the organism is gone. If it isn't, then we'll begin further treatment. Is there anything about any of the recommendations that you feel you may have difficulty doing?

> *Ms. Hernandez:* How expensive do you think the medicine is? I've just quit my job and become a full-time student. My money is really tight now. I don't think I can afford both the medication and the return appointment.

Physician: Let me see if we have some free samples of Bactrim DS. If not, I can give you samples of a comparable medication that I know that we have in stock, and it's just as effective. Both the medication and the return appointment are very important. Since you're a student, though, didn't you pay a health fee to cover visits to the student health service?

Ms. Hernandez: Yes, I did.

Physician: Then at the end of the 10 days, why don't you go there and have your urine retested. The visit will be free there. I'll call Dr. Martin at the health service and make the arrangements.

The physician organized the teaching plan based on preliminary assessment of Ms. Hernandez's needs. Ms. Hernandez was made aware of the importance of taking the medication as directed and was taught measures of prevention. During the teaching interaction, however, barriers to carrying out the instruction were identified. By maintaining flexibility, the physician was able not only to include alternative recommendations for treatment but also to teach Ms. Hernandez how she could carry out the plan despite the barriers. The physician consequently helped increase the probability that the time spent in patient teaching would have a positive outcome. A summary of the problem-solving approach to patient education may be found in Table 4-3.

DOCUMENTATION OF PATIENT TEACHING

Communication between members of the health care team is essential if there is to be a coordinated, consistent approach to patient teaching. Although some communication takes place through word of mouth, another method occurs through documentation in the patient records. Such documentation not only communicates that patient teaching has been done but can also communicate what has been taught, the patient's level of understanding, and what further teaching or reinforcement of information may need to be performed. Such information prevents redundancy and can assist in the evaluative process as well.

For example, by charting the teaching interaction, the nurse who taught Mr. Oliver about his discharge instructions in the earlier example might specify barriers that would decrease Mr. Oliver's ability to carry out the regimen, as well as specifying plans that have been made to overcome those barriers. In the case of Mr. Oliver's work schedule, which may make it difficult to take the six small meals as prescribed, the nurse may make note of the problem and document the strategy implemented to overcome the barrier. In this instance, the plan may be to have the dietitian discuss types of foods that may be incorporated into the six small meals. Unless the dietitian has previously been made aware of the potential problem with regard to Mr. Oliver's schedule, however, much time is wasted in initial teaching sessions rediscovering the barriers that have already been revealed. Thus, extra time is devoted to patient teaching that could have been saved, making the process more efficient.

TABLE 4-3	A Problem-Solving Approach to Patient Education

1. Set preliminary goals for patient teaching in terms of specific patient behavior.
2. Identify factors that influence patient behavior.
   A. *Individual factors*
      knowledge
      skill
      attitude
      past experiences
   B. *Social factors*
      system of social support
      attitude and belief of family, peers, employer
      cultural values
      religious influences
   C. *Environmental factors*
      geographic location
      living arrangements
      financial status
      daily schedule
      employment
   D. *The medical regimen*
      complexity of the regimen
      side effects
      cost/benefit
      duration
3. Identify which factors listed above facilitate the patient's reaching the desired goals.
4. Identify which factors listed above may hinder the patient from reaching the desired goals.
5. Identify which factors can be modified through patient teaching or use of appropriate alternatives or resources.
6. Arrange original goals according to priorities.
7. Develop a patient education plan based on factors identified above and on prioritized goals.
8. Implement the plan.
9. Monitor the effectiveness of the plan in terms of the extent to which it has helped the patient reach the desired goals.
10. Modify the original plan as needed.

Documentation of patient teaching helps other health professionals reinforce information given, also providing an opportunity to gather further information or to identify additional problems that may arise. In the case of Mr. Oliver, for example, the physician, noting documentation of patient teaching on the chart, may check the effectiveness of the teaching in terms of patient understanding and acceptance of the recommendations and may also identify additional patient information needs as well. The interaction between the physician and Mr. Oliver may be as follows:

Physician: I see both the nurse and the dietitian have been talking to you about your instructions for going home. How have things been worked out with regard to the six small meals a day, even though you're on the road a lot?

Mr. Oliver: Well, I thought that might be a problem, but the dietitian helped me plan some carry-along, brown-bag type of meals that I can just take with me in the car, so I don't think that will be a problem now.

Physician: Good. This will only be necessary for the first 6 months or so. It's important that you avoid overeating but still receive adequate nutrition. That's the reason we spread the meals out. I see the nurse talked with you also about relaxation techniques. How are those going?

Mr. Oliver: Oh, fine I guess, but I'm not sure I need them or see the point in doing them. I don't really know what that has to do with my diet.

Physician: Well, it actually has more to do with your condition in general. Even though you have a special diet and eat six meals a day, emotional factors also have a definite effect on food digestion. I know you're under a bit of pressure at work. Learning ways to help reduce the effect that such pressures have on our bodies can be helpful in preventing a lot of conditions.

Mr. Oliver: I hadn't thought of it that way. I guess I can try the stress-reduction techniques, but I really don't think I'm very tense.

Physician: I'll be seeing you for follow-ups periodically in the office. Why don't you try the stress-reduction techniques just until our next office visit and see if you can notice any difference?

The physician, because of the documentation on the chart, knew what Mr. Oliver had been told and was able to reinforce information and identify further patient needs that could be incorporated into teaching in the future. Through the physician's assessment, Mr. Oliver's lack of awareness of the influences of the pressures at work was identified. Through documentation, the physician alerts other health professionals that a potential problem has been identified and indicates that follow-up and additional teaching will be continued through follow-up office visits. The teaching plan that the physician establishes for follow-up visits might include time set aside for helping Mr. Oliver talk about his feelings about and reactions to work. The physician in the original interaction did not contradict Mr. Oliver about his reported lack of tension nor insist that the only solution was stress reduction. Through team communication and documentation, however, as well as through flexibility, the physician was able to bridge the transition from inpatient to outpatient teaching with a plan that remains consistent with the information and approach that had been used in the hospital setting.

Documentation is also relevant in the outpatient setting. In the case of Ms. Hernandez, unless the physician documents what Ms. Hernandez was told about her regimen, others will have little opportunity to reinforce patient teaching or evaluate the extent to which Ms. Hernandez carried out the plan.

In other instances, in the outpatient setting, especially when patient teaching may continue through several clinic visits, documentation helps remind the health professional what has been covered at previous visits and what needs to be covered in the future. Such might be the case with the prenatal patient, for whom some patient teaching extends throughout pregnancy. Although patient teaching in this instance may be determined partially by the trimester of pregnancy, every patient has different information needs and priorities. Thus, teaching at outpatient visits may not follow the same pattern for every patient. By documenting information that has been provided at every visit, the health professional is able to organize teaching according to patient needs and priorities, avoiding the risk of neglecting to give the patient pertinent information that may not have been provided earlier.

To be useful, documentation need not be elaborate, nor need it take an inordinate amount of time. In some instances, when information is complex or is given often to many patients with similar conditions, such as with prenatal patients, documentation may consist of a simple checksheet that can be placed on the chart with space for comments about individual patients. In other instances, documentation may consist of a simple note on the patient's chart as part of the regular records. In either instance, documentation is an important component of the process; it also helps make patient education effective by providing a means of communication and documentation between health professionals about what patient teaching has been delivered.

EVALUATION

Patient education is effective if it reaches the goal it was designed to accomplish. As part of the process, goals or desired outcomes must be established before they can be evaluated. Unless patient teaching is evaluated, there is no way of knowing whether or not it was effective. Conducting the exercise of giving patients information without also determining whether or not the teaching was effective is as inefficient as giving patients information without first assessing patient needs and priorities, or without assessing their learning readiness. Evaluation is essential to patient education.

Evaluation consists of measurement of the effectiveness of patient teaching on a short-term as well as a long-term basis. Evaluation of the effectiveness of patient teaching on a short-term basis measures only the effectiveness of the immediate interaction in reaching the goals established for that particular interaction. For example, in a total teaching plan for a newly diagnosed diabetic, one teaching session might be devoted to teaching the patient how to draw up and inject insulin accurately. If the health professional asks the patient to give a return demonstration at the end of the teaching session, and the patient is able to perform the behavior accurately, then the teaching session could be said to be effective. If the goal for patient teaching is to provide the patient in an outpatient setting with a clear understanding of when to take prescribed medication, and, at the end of the clinic visit, the patient is able to tell the health professional how the medication is to be taken, the teaching session might also be said to be effective on a short-term basis. The ultimate goal of patient education, however, is not merely to enable patients to perform a behavior accurately in the presence of a health professional or to repeat information to test understanding of the material presented. The ultimate goal of patient education is to enable patients to carry out recommendations in their home environment, when they are not under the supervision of the health professional conducting the patient teaching. The long-term evaluation of the effectiveness of patient teaching, then, is the extent to which the patient actually follows the recommendations given.

Short-term goals for patient education must be established and evaluated if long-term goals are to be reached. For example, for the patient with diabetes, a long-term goal might be to reduce hospitalizations. In identifying reasons for repeated hospitalizations, it maybe discovered that most of these relate to faulty foot care. Short-term goals for patient education in this case might be as follows:

- The patient will wash feet daily with soap and lukewarm water.
- The patient will dry feet thoroughly, especially between the toes, but not rub them hard.
- The patient will cut toenails after a bath when the feet are clean.
- The patient will cut the nails straight across, never cutting back the sides.
- The patient will wear properly fitted shoes, breaking them in gradually.
- The patient will avoid walking barefoot.
- The patient will avoid cutting off corns and callouses.

If the patient does not have a clear understanding of what is to be done and why it is important, or if the patient cannot perform the desired behaviors in the presence of the health professional, it is unlikely that the individual will be able to carry out the recommendations at home. By evaluating the patient's understanding of the information at the end of the teaching session, the health professional can determine whether additional teaching is necessary to enable the patient to reach long-term goals.

Evaluation of the teaching interaction can be accomplished in a variety of ways. If the patient is to perform a behavior, return demonstration is the most logical way to evaluate how well the patient understood the information given. If the session was directed toward teaching about the schedule of medication administration or other treatment regimen, the patient's understanding can be assessed by asking him or her to describe that regimen. In some instances, if the purpose of teaching is to increase the patient's cognitive knowledge of his or her condition, assessment may be made by having the patient complete a questionnaire or paper and pencil test that includes key points of information. The purpose of evaluation in each of these instances is to enable the health professional to identify lack of knowledge or areas of misunderstanding that need to be remediated before long-term goals can be reached.

Informal means of short-term evaluation may involve conversations with the patient or with other health professionals who have interacted with the patient in areas where misunderstanding of misinformation have been identified. Although the patient may have appeared to understand the information in the immediate evaluation of teaching sessions, statements made later may indicate a need for additional information. Reassessment of the extent to which immediate goals were reached may supplement, validate, or invalidate the original evaluation of effectiveness. Such information enables the health professional to identify problems and to provide additional information, assistance, support, or resources to enable the patient to carry out recommendations.

Not all health professionals have the opportunity to evaluate formally whether or not patients have complied with recommendations. In a hospital situation, a nurse who has conducted patient teaching may not see the patient again after discharge to determine whether or not the teaching was effective. If there has been adequate communication between health professionals, however, evaluation may still be conducted. For example, the patient's physician, if aware of what teaching the patient received in the hospital, should be able to evaluate the extent to which the patient followed recommendations when seeing the individual for a regular clinic visit. Although the nurse may not have a direct means for evaluating teaching effectiveness, consequent readmissions of the patient for the same condition may be an indirect means of evaluation. Other means of evaluation available to health professionals in a hospital setting might be telephoning the patient after discharge or contacting the patient's physician or clinic nurse for follow-up.

Teaching conducted in an outpatient setting may be more easily evaluated if the patient is seen regularly. If patient teaching has been documented, then compliance can be assessed at subsequent visits. Methods of evaluation are varied. In some instances, objective methods of measuring effectiveness may be used, whereas in others, evaluations may be more subjective. If the dietitian has taught a patient about a weight-reduction diet and, at subsequent clinic visits, the patient's weight continues to drop at the anticipated rate, the dietitian may evaluate the teaching as having been effective. If the physician conducting prenatal teaching stressed the importance of prenatal care and notes that the patient regularly returns for prenatal visits, teaching may be said to be effective. In instances when measures are not as readily observable, other techniques may need to be used. If the person with diabetes continues to have elevated blood glucose levels despite alterations of insulin dose, the health professional may suspect that the patient has not followed the regimen as instructed and, thus, that patient teaching has not been effective. Further assessment of patient knowledge, skill, or attitude may help the health professional determine where the problem lies and what type of remediation may be necessary. Health professionals must be aware, however, that other factors may also influence patients' failure to reach the treatment goal. Are there complications of the condition or treatment that were unforeseeable? Was the patient correctly diagnosed and treated?

Evaluating teaching effectiveness by assessing the degree to which patients followed recommendations is productive only if accurate information is gained. Frequently, if patients are simply asked whether or not they actually followed the treatment plan, an affirmative answer may be obtained no matter what their compliance was. Such evaluative techniques not only provide little useful information but also close the door to further information that could be helpful in assessing barriers that prevented the patient from following the plan. Unless barriers are actually identified, alternatives cannot be provided. Less direct questioning of patients can yield useful information and can continue to build the trust and rapport needed between patient and health professional if teaching is to be effective. In addition, if done in a nonjudgmental way, such evaluative techniques communicate to patients that the health professional is interested in helping them to carry out the recommendations and that those recommendations truly are important enough to follow up.

Remarks such as "Tell me how you've been taking your medication," "How many pills do you have left?" or, in the case of diet instruction, "Tell me what you had for breakfast this morning and for dinner last night" can yield much more information than questions such as, "Are you taking your medications?" or "Are you following your diet?"

Evaluation of patient education is conducted to identify problems that may prevent patients from following the regimen. It is important for health professionals to remember that the purpose of patient education is to teach patients the knowledge, skills, or attitudes that will enable them to carry out recommendations. Patient education is not conducted to coerce patients into following the advice given. Positive health outcomes from patient teaching are more likely if health professionals and patients work together as a team and maintain a relationship of mutual respect. Evaluation is a means of reassessing the effectiveness of the teaching plan. If the original teaching plan was not effective, then new strategies must be incorporated to assist the patient in reaching the goals that are to be accomplished by patient education.

REFERENCES

Bartlett, E.E. 1982. Behavioral diagnosis: a practical approach to patient education. *Patient Counseling and Health Education* 4(1):29–35.

Bloom, B.S. (Ed.). 1956. Taxonomy of educational objectives: the classification of educational goals. Handbook I: Cognitive domain. New York: David McKay Co.

Leventhal, H. 1971. Fear appeals and persuasion: the differentiation of a motivational construct. *American Journal of Public Health* 6:1208–1224.

Rudd, P. 1995. Clinicians and patients with hypertension: unsettled issues about compliance. *American Heart Journal* 130:572–579.

Life Stages and Patient Teaching: 5

A Developmental Perspective

DEVELOPMENT AS A LIFELONG PROCESS

There has been considerable study of the development of children but, until recently, little realization that development is a continuing process reaching through adulthood as well. A concept of development is integral to understanding patients and, subsequently, to understanding how to conduct patient education effectively. The patient, rather than the disease, should be the focus of attention in patient education. Knowledge of development is therefore fundamental to effective patient education. Such knowledge enables health professionals to use special strategies appropriate to the individual, rather than conducting all patient teaching the same way regardless of the patient's age.

Each stage of life has its own particular stress or problems apart from those that may be experienced because of illness. When people become ill, they experience additional stress. Patients' reaction to illness and the type of stress experienced may vary according to their developmental stage. Children obviously differ from adults—not only physiologically but in their reactions to illness. The proper approach to patients differs at particular phases of development. Information needs may also differ at various developmental phases. Patients may react to illness in different ways at various life stages. Thus, the approach to patient education cannot be the same for patients who are at different stages of development, though their conditions may be similar. Teaching a child with cancer is certainly different from teaching an adult with cancer. In most instances, not only will language ability differ but also the ability to understand concepts surrounding the condition and its treatment. The person who has had a myocardial infarction at 40 will require a different educational approach than a patient who has a myocardial infarction at 80.

Life style, responsibilities, and attitude can often be different at middle age than at older age. These contrasts affect not only patients' reactions to their condition but also their reactions to and motivation for carrying out recommendations.

The approach to teaching patients about prevention or providing them with information about potential problems they may encounter also varies among different age groups. Prevention teaching for a toddler, for instance, may involve talking with the parents about child safety, whereas prevention teaching for adults may range from awareness of health risk factors to stress reduction. An understanding of the developmental process helps health professionals to recognize specific patient needs at various life stages, enabling them to give support in accord with particular needs. Using a developmental approach to patient education can help health professionals:

- understand and anticipate patients' reactions to illness
- alter the approach to patient education in accord with individual needs
- identify aspects of patient education that maybe associated with a particular life phase, in addition to education about specific disease entities

Because all aspects of development are related, each life stage must be understood within the context of the patient's past experience and social support system. Development is a continuing process without clear lines of demarcation between varying life stages. For purposes of discussion in this chapter, the life stages will be delimited by category; however, phases of development for each individual, of course, are not separated nearly so clearly.

THE PRENATAL PERIOD

One of the most important phases of an individual's life occurs before birth. Much of what happens *in utero* affects the remainder of the individual's life. During the embryonic period, the individual is vulnerable to many potential hazards that influence development and health potential not only *in utero* but also over a lifetime. Because growth and development of the fetus are so dependent on the mother's health and well-being, the prenatal period is an extremely crucial time. Although health professionals obviously cannot deal with the fetus directly, effective education of the prenatal patient holds paramount importance for the well-being of the fetus. Health professionals must be aware not only of patient education, which is crucial to this life stage, but also of parents' reactions to pregnancy.

Pregnancy, even if planned and wanted, can be stressful. A variety of physical and emotional changes are part of pregnancy. In addition, there is the knowledge of the probability of a considerable change in life style that will likely result after birth of the child. Health professionals should be aware of pregnancy as a source of stress and should be able to identify factors in patients' life situations that may cause additional stress, subsequently giving information and support as needs dictate.

Most parents have some ambivalence toward pregnancy and parenthood during the prenatal period, no matter how much the pregnancy is desired. Having total responsibility for another human being may seem awesome. The realization that parenthood means giving up certain freedoms and fantasies may also cause some reflection. Although such ambivalence is natural and normal and is usually resolved, not all expectant parents recognize it as a normal phenomenon. Consequently, such feelings may cause them considerable guilt. Health professionals can relieve stress by helping parents express their feelings about the pregnancy and by reassuring the couple that such feelings are common. Additional reassurance can be given by helping them prepare for their role as parents. Much can be accomplished with patient education. Prospective parents can be taught about issues such as aspects of infant care. If there are other children, the process may involve teaching parents how to tell siblings about pregnancy and birth.

Stress may also be generated from the unknowns in pregnancy. Expectant parents vary in their sophistication and knowledge about pregnancy, labor, and delivery. Health professionals can do much to alleviate stress by teaching prospective parents about the emotional and physical changes to be expected during pregnancy and about what to expect during labor, delivery, and the postpartum period. Although health professionals may have more contact with the prenatal patient herself, the impact of other people in her life should not be underestimated. Including the expectant father promotes a feeling of inclusion for him in the prenatal and birthing process and can do much to reduce stress between the couple if there is a common understanding of changes to be experienced and what to expect. Not all prenatal patients have a partner supporting them through pregnancy. In such instances, health professionals must be aware of the additional stress this may cause and its impact on the patient's health behavior, as well as other potential sources of social support that may help the patient in carrying out the recommendations made in patient teaching.

Health professionals' approach to prenatal patients and significant people in their lives should be open-minded, with no preconceptions. Health professionals should be aware of parental attitudes about pregnancy and be alert to potential adjustment problems. When developing a teaching plan, health professionals should also be aware of patients' current life situation, knowledge level, misinformation, and any other barriers to effective education.

Common educational content areas for most patients in this life phase are the normal changes associated with pregnancy, both emotional and physical; sexual activity during pregnancy; preparation for the newborn; diet counseling; preparation for parenting; and what to expect during labor, delivery, and postpartum. As with all patient education, more than content must be considered.

Especially in this life phase, patient education may include a high degree of emotional support and awareness of barriers that interfere with compliance with recommendations that are crucial not only to the patient's own health but also to the growth and future development of her infant.

TEACHING PARENTS

Children should be included as much as appropriate for their age level in the teaching process when they are the patients. However, the fact remains that in most instances it will be the child's parents who will be supervising the degree to which the treatment regimen or recommendations for prevention related to their child's care are followed. The health professional's ability to work effectively with parents is crucial to the effectiveness of the patient education interaction.

Health professionals conducting patient teaching must establish rapport not only with the child as the patient but with the parents as well. Not only must the child's learning readiness be assessed, so must the parents'.

In preparation for patient teaching, the health professional should assess the quality of relationship between parent and child and take it into account in the teaching process. Although some parents are open and honest with their children, and foster independence, others do not. Some parents provide structure and guidance while allowing their children the latitude to make some choices of their own, whereas other parents are rigid and controlling, allowing their children little freedom of thought or expression. In other instances, parents provide little structure or guidance, enforcing no rules and essentially abandoning the child emotionally. The approach to patient education the health professional takes in each of these instances will differ. Child-rearing practices can be a source of conflict and controversy. Rather than being critical, health professionals should use the relationship between the child and parent to its maximum advantage for patient teaching to be most effective.

In addition to the parent/child relationship, the degree of parent involvement in patient teaching will depend not only on the cognitive ability and learning readiness of the child but also the ability of the parents to grasp the concepts. This ability can be hampered by parents' limited intellectual ability, their own degree of emotional maturity and responsibility, and, in some instances, their level of anxiety. Some parents, although concerned and well meaning, may have difficulty understanding information presented or directives that are to be carried out. In this instance, health professionals should alter the approach to patient teaching to meet the parents' as well as the child's level of ability to understand. Health professionals should also be sensitive to the parents' perception of the child's condition and deal with their concerns and anxiety as much as possible.

TEACHING CHILDREN

When conducting patient education with children, the parent or caregiver is the recipient of patient education information as well. Health professionals should keep in mind, however, that under these circumstances, the patient is still the child. Consequently, health professionals should direct patient education to the child in an age-appropriate manner.

When first initiating patient teaching with the child, health professionals should introduce themselves to the child as well as to the parents or caregiver. To place the child at ease and to build rapport, health professionals should engage in friendly conversation about topics of interest to the child. When talking with children, health professionals should make an effort to speak with them at eye level. Children should be allowed the opportunity to express their concerns, as well as to ask questions.

Because health recommendations given to a child necessitates involvement and cooperation of a caregiver, health professionals should, as much as possible, present information in such a way as to establish a "team effort" involving parent or caregiver, child, and health professional. Having an understanding of development of children at different ages and what generally can be expected behaviorally and cognitively at each stage will assist the health professional to tailor patient teaching to best meet the individual child's patient education needs.

INFANCY

It may be difficult for health professionals to consider infancy significant when talking about patient education from a developmental perspective. It is hard to imagine a health professional teaching an infant about care. The infant, of course, does have a parent to whom considerable information about the infant's health and care may be given. Patient education for infancy may involve little time spent teaching about illness but considerable time spent teaching aspects of prevention. In addition to helping parents learn what they should expect from their infant in the first year of life, such preventive teaching as infant safety and the importance of immunization is an important part of patient education.

Infancy is a time of rapid growth and development. Many normal aspects of infant development may be misinterpreted by new parents as a deviation from the norm. Parents with little experience in child care may also experience considerable insecurity in caring for their infant. Much of this can be alleviated by informing them of what to expect.

Infant development, although occurring at a rapid rate, does not occur at the same rate for all infants. Unless new parents are aware of this, they may experience considerable anxiety when comparing their infant to others who may be developing more quickly. Teaching parents about normal infant development, as well as the range of individual differences, can relieve unnecessary anxiety and increase parents' enjoyment in watching their infant reach various milestones.

As the infant develops more physical skills, the importance of exploration of self and the environment becomes paramount in stimulating further infant development. Patient education may also involve increasing the parents' awareness of the importance of stimulation for their infant. Parents may be taught means of providing such stimulation at home, such as holding and talking to the infant or hanging colorful mobiles above the crib.

Infants' psychosocial development consists of building a basic trust that their needs will be met. Parents should be helped to understand the importance of consistency in meeting their infant's needs but also to realize that the infant can gradually be helped to adjust to the parents' schedule as well.

Again, if patient education is to be effective, health professionals must consider affective as well as cognitive and psychomotor aspects of patient teaching. Parents' strain has an impact on the health and well-being of the infant as well. Health professionals who are alert to clues indicating potential or actual problems can do much to alleviate strain by providing information to help prevent problems from occurring. In other instances, health professionals can work with parents to find alternative solutions to problems that already exist. Health professionals may need to stress the importance of the couple still finding time for themselves alone and time to give other children individual attention as well. In the same vein, talking with both parents can be an opportunity to emphasize the need for the new mother to have some time alone away from the baby. Strain can be ameliorated if health professionals reassure the parents that it is normal to have feelings of frustration in caring for a newborn.

Being aware of the insecurity of new parents, sibling rivalry, and other sources of parental stress helps health professionals adapt an approach based on patients' individual needs. Supplemental information can be given as needed to alleviate stress and enhance the parents' ability to carry out recommendations.

THE TODDLER

Development proceeds rapidly in the toddler phase of development as well as in infancy. Consequently, health professionals have numerous topics of patient information that can be shared with parents. Information can be given during any contact with the parents and child. Patient education need not only be illness-related.

During the toddler stage, children rapidly acquire language skills. Health professionals can help parents foster this aspect of development by encouraging them to talk with their child, as well as listen.

The toddler stage is also a time of increased autonomy. At this stage, toddlers recognize themselves as individuals different from their mothers. Their newfound independence may be asserted through negativism, frequently referred to as the "no" stage. Children in this stage may have difficulty making up their minds and may be prone to temper tantrums. Such behavior can be a source of irritation for parents, especially if they fail to realize that such behavior is common to children in this age group. Health professionals can teach parents about normal development, helping them learn what behavior to expect as well as teaching them what steps to take to handle their toddler's behavior. Appropriate, consistent techniques of discipline and limit setting, without being overly restrictive, are important aspects of patient education in this phase.

Another important area involves child safety. The toddler has become more mobile, as well as more curious and interested in exploring the environment. Parents may be unaware of safety hazards and may need help in learning ways to child-proof their home.

The toddler stage is also characterized by toilet training. Toilet training is commonly an emotional process in which parents place considerable pressure on themselves and their child to perform. By teaching various ways to implement toilet training and by emphasizing individual rates of development, parents may be helped to accomplish the task with considerably less stress for themselves and their child.

Although most patient education will still be provided to parents, children in the toddler stage are capable of some degree of understanding of procedures they may experience. Health professionals should establish rapport with the child through simple patient teaching that can also enhance cooperation from the child. The health professional's approach to the child should be warm and matter-of-fact. Although children this age are able to comprehend at least 400 words, they are still unable to reason. Many things are taken literally. Therefore, when giving explanations to children in the toddler stage, health professionals should avoid analogies and give the explanation in accurate, simple terms.

PRESCHOOL

Preschool children continue to develop their own identities and to expand their world through involvement with others outside the family unit. In previous stages, although the child might have played alongside another child, there was little actual interaction between the two. In the preschool period, children actually begin to interact with others in cooperative play. The preschool child also engages in imaginary play and may develop imaginary playmates.

Health professionals' interaction with preschool children and their families may be sporadic, occurring only when there are medical problems. As well as teaching parents about their child's condition, illness, or medical recommendations, health professionals may use this interaction to incorporate health promotion, reassurance, and guidance.

Children in the preschool stage begin to develop a sexual identity. As part of the development of gender identity, the preschooler becomes aware of differences in the opposite sex and has increased sexual curiosity. Such interest and subsequent questioning may bring about considerable anxiety in parents who do not know how to respond to their child's questions or who question whether their child's sexual curiosity or even masturbation is normal. Health professionals, although perhaps not directly involved in the sex education of the preschool child, can facilitate the parents' role in this matter by teaching them about normal developmental processes at this stage, by reassuring them, and by teaching them ways to respond to their child's questions. Parents should be reassured that sexual curiosity is normal. They should be helped to provide simple, straightforward responses in a relaxed manner.

In recognizing approaches to children at this age, health professionals facilitate communication between parent and child as well as their own relationship with the children. Children have a vocabulary of approximately 2,000 to 2,500 words by the time they are 5 years old. Teaching children about procedures to be performed should, therefore, become a routine part of the interaction with children as patients. The preschool child, although having developed a fairly extensive vocabulary, may not be able to recognize someone else's point of view. Reasoning with children at this age by explaining the purpose of a procedure and why it is important is therefore probably of no avail. Explanations should be kept simple and matter-of-fact. Preschool children fantasize and are quite vulnerable to fear of pain and bodily harm. It is therefore important for the health professional to help children to express their fears and to deal with them openly.

LATER CHILDHOOD

A great change comes about when a child goes to school. Although there has been a gradual expansion of their world since birth, children at this stage begin to establish their self-concepts as members of a world larger than their own family. School facilitates children's sense of responsibility and reliability. The experience also helps them form their own values, comparing family values to those of the outside world. The child enlarges the extent of intimacy beyond family to include a special friend, forming special groups, cliques, or clubs.

Although children in later childhood may still engage in some magical thinking, they are capable of concrete logical reasoning. The child may experience a need for some ritualistic behavior. Throughout this phase of development, children decrease their dependence on family, becoming more social beings by learning how to handle strong feelings and impulses appropriately.

Including children in the patient education process, especially about procedures, becomes even more important as they increase their ability to comprehend. Health professionals should explain procedures, as well as the reasons for them, in a simple, logical way and with confidence and optimism.

Health professionals still, of course, will spend considerable time teaching parents. In addition to teaching them about the child's illness and treatment plan, parents may also be encouraged to foster the child's independence and to praise his or her accomplishments. Specific problems arising during this phase of development that may come to the health professional's attention are behavior disorders, hyperactivity, learning disorders, and enuresis. Any of these problems may cause stress for the child as well as the family and may require extensive teaching to enhance both the parents' and child's understanding of the condition and the methods to be used in dealing with it.

In all stages of childhood, when patient education is done because of illness, it is important to keep the child's developmental stage in mind and to encourage parents to foster the child's normal development despite limitations that may be imposed by illness.

Health professionals are increasingly able to establish a one-to-one relationship with patients in later childhood. At this stage, children are able to report symptoms fairly accurately. They are capable of reasoning and are more autonomous than at previous stages and are emerging as more distinct individual personalities.

ADOLESCENCE

Adolescence is a stage marking transition from childhood to adulthood. Adolescents are capable of abstract thought and logical reasoning; therefore, they are capable of understanding and general comprehension of explanations given as part of patient teaching. Although health professionals must still include the family in education, adolescents themselves are a major focus of teaching because they have considerable independence and are, consequently, in more control of the degree to which recommendations will be carried out.

Understanding characteristics of the adolescent phase of development is crucial if patient education is to be effective with this group. Although considerations of the family and solicitation of its support of the patient in following recommendations is always important, facilitating the relationship between the adolescent and the family in following recommendations is perhaps more important than at any other time.

Adolescence is a time of marked change. Adolescents are in the process of forming their own identity, emancipating themselves from parents, and adapting to a rapidly changing body. As part of the need to establish themselves as independent individuals, adolescents may rebel against authority and become disillusioned with parents or other authority figures. Bodily changes may bring about a strong preoccupation with body and appearance. Sexual adjustment and a strong desire to express sexual urges become paramount.

Educational needs of the adolescent are wide and varied. Whether or not health professionals see adolescent patients because of illness or injury, an understanding of adolescents themselves is crucial to effective patient education. Adolescents have difficulty imagining that they can become sick or injured. This alone may contribute to accidents because of risk taking or poor compliance in following medical recommendations if disease is present. Because of adolescents' strong preoccupation with body and appearance and their strong need for peer acceptance and support, health recommendations that they view as interfering with their concept of themselves as independent beings may be less likely to be followed. In their need to establish themselves as independent beings, adolescents may rebel against following recommendations that they consider authoritarian. The consequence of noncompliance is, of course, a function of the seriousness of the disease or condition for which the patient is being treated. In any instance, health professionals who are concerned about effective patient education would do well to consider these points.

Numerous other areas are potential topics of patient education during adolescence. Because this phase of development is marked by sexual adjustment and strong sexual urges, health professionals' one focus of patient education will probably be about sexual issues and contraception. Adolescents develop at different rates. Health professionals may need to reassure those teens who mature either "too late" or "too early" in comparison with their peers. Patient education may also involve dispelling misconceptions adolescents may have about sexual development or sexual behavior. Teaching them about sexuality requires a special sensitivity and understanding. Regard for the adolescent's modesty and privacy is important in providing an atmosphere of openness and trust so these issues can be addressed.

Other important areas for patient education at this stage are alcohol and drug use and abuse as well as general health and safety measures. No matter what the topic, the likelihood that patient education will be effective is higher if health professionals establish trust by respecting adolescents' needs and showing empathetic understanding. Patient education should take the form of guidance, not lecturing. Adolescents should be treated neither as adults nor children; the approach should be modified according to the individual reaction. Health professionals who want to gain credibility with an adolescent must establish themselves as advocates of the adolescent rather than representatives of the parents.

Although much patient education is done directly with the adolescent, health professionals may enhance teaching effectiveness by considering the family as well. Health professionals may give guidance and support to family members, enabling them to understand adolescent behavior. Parents should be encouraged to set realistic limits for adolescents while at the same time fostering their independence. Adjustment to an adolescent's gradual independence may be difficult for parents, who must now also begin to redefine their role as parents. Patient education of adolescents can be enhanced if health professionals can identify potential sources of stress in the family and support parents in their own readjustment. Because of the ambivalence of the stage between childhood and adulthood, health professionals should be aware of the importance of considering both adolescents and their parents when conducting patient education.

YOUNG ADULTHOOD

For many individuals, young adulthood is a time for forming a long-term intimate relationship with another individual and subsequently learning to adjust life styles to live with that person. For many, this period may involve establishing and managing a home, becoming established in an occupation, and beginning a family. All these changes, though probably happy events, can also be a source of stress. Knowledge of patients' individual life changes can help health professionals conduct patient education. Identification of particular aspects of change may, for instance, be a cue for specific aspects of patient education. If an individual is planning marriage, some teaching about contraception or marital adjustment may be needed. If the patient becomes pregnant, obviously, prenatal teaching, newborn care, and numerous other topics related to child care need to be covered during the next years of interaction.

Identifying the specific significant persons in the patient's life can help the professional determine sources of support for the individual in carrying out treatment recommendations as well as determining sources of stress that may influence how well the patient carries out recommendations. Health professionals should refrain from making assumptions. Questions about patients' significant others should be approached in a direct, neutral, and sensitive way. Not all patients live in a traditional family setting. Data suggest that 4% to 9% of the population is primarily homosexual (Harrison and Silenzio 1996). Although homosexuality is becoming more visible, many individuals are still reluctant to identify themselves as such because of fear of discrimination or, in some instances, fear of physical or emotional abuse (Greco and Glusman 1998). Consequently, patients may not always be forthcoming about sexual preferences. Making assumptions about individuals' life style or sexual preference without checking with patients themselves not only serves to alienate patients but also can cause missed patient education opportunities. Just as patient education about sexual practices or sexual problems is important with heterosexual patients, the same is true of homosexual patients. Although sexual issues should be addressed, as with all patients, patients who are homosexual also have the same need for patient education information in other aspects of their lives as do individuals who are heterosexual. Homosexual patients may also be parents. They may have job-related stress or have the need for the same type of prevention or disease management information as heterosexual patients. Discussing issues of sexual orientation openly helps health professionals build rapport and trust with patients. As with all patients, frank and open discussion helps health professionals determine patient education needs. Patients who trust the health professional are more likely to follow recommendations given (Greco and Glusman 1998).

Knowledge of all aspects of an individual's life helps professionals determine patient responsibility and potential barriers to carrying out treatment recommendations. Financial constraints, family responsibility, and work schedule may all be common factors in this stage that can influence the individual's ability to comply with a treatment regimen.

Health promotion issues, although often neglected, may be especially important to address at this life stage. Stress may contribute to further illness, and much of the individual's future health may be determined by health practices established now. Helping patients learn to cope with stress, talking with them about health risk factors, and helping them establish good health practices may all be important in preventing many of the health problems that may otherwise occur in the future.

MIDLIFE

Just as adolescence is the link between childhood and adulthood, so is midlife the transition period between young adulthood and the later years. During these years, many individuals have reached the peak in their career. They may also begin to reexamine and question former goals and values as well as their perceived degree of achievement. During this personal assessment, people may begin to modify aspects of their lives that they consider unsatisfactory. They may begin to adopt a new life structure that is perceived as a solution to many dissatisfactions they may be experiencing.

Persons in the midlife phase of development, if in a family group, may find themselves reappraising not only their marital relationship but that with their children as well. As their offspring begin to leave home and establish their own families, parents also need to adjust their roles. At the same time, people in midlife may grow increasingly responsible for their own parents, whose health may be failing. Recognizing their own physical changes, their parents' declining health, and their own goals and values, middle-aged people may become especially aware of their own mortality. This realization may either motivate the individual to follow recommendations more closely or, if the prospect of mortality is especially threatening, to deny illness or abandon health promotion and prevention practices.

Depending on the individual's situation, there may be many areas of stress and a variety of reactions that can contribute to illness behavior as well as acting as barriers to effective patient education. Health professionals should be aware of potential problems and approach patients with a nonjudgmental attitude. In addition to teaching about specific medical recommendations, teaching may also involve health risk factors, stress reduction, and identification of misconceptions or misinformation that may be present. Misconceptions regarding physical changes such as menopause and other changes may be especially prominent. Helping persons in midlife cope with stress can do much to enhance education and to enable patients to live happier, more productive lives as well.

THE LATER YEARS

Patient education for older patients may be viewed by some as a futile task. Chronic diseases become more apparent in the later years for many people, so much patient education may revolve around illness and disease with aspects of prevention being neglected. Patient education of the older patient may, for some health professionals, seem more of a formality than of actual benefit to the patient. Health professionals' attitudes as well as inadequate understanding of later life stages may well be the greatest barriers to effective patient education for this group. Working with older patients may elicit fears in health professionals of their own aging and death; therefore, interaction with older patients may be avoided. Health professionals may believe myths about aging and approach older adults with those stereotypes rather than approaching them as individuals. Patient education with older patients can, however, be of great benefit to the patient and rewarding to the health professional as well.

Older patients may experience various degrees of loss and therefore may have considerable anxiety. There may be the loss of spouse or friends or the loss of physical capability. Depending on the degree of loss, there may also be decreased independence, with resulting loss of self-esteem and self-satisfaction.

Health professionals conducting patient education should approach each patient without stereotypes. As in all other life stages, not all changes of aging occur at the same rate, and not everyone in the same age group has the same experience or life circumstances. Aging should be viewed as a multidimensional process in which the individual's function and health status are related to multiple factors. When conducting patient education, the health professionals should treat older adults as individuals and with the same interest and respect as any other patients with whom patient education is being conducted. For instance, health professionals should not use first names in teaching interactions unless invited to do so. Patient education with older people should be conducted with the same conviction with which it would be delivered to patients at any other age.

When communicating patient education information, health professionals should position themselves close to the older person and speak clearly and concisely, remembering that raising the loudness of the voice does not necessarily contribute to the listener's better hearing. Patient education should be realistic but hopeful. Pat phrases, such as, "What do you expect at your age?" or "You'll live to be 100," are inappropriate and should be avoided.

Patient education need not be confined to illness with older individuals any more than it is with younger patients. Patient education issues to be addressed in addition to those that deal with specific disease entities or treatment recommendations might include sexuality, exercise, nutrition, and a variety of other topics that are oriented toward prevention and enhance the quality of life.

Barriers to independence should be assessed to help the patient find ways to maximize strengths and independence. Older patients should be helped to learn how to make optimum use of their skills and functions. Because of problems that may exist in this life phase, health professionals should be especially aware of compliance problems due to misunderstanding, physical limitations, or financial barriers. Health professionals may be able to enhance patients' ability to follow medical recommendations by providing information, considering patients' individual needs, and building an awareness of community services and resources that can help them follow recommendations given.

A LIFE-CYCLE–CENTERED APPROACH

Conceptually, a developmental approach to patient education helps health professionals consider patients in the context of the biologic, psychologic, and social environment and the interaction of these areas at a particular point in an individual's life. Throughout life, people experience events that lead to a variety of changes. These changes influence the individual's attitudes, perceptions, actions, and behaviors. Although developmental changes may be more apparent in childhood, such changes occur in adulthood as well. Knowledge of changes that can occur at various life stages can enhance health professionals' ability to teach effectively, as well as helping them identify topics of education that may be presented to patients, along with specific recommendations about patients' diseases or conditions. Opportunities for patient teaching exist whether or not illness or injury does. Examples of health-related topics that may be covered at various life stages are illustrated in Table 5-1. The list, although not all-inclusive, points out a variety of topics that may be discussed whether or not the patient is seeking advice for a health problem.

During early phases of the life cycle, most patient teaching is conducted with parents rather than children themselves. As the individual moves through the life cycle, more interaction obviously will occur directly between the patient and the health professional. Although health professionals should always approach each patient as an individual, a knowledge of general human characteristics at various stages of development can be helpful. Table 5-2 offers suggested approaches for use with patients at various stages of development to make the teaching interaction more effective.

TABLE 5-1	Potential Patient Education Information During the Life Cycle
Prenatal	Normal changes associated with pregnancy, both emotional and physical; sexual activity during pregnancy; preparation for the newborn; diet counseling; preparation for the role of parenting; process and procedures during labor, delivery, and postpartum
Infancy	Normal infant development, individual differences, immunizations, infant stimulation, infant feeding, safety issues, teething, family interactions
Toddler	Child development, safety, toilet training, discipline and setting limits, nutrition
Preschool	Importance and role of play, dealing with sexual curiosity and questions, general health practices, school adjustment, sleep problems
Later childhood	Importance of fostering independence and praising accomplishments, sex education, general health practices
Adolescence	Normal development patterns and individual differences, emotional and physical; sex education; skin problems; nutrition and other health practices; safety; drug and alcohol use
Young adult	Stress reduction; health maintenance and promotion; for some individuals, marital adjustment, prenatal teaching, child-rearing practices
Midlife	Physical changes, such as menopause; health risk factors; changes in family relationships; stress reduction and health promotion
Later years	Adjustment to retirement, nutrition and exercise, adaptation to loss, modification of environment to promote independence as necessary, sexuality

TABLE 5-2	The Health Professional's Approach to the Patient for Teaching During Various Phases of the Life Cycle

Life State		Approach of Health Professional
Prenatal	Parents:	Use an open-minded approach with no preconceptions; nonjudgmental; give emotional support to both parents; work within parents' framework.
Infancy	Parents:	Foster security by giving positive feedback regarding parents' ability to care for child; no nagging or lecturing; take what may appear to be small problems seriously.
Toddler	Patient:	Encourage child in warm, matter-of-fact manner; use no analogies when giving explanations; give explanations in accurate, simple terms.
	Parents:	Use a nonjudgmental approach; continue support and positive reinforcement.
Preschool	Patient:	Encourage child to express fear; give no false promises; explain procedures before doing them.
	Parents:	Provide guidance and encouragement.
Later Childhood	Patient:	Give explanations in simple, logical way; approach child in confident, optimistic manner.
	Parents:	Give continued guidance and support.
Adolescence	Patient:	Treat neither as adult nor child, but rather modify approach depending on expectations and reactions; demonstrate empathetic understanding and respect; show regard for modesty and privacy; Identify and dispell misconceptions; provide guidance regarding sexual issues as appropriate.
	Parents:	Provide guidance and support to help parents understand adolescent behavior; encourage parents to set realistic limits; support parents in their own readjustment.
Young Adult	Patient:	Use an empathetic, nonjudgmental attitude.
Middle Age	Patient:	Use an empathetic, nonjudgmental attitude.
Later Years	Patient:	Approach patient as unique, not stereotyping because of age; keep awareness that aging is a multidimensional process in which multiple factors affect functioning; capitalize on patients' strengths; refrain from using first names unless invited to do so; speak clearly and concisely; avoid patronizing.

REFERENCES

Greco, J.A., Glusman, J.B. 1998. Providing effective care for gay and lesbian patients. *Patient Care* 32(12):159–162,167–168,170.

Harrison, A.E., Silenzio, V.M.B. 1996. Comprehensive care of lesbian and gay patients and families. *Primary Care* 23:31–46.

The Family in Patient Education and Patient Compliance

6

ROLE OF THE FAMILY

Education of the patient about health, life style, and health care begins at home with the family (Lipkin 1996). Many of the health practices and health beliefs patients hold stem from what they have been told, have experienced, or have observed as part of their family system. It should be obvious then, that the family has considerable influence on patients health practices and, consequently, should be an important aspect of effective patient education in health care settings.

As patients' primary support system, families often affect patients' decision making about health and health care. Families often help patients make decisions about how and when to enter the health care system, whether entry involves emergency care, seeking care for acute or chronic disease, or for general health maintenance (Reust and Mattingly 1996). Families may also influence the extent to which patients follow recommendations, from influencing whether or not patients take their medication, follow the prescribed diet, or have recommended diagnostic tests or surgical procedures to determining end-of-life decisions or nursing home placement (Jecker 1990). Understanding how families contribute to patients' ability or willingness to follow recommendations given by health professionals can be a valuable asset in conducting patient education.

Although consideration of the individual is important in patient education, the patient's family is also of central importance if teaching is to be effective. For the individual patient, the family constitutes the social context in which illness occurs. Illness and treatment affect the family as well as the patient. It alters the context of daily living and utilizes additional time and energy of family members. Illness and treatment of patients can disrupt employment or school patterns of family members and cause financial hardships. In addition, illness and treatment can enhance or threaten family relationships or alter roles its members play (Reust and Mattingly 1996). Likewise, the family unit contributes to the health and health behavior of the patient. The happiness and health of each individual depends, to a significant degree, on the nature of his or her interaction with other members in the family unit. How a family functions influences the health of its members as well as how an individual reacts to illness. Teaching the patient without considering the family may result in less-than-adequate compliance with recommendations. Health professionals' ability to teach the patient how to maintain or restore health depends on their insight into the patient's relationship with family members. Health professionals should capitalize on how family members can help the patient, assisting them to encourage the patient and help them with things that may be difficult. The family should be helped to feel a part of the teaching plan. What good does it do to teach a middle-aged man about his diet if his wife does all the cooking and is excluded from the teaching? Likewise, it may be difficult for a husband to be supportive of his wife's blood pressure treatment program if he does not understand the reasons for the recommendations and the consequences of not carrying them out.

Just as it is important to consider the influence of family members and to include them in patient education, it is also important to remember that not all families can meet expectations of health professionals. Not all patients receive the support and encouragement needed from their families. Not all families have the emotional stability to cope with long-term illness. If the relationship between family members was not stable before the patient's illness, or if the relationship was strained, the additional stress of illness may cause even more problems. In other instances, family members may have conflicting obligations. They may have roles and obligations to fill in addition to their roles within the patient's family unit, and some roles and obligations may conflict with the patient's needs. For example, children of an older patient may have families of their own. Although they may feel concern and responsibility for their aging parent, the health professional cannot realistically expect that they will sacrifice their own family to help their aging parent carry out the recommendations given.

Long-term illness, even in the most stable of family units, is bound to bring about changes in family relationships. Illness itself changes patients' role within the family. Such change naturally produces some disequilibrium within the family structure until adjustment occurs. For instance, if the head of the household and chief breadwinner has been the husband, a disabling illness that prevents him from working may change his role in the family. His wife may have to assume the role of chief breadwinner while he assumes the role of a dependent. If the health professional does not recognize this change, what the change might mean to the patient and family, and how it might affect the patient's willingness and ability to carry out the recommendations, the effectiveness of patient education may be diminished.

When teaching the patient and family, it is important for health professionals to identify patterns of relationships and to be alert to attitudes of family members. Health professionals may also be able to identify resources within the family group and help family members mobilize their resources to help the patient.

When gaining support from family members that facilitates the patient's ability to follow recommendations, health professionals must also remember that family members are just that—family members—and not health professionals. The purpose of involving families in patient teaching is to gain their support by helping them to be better informed, not to prepare them as spies to monitor the patient in the health professional's absence.

When conducting patient teaching with family members it is important for health professionals to be alert to some of the same barriers in family members that act as a barriers to effective patient education with individual patients. Illness in a family member tends to raise the anxiety of all those close to the patient. Anxiety may be misinterpreted by the health professional as lack of interest or as reluctance on the part of the family member to provide the patient with help and support. The more health professionals can be aware of these reactions and help family members deal with their feelings, the better able the health professional will be to teach family members about the patient's condition and treatment and to mobilize their support.

While it is important to understand how devastating illness can be to a patient, it is also important to understand that illness causes a strain on the family as well. If the family is already under stress, illness will most probably subject both patient and family to additional emotional pressures. Information about the family function, stress, transition, and expectations can be invaluable in developing a teaching plan that will be most effective for patient and family alike. Although health professionals focus attention on the patient, an increasing awareness of the impact of the family on interactions and management of the patient's condition is also needed.

FAMILY STRUCTURE AND STYLE

Commonly, most health professionals think of family in terms of the nuclear family—a group in which there are parents and children—or in terms of the extended family—which includes parents, children, grandparents, aunts, uncles, and the like. Although these two family groups are traditional, a modern interpretation may be useful to health professionals when determining who is the most influential in the patient's life. Expanding the definition of *family* may be important when developing a teaching plan rather than narrowly viewing the family only in the traditional manner. People's emotional effects on one another need not be limited to blood relations. If perceived this way, a family might include two people living together with or without sexual attachment, single-parent families, remarried families with children and/or stepchildren, and a host of other family forms.

The family is the social network from which the patient derives some of his or her identity, with which the patient has strong psychologic bonds, and in which each individual has a specific role. The family influences health behavior through interactions and reactions, through past experiences and attitudes, and through the family's relationship to the community in which its members live. For example, an individual whose family is in a socially isolated, rural area will probably hold different attitudes and perform different practices of health and illness behavior than individuals whose families live in a suburban metropolitan area. The child whose father is a physician will probably have different reactions and attitudes toward health and health care than the child whose father is a farmer.

Not all families function the same way, nor do all families have the same structure or style. As each individual in the family unit goes through his or her own stages of development, the structure, composition, and role of the family change. Just as illness may have a different impact on individuals at different phases of development, so it has a different impact on families at different stages. Awareness of this changing impact helps health professionals approach patient education more appropriately. Health professionals can gain this type of information by talking with the patient and through observing family interactions. Who does the patient talk about most? What is the patient's reaction when talking about the family and individuals in it? Who comes to visit the patient in the hospital? Who accompanies the patient in an outpatient setting? What is the interaction between the patient and individual family members like? What sources of stress were family members experiencing prior to illness as a result of their stage of development? Are there children in college causing additional financial burden? If the family is a young, newly married couple, are the patient and spouse struggling to adjust to their new roles within the marriage?

Illness during the early stages of married life, for example, may cause additional strain because of economic considerations, interruptions in career development, and/or the marital adjustment process itself. If the patient is a young child, there may be additional strain to the family if there are other children whose needs also must be met. Illness in the middle stage of family life, when adolescents may be attempting to emancipate themselves from family ties, while at the same time their parents are experiencing their own midlife transitions, may place further strain on what already is a tumultuous time for the family. Illness in either parent or child may interfere with the mutual weaning process that should be occurring at this stage. Illness in later age may have an impact not only on grown children but may occur when the older couple had anticipated a time of enjoyment together and are less able to care for each other because of their own physical limitations that may be associated with aging.

When patient education, especially regarding illness, is conducted, health professionals will be more effective if they are able to identify the family's predominant lifestyle and find ways to sustain and incorporate recommendations into it rather than trying to impose a different pattern. For instance, some families exhibit a high degree of structure, while others exhibit little structure, appearing to be in a constant state of chaos. If aware of the system by which the family operates, health professionals can work within the system rather than trying to fight it. Again, the most effective patient education is that which fits into the patient's frame of reference and with which the patient feels most comfortable.

If health professionals can identify relationship patterns and attitudes within the family unit, such factors can be incorporated into the teaching plan. These factors can then at least be considered when estimating the patient's potential for following through with recommendations. An example of family influence is illustrated by the following case.

Mrs. Roberts was pregnant with her first child. She and her husband lived in the same small community in which they had grown up. Their extended family was quite large. Mrs. Roberts regularly attended prenatal classes offered at the local hospital. At one session, the topic was breast-feeding versus bottle feeding. The pros and cons of each were discussed. It appeared to Mrs. Roberts that there were obviously more benefits to the infant from breast-feeding than bottle feeding.

At her next prenatal visit, she discussed breast-feeding with her physician, and it was agreed that she would breast-feed her infant. After the birth of her baby, Mrs. Roberts had considerable difficulty breast-feeding. After two weeks, she visited her physician, stating that she would have to bottle feed instead. She was obviously upset, perceived herself as failing, and worried that the transition from breast to bottle would affect her infant. The nurse in the physician's office took time to talk with Mrs. Roberts about her feelings and discovered that Mrs. Roberts' mother and mother-in-law had both been quite opposed to her breast-feeding, feeling that in their day breast-feeding had been done out of necessity. They were anxious for their children to have it easier than they did and strongly encouraged the use of modern conveniences—in this case, premixed formula. In addition. Mr. Roberts also had concerns about breast-feeding and the effect it would have on his wife's figure. He also perceived it as imposing severe limitations on his wife's ability to be away from the baby for any length of time.

Mrs. Roberts had had little support or encouragement from family members in her efforts to breast-feed. Under the circumstances, even the best information about breast-feeding was bound to be less than effective in helping her attain her goal. The family's influence might have been identified earlier. Mr. Roberts might have been included in more of the patient teaching, which might have addressed many of his fears. The nurse, knowing the attitudes of the couple's mothers, might also have provided more individual support and suggestions to Mrs. Roberts. Not surprisingly, the family's attitudes and support, or lack of it, have a far greater impact on the degree to which patients follow health advice than mere information presented by a health professional. These influences must be considered if teaching is to be used effectively to help patients follow recommendations.

The family may also influence the individual's beliefs about the severity of various illnesses and the benefits and costs of treatment. If family members fail to realize why a certain medicine is ordered to treat a specific disease or fail to see the cure or effects they expected of treatment, their attitudes may be a direct barrier to patient compliance.

FAMILY AND ILLNESS

Illness disrupts the family. Each individual within a family—whether child or parent—plays a certain role that the family incorporates within its basic everyday function. When a family member becomes ill, other members must alter their life style and make some allowances for role changes for the individual who is ill, as well as changes in their own functioning. The illness of an individual within a family may cause all other members to experience some degree of strain, whether the illness is acute or chronic. A child who is ill with otitis media and is up most of the night, or who must stay home from school, requires parents and perhaps even other children to reorganize some of their regular activities. If a husband who is the breadwinner suffers a myocardial infarction, his wife may have to return to work to supplement, or bring in, income for the family. A grown child whose aging parent becomes chronically ill may need to alter daily living patterns to accommodate care of the parent.

The extent of disruption of a family, of course, is dependent to some extent on the seriousness of the illness. It is also dependent on the family's level of functioning before the illness, on socioeconomic considerations, on the emotional dependency of others, and on the extent to which the role of the person who is ill can be absorbed by other family members. In some instances, major illness brings a family closer together; in others, even a minor illness causes significant strain. When conducting patient education, health professionals should assess the impact of illness on the family because the group's reaction can have a significant influence on the patient's motivation to recover and cooperate with the treatment recommended. As mentioned previously, health professionals can gain this type of information by talking with, listening to, and observing the patient and family and then altering the teaching plan accordingly. Take, for example, the health professional teaching the wife of a patient with a recent amputation about stump care. The health professional may note the wife's reluctance to look at the stump or touch it. The professional may also notice the wife grimacing when procedures in stump care are discussed. At this point, an alteration in the teaching plan may be needed. The health professional may need to take time to talk privately to the wife about her feelings. If the wife's feelings cannot be altered, then the health professional may have to develop alternative methods to help the patient with stump care at home. In any case, the health professional should be aware that the wife's attitude can well affect the degree to which the patient is willing to follow recommendations.

In this context, it is important for health professionals to identify the meaning of the illness not only to the individual but also to the family. The family's perception of illness is often more important than the type of illness for which the patient is being treated. The following two cases illustrate this point.

Michael was a four-year-old boy with many allergies and asthma. Although Michael's mother brought him to the health clinic when he had asthma attacks and had received teaching about how to clear the home of many of the allergens thought to precipitate his attacks and about what to do to lessen their severity, Michael continued to have frequent attacks. During one visit, the physician began to question Michael's mother about the changes she had made in the home to help reduce allergens in the environment. Many of the recommendations had not been followed for a variety of reasons, none of which seemed substantial to the physician. Michael's mother concluded by saying: "Well, if I wasn't working, I'd have time to do all the things I need to do. Our child's health is suffering because my husband insists I supplement our income. I never wanted to work outside the home. Now we're seeing what the consequences are."

The physician gained some insight into the meaning of Michael's asthma attacks. The boy's attacks provided his mother with an excuse to stay home as well as leverage to quit her job. Although her feelings were no doubt unconscious, they appeared to be a strong contributing factor in Michael's continued illness through lack of compliance with the recommendations provided. Through identifying the meaning of Michael's illness to his mother, the physician was able to take a different approach to patient teaching and to begin to help Michael's parents start to discuss openly some of the issues that were interfering with their son's treatment.

In a second case, Mr. Arnett, a 65-year-old retired businessman with arteriosclerosis, had had a mild stroke with some residual paralysis. Both Mr. and Mrs. Arnett received extensive teaching about his care and rehabilitation, ways to prevent complications, and information about arteriosclerosis itself. Upon follow-up visits, the nurse noted that although Mr. Arnett appeared to be progressing well physically and his degree of compliance with recommendations appeared excellent, he seemed somewhat sad and withdrawn. Observation of the interaction between Mr. and Mrs. Arnett alerted the nurse to the possibility that their relationship had become somewhat strained. Further investigation indicated that Mrs. Arnett demanded that her husband comply rigidly with every recommendation and enforced many of them quite literally, until Mr. Arnett had very little freedom to live his life to its full potential. After talking with the couple in several consecutive visits, the nurse learned that Mrs. Arnett felt that Mr. Arnett's illness was a great threat to his life. She feared being left alone and became so frightened at the possibility that she had virtually made him a prisoner of health advice. After Mrs. Arnett's beliefs were revealed, the nurse was able to help her establish priorities in carrying out the teaching recommendations, demonstrating which were crucial and where there could be more flexibility.

In other instances, illness may place individuals in a family role that they prefer over the old role. For example, a patient who has craved dependence and attention in the family, rather than functioning in an independent role, may have less incentive to get well. On the other hand, if the illness of a dominant person within the family enables another family member to assume the more authoritative role that they desired, there may be less support and encouragement to help the patient become well.

THE HEALTH PROFESSIONAL AND THE FAMILY

Health professionals' patient education efforts will be more successful if they are able to recognize the impact that illness has on the family and take steps to include the family in the teaching process. Much information about the family can be gathered through simple observation. Who appears the most concerned and interested in the patient? What type of interactions are observed among family members? Who talks to whom and in what way? What is the family's general life style? What activities appear important to them?

Health professionals should also be alert to family reactions to learning about the patient's condition and treatment. Do family members appear apprehensive about learning skills to be used in caring for the patient at home? Is there virtually no response from family members in patient education interactions? What stresses are present in the family? How has the family coped with stress in the past? How are they coping now?

When conducting patient education that includes the family, health professionals should identify conceptual problems through appropriate data gathering. The meaning of the patient's illness to the family may be assessed by asking members what they consider to be major problems. Health professionals should develop a sensitivity to reactions and behaviors associated with different areas of patient teaching by observing verbal and nonverbal indications. Does the family appear responsive to patient teaching? Is there dominance of conversation by one family member? Are there numerous disruptions of patient teaching from the family?

When including the family in patient teaching, health professionals should use open and factual terminology and remain calm and unreactive. There should be no unwarranted optimism or pessimism. Various goals in patient treatment should be discussed so the family as well as the patient knows what to expect. Patient responsibility should be clearly established, but the importance of the family's supportive role should also be stressed.

If particular problems are uncovered, they should be discussed, along with ways in which they might be solved or at least alleviated. Families themselves can be helped to generate options. Family values should be accepted rather than criticized. Family members should receive help in recognizing and ventilating their own feelings. Only after health professionals have identified feelings and problems within the family can help be given to the family in working toward solutions. Is lack of family support a barrier to patient compliance? Can the lack of support be changed through intervention? If not, can the health professional provide additional support or refer the patient to other sources of support? Can the health professional help the family identify outside resources that will increase the patient's potential for following recommendations?

Health professionals should also be aware of the tendency of family members who are anxious and under stress to misunderstand or misinterpret what they are told. It is not uncommon for people to distort information, turning it into what they want to hear. Such occurrences can cause conflicts between the patient and the family and can contribute to noncompliance as well. It is often helpful to assess family members' understanding of what they have been told so that any misinterpretation can be corrected early. Although information should be given in a positive way, it is also important that health professionals help family members develop realistic expectations. Giving the patient and the family written information to read at a later time and then having them return to discuss it may be helpful.

Using a family orientation style in patient education in which the family is viewed as the unit of care can help health professionals provide more effective patient education (Gotler et al. 2001). Getting to know the patient in the context of their family can be important in helping patients meet their health goals. Health professionals can do much to facilitate the effectiveness of patient teaching by fostering discussion among family members. If health professionals have continued contact with the patient and the family, they may check on the progress of the patient with the regimen and identify any new problems or strains that interfere with compliance, helping the patient and the family find new solutions and resources to maximize the potential for compliance.

REFERENCES

Gotler, M.A., Medalie, J.H., Zyzanski, S.J., Kikano, G.E., Stange, K.C. 2001. Focus on the family. Part II: Does a family focus affect patient outcomes? *Family Practice Management* April:45–46.

Jecker, N. 1990. The role of intimate others in medical decision making. *Gerontologist* 30(1):65–71.

Lipkin, M. 1996. Patient education and counseling in the context of modern patient-physician-family communication. *Patient Education and Counseling* 27:5–11.

Reust, C.E., Mattingly, S. 1996. Family involvement in medical decision making. *Family Medicine* 28(1):39–45.

7

Multicultural Issues in Patient Education and Patient Compliance

A HISTORICAL PERSPECTIVE

Some cultures have experienced a history of subjugation, decimation, and discrimination by people from other cultures. In some instances, policies and procedures have been used to control and force dependence on other cultures. As a result, individuals from cultures that have experienced a history of this type of oppression or discrimination may have difficulty trusting the motives and recommendations made by individuals of other cultures. This perception can lead to psychological barriers, which, in turn, affect the success of patient education interactions.

Directives from the health professional maybe viewed as a tool of oppression, domination, and social control. Patient education information given may be viewed with suspicion. Patients from cultures with a history of suppression or domination may doubt that the recommendations given are in their best interest or that the recommendations will enhance their well-being. Consequently, they may be reluctant to follow through with the patient education information.

Although each patient must be considered individually, it is also important for health professionals to have an understanding of the historical perspective that may have in part shaped the perspectives of patients from different cultures. It is especially important to understand how historical events may have shaped individuals' views of the health professional's culture, and why those from other cultures may be reluctant to accept the advice and recommendations of those from the new culture in which they find themselves.

Some cultures, for example, have experienced decimation due to war and disease brought on by people from other cultures. In other instances, ethnic minority groups have been relegated to special areas with regulations imposed, experiencing not only prejudice due to cultural differences but hate because atrocities of war were attributed to the culture as a whole. At times, traditions of various cultures have been undermined and treaties have been broken. In other instances, cultural groups immigrating to other countries have been used as cheap labor while being denied the right to citizenship. Many culturally different groups have been forced to live in substandard conditions and have often had violence directed toward them by members of different cultures. In still other instances, discrimination based on color has prevented individuals from receiving the same education, employment opportunities, health care, and living standards as most other individuals living in the same country.

Individuals born in a country different from their cultural heritage or ethnic origin cannot help but internalize the experience of their ancestors and may continue to feel prejudice. Some individuals may have experienced a perilous journey during immigration and as a result may experience considerable residuals of stress. Because of their immigrant status, living and work standards in the new country in which they find themselves may be considerably lower than they had experienced before, further contributing to the stress of their new situation. The existence of stress, prejudice, and violence may produce a variety of survival mechanisms among individuals assuming a place in a new country. In addition, immigrants are exposed to both standards of the new culture and standards of their own culture, which in some cases may be in conflict. These stresses and adaptive behaviors may present considerable barriers to effective patient education unless health professionals are sensitive to their origins and meanings and are willing to take them into account when working with individual patients.

Views and adjustment of individuals may be influenced by their experience in minority status. Individuals who have experienced discrimination and hostility may come to expect negative reactions especially by those perceived as having power or authority. As a result, health professionals of a different culture may have difficulty understanding the patient's apparent hostile or defensive response that would appear to be unjustified. Because of the patient's previous experience, however, expectations may be such that negative meanings are attributed to even the most helpful messages. By taking time to investigate patients' previous experiences and by attempting to understand the role these experiences can play in the patients' current response, health professionals begin to build rapport with the patients, a necessary and basic component for effective patient education.

The credibility of health professionals is very dependent on the frame of reference of patients from a different culture. Understanding the patients' frame of reference may facilitate health professionals' ability to use social influence needed to help patients incorporate medical information into their own lives. Whether or not patients accept or reject the information given by health professionals will be based on whether they perceive the information as truth, whether in their mind it is an accurate representation of reality, and whether they believe health professionals have their best interest at heart.

CULTURE

Culture is an integral part of everyone's life. Every personal interaction is affected by cultural factors. Values, beliefs, and traditions that are observed in various cultural groups have deep roots that affect individual behavior and reaction to different situations and events. As technology has made travel and thus mobility possible for larger numbers of people, few countries remain culturally homogenous. Consequently, many societies have become more pluralistic, and their populations have become more culturally diverse. Such cultural diversity has implications for all segments of society, but especially health care delivery, and patient education in particular. Every patient education interaction has a cultural dimension.

Individual development within a population is dependent on heredity, the environment to which individuals are exposed, and the society in which they live. Every society has standards to which individuals are expected to conform. The influences of society on an individual are known as culture. Culture comprises many elements, including language, customs, beliefs, traditions, modes of communication, and elements such as tools, art, buildings, and technology.

Culture is the characteristic pattern of attitudes, values, beliefs, and behaviors shared by members of a society or population. Members of a cultural group share characteristics that distinguish them from other groups. These characteristics include patterns of communication and interaction that are used to interpret and process messages and to arrive at conclusions. Culture gives individuals a sense of belonging to a group and creates parameters or boundaries within which individuals in the particular culture function. Culture is learned, and, for the most part, cultural concepts are communicated from one generation to another by specific groups within the culture. Examples of these groups are cultural institutions, such as the family, or social organizations, such as tribes or religion. Individuals are socialized within the cultural group or social organization to follow norms or shared values of the culture. Customs, or the habitual practices of the group, regulate the social life within a culture and include specific ways of thinking or behaving that are common to members of that group. All cultures have some taboos, or prohibitive norms. In addition, certain traditions are followed that are important to the culture.

Culture affects individuals' attitudes, beliefs, and behaviors in many areas of life, including health and illness. Individuals' views of what constitutes health and how to react to illness can be influenced strongly by cultural factors.

Cultural characteristics of patients obviously have implications for patient education. Although it is easy when considering cultural issues and their relation to patient education to focus on language differences that may impede effective exchange of information, cultural differences extend beyond language. Culture is a multidimensional concept that affects values, attitudes, and behaviors of individuals within a given group. Every culture has views, practices, and beliefs that relate not only to life style, gender roles, and world view, but also to health and illness. Each culture has a belief and value of what constitutes health and illness, how each should be managed, and what priority each has. Every culture has managed to survive in part because it has developed some method to deal with health problems to some extent. In doing so, some practices have become deeply rooted in the culture and, although perhaps changed to some degree over time, remain to some extent imbedded in the beliefs and actions of people within that culture. The extent to which patients perceive patient education as having cultural relevance for them can have a profound effect on their reception to the information provided and their willingness to use it.

The degree to which individuals choose to follow health advice, regarding activities related to either prevention of disease or treatment of illness, can be affected significantly by the norms imposed by their cultural environment. Patients from a cultural group different from that of the health professional may find the mode of health care or type of patient education information incompatible with their own notions of health and illness. Different cultures may have different priorities. Those things highly valued and prioritized by health professionals may be ranked differently by patients from another culture. Although good health and preventive health practices may be valued highly in some cultures, other cultures may view such practices as a luxury, focusing more on day-to-day survival, which involves attaining basic necessities such as housing, food, and transportation, or economic survival.

Cultural norms may also influence how much personal responsibility individuals take for their health. Cultural expectations influence individual beliefs about the degree of control they have over their lives. If, for example, patients believe that the source of illness is spiritual, they may see no need or relevance for patient education information.

Culture determines, in part, beliefs about what constitutes illness, when health care should be sought and by whom, and how to behave when sick or injured. In some cultures, seeking help from health professionals may be considered a sign of weakness, or it may be viewed as a practice to be taken only as a last resort. Some cultures have a variety of levels of health practitioners who have different skills that are sought for different perceived needs. For example, in some cultures, when someone becomes ill, a pharmacist may be consulted first for a prescription for the symptoms rather than a physician. In other cultures, women would seek most health care advice from older women in the group rather than from another level of health care practitioner. Consequently, for individuals from some cultures, seeking care from a physician may not be the first step thought of when illness occurs. Treatment may be sought from other levels of health practitioners first.

In addition, some conditions may be thought to be better treated with folk remedies than with remedies prescribed by health professionals. Take, for example, the case of Mrs. Mantea. At an office visit, Dr. Kaster noticed that Mrs. Mantea had several warts on her fingers. Dr. Kaster suggested that the warts should be removed, and that if she would like, an appointment could be made in the next week to have it done. Mrs. Mantea replied that there was no need to go through such a procedure, which may cause pain and scars. Instead, she stated a better solution would be to buy a new silk ribbon and tie as many knots in the ribbon as she had warts. The ribbon, she explained, would then be dropped in the neighborhood, and whoever picked it up would also receive her warts. Under these circumstances, for Dr. Kaster to dispute Mrs. Mantea's remedy or to attempt to discount her belief could reduce his credibility and make future patient education attempts less than effective.

Culture is closely allied to the patient's immediate environment and includes all the social, moral, religious, and cultural groups with which the individual comes in contact. Cultural factors influence specific beliefs or interpretations regarding the body, its normal functioning, causes and consequences of illness, help-seeking, treatment, compliance, and many other related issues. Many cultures maintain at least a portion of their own folkways and remedies. To deal effectively with patients, health professionals must understand the impact of culture on patients' health and health care. To conduct effective patient education, health professionals should be prepared to address specific concerns and beliefs of patients from different cultures.

ETHNICITY

Embodied in culture is ethnicity. Ethnicity is biological and racial, and although tied to culture, may also be separate. For example, Ms. Liu's ethnic background is Chinese; however, her family had immigrated to another country several generations ago. Consequently, Ms. Liu largely ascribes to and identifies with the culture of the adopted country and is more strongly influenced by the culture in which she grew up and currently lives rather than the culture of her ethnic background. Under these circumstances, for the health professional to assume, without gaining further information, that Ms. Liu holds the same traditions and customs as those of her ethnic background would be as erroneous as assuming that an individual who recently immigrated to the health professional's culture had automatic acceptance and understanding of that culture. Likewise, in some instances, even though individuals have lived within a culture for generations, they may still hold a strong ethnic identity with their native culture, which is separate from the culture in which they now live.

ACCULTURATION

Distinct from ethnicity is acculturation, a term related to the individual's adaptation to the customs, values, and behaviors of a new culture. The degree of acculturation any one individual experiences may be dependent on a number of factors. In some instances, individuals who have immigrated to a new country may reject the beliefs and behaviors of their culture of origin and take on those of the new culture. When this is the case, the individual is said to be acculturated. The length of time in a new country, however, is not an indication of the individual's degree of acculturation. Some individuals may live in a new country for their entire lives but still hold fast to the traditions, values, and beliefs of their own culture.

The amount of acculturation that takes place is affected to some degree by the patient's age at the time of immigration. For instance, children may have a greater tendency to acculturate than older adults. Acculturation is also affected by family influences. For example, individuals in a close, socially isolated family may have less exposure to outside influences and thus receive more family support for holding onto traditional values. For example, Mrs. Santos had immigrated to a new country with her family when she was 2 years of age. Her family, however, was quite close and moved to a city community in which many others from Mrs. Santos' own culture lived. Mrs. Santos' family never traveled, and the school she attended was made up mostly of people from her own ethnic and cultural background. Immediately after high school, she married a classmate of her own ethnic background. They settled in the same community in which they had been raised. Although Mrs. Santos has lived in her adopted country nearly 20 years, she continues to ascribe to the traditions and values of her culture of origin.

Education and socioeconomic class also influence acculturation. Those individuals who have broadened their perspectives through education, travel, or wider experiences with others from different countries may acculturate more easily than those individuals who have had little exposure to other cultures. For example, as a child, Mr. Pachesque had been sent to boarding schools located outside his native country. Although during his school years he frequently returned to his country of origin, after completing college he moved to another country to live and has adopted most of the traditions and practices of the new country.

CULTURAL DIFFERENCES AND THE HEALTH PROFESSIONAL

When working with patients from other cultures, health professionals must consider more than patients' cultural background alone. The culture of the health professional must be considered as well. Both patients and health professionals bring their own cultural values, attitudes, and behaviors to the patient education interaction.

Cultural differences between health professionals and patients can be a potential impediment to effective patient education. Many health professionals hold a cultural perspective that may not be shared by patients from a different ethnic group. Based on one's frame of reference, such differences or diversity can take many forms. The health professional's lack of understanding of specific cultural variables and their impact on patients' lives can create barriers to effective patient education and be a source of conflict and misunderstanding. Health professionals' preconceived notion of patients' culture may affect the definition of the problem and assessment of the situation.

Health professionals who are unfamiliar with certain cultural groups and have limited or no experience with members of the patients' culture may hold various myths and stereotypes about the group as a whole. It is important that health professionals avoid projecting their own unconscious myths or stereo-types. Health professionals might hold a pervasive and inaccurate stereotype that individuals from a certain culture are a homogenous group without acknowl-edging the diversity that exists within all cultural groups. In other instances, myths about a group and its beliefs and practices affect patient teaching.

Myths are beliefs that are not based on fact. Stereotypes are rigid precon-ceptions about all people who are members of a particular group. Health pro-fessionals unfamiliar with variations within each culture may have a tendency to treat all people within a cultural group as if they were the same, not allowing for individual differences. Rather than forming impressions based on experience with patients as individuals, health professionals may form opinions based on preconceived ideas, myths, and/or stereotypes held for that ethnic group. Consequently, rather than considering individual differences, all incoming infor-mation becomes distorted to fit health professionals' own ideas of what the par-ticular ethnic group is like.

Myths and stereotypes that health professionals may have are obviously bar-riers to effective patient education. For example, Mr. Perez was a patient of His-panic background who had been recently hospitalized because of gastritis. He was referred for patient education regarding diet. The health professional discussed the possibility that spices may irritate the condition and specified that even though she knew Hispanics liked hot and spicy foods, Mr. Perez would have to become accustomed to a more bland diet. When later, Mr. Perez was asked by another health professional if he had found the patient education information helpful, he replied, "Not really; where I am from, the foods we eat are only lightly seasoned, and I personally have never cared for spicy food anyway." The health professional conducting the patient education had presented informa-tion based on stereotype and did not account for individual differences within a culture or differences of various regions or areas within the country from which the culture originates.

Categorizing individuals into a group perpetuates exaggeration of differ-ences between groups and can minimize distinctions of individuals within the group. There is great intracultural variability among individuals in every cul-tural group. Variation may occur because individuals have different levels of education, have different socioeconomic status, have different levels of accul-turation, and have different values based on generational differences or urban or rural backgrounds.

Cultural groups are represented at all economic and educational levels. The same differences exist between individuals in all cultures. There can be great diversity of thought and behavior within any cultural group. Lumping all persons from one culture together ignores significant differences between groups and vio-lates the patient's identity. Failing to realize that not all individuals from the same culture necessarily ascribe to all of the values, customs, or beliefs of their cultural group can interfere with rapport-building, which is necessary for effec-tive patient education. In this case, health professionals may fail to individualize patient education according to patients' specific needs, focusing instead on beliefs about the patients' cultural group as a whole. Health professionals must explore their own beliefs regarding certain cultures, separating fact from myth and prejudice, and recognizing differences in priorities and value systems in patients' cultures from their own.

When conducting patient education with patients from a different culture, health professionals may experience feelings of inadequacy, frustration, or resentment. If health professionals know nothing about the patient's culture, some of the patient's behavior or beliefs that are unfamiliar may be viewed as bizarre, uncooperative, or strange, even though in the context of the patient's culture, the behaviors or beliefs are totally appropriate. For example, Ms. Holmes had been a nurse on the diabetic unit for several years and had generally been thought of as having exceptional patient education skills. However, she found one patient, Mr. Sayyid, a patient from Afghanistan, extremely difficult to work with. Finally, one day in exasperation, Ms. Holmes stated, "I give up—you can lead a horse to water, but you can't make him drink. I've tried everything, but Mr. Sayyid misses appointments, doesn't appear to have followed through on recommendations we discussed, and at the last session couldn't even remember what we had talked about the session before. He is unmotivated, so until he decides to help himself, there's nothing I can do."

The nurse working with Mr. Sayyid's physician said, "Let me talk to him and see what the trouble is." At his next physician's appointment, the office nurse, while preparing him for the exam, said, "You've been going to patient education for awhile now, haven't you? How's it going?"

"Terrible," said Mr. Sayyid. "Ms. Holmes is very nice, but I know she doesn't like me. When I try to explain to her why I can't do some of the things, she says, 'Of course you can; it's easy.' I want to be a good patient and to learn, but it's very hard. She doesn't understand."

"Maybe you could give her one more chance," the office nurse encouraged. She then reported back to Ms. Holmes, who had been unaware of her abrupt and insensitive attitude.

At the next session, Ms. Holmes said, "You know, Mr. Sayyid, I've been thinking, I really don't know very much about your culture. With all the talking I've been doing, I haven't taken the time to consider that some of the things we're doing may be difficult for you. Tell me a little bit about some of your customs."

Mr. Sayyid seemed pleased and proceeded to explain some basic beliefs and traditions that he held dear. After that, adjustments could be made in his patient education plan so that he was better able to follow through with treatment recommendations.

GAINING CREDIBILITY

When developing a relationship with patients from other cultures, it is a mistake for health professionals to assume that patients will automatically accept patient education information as accurate or important because of the health professionals' qualifications or professional preparation. Although certain credentials may be perceived to indicate a level of expertise and legitimacy, the same credentials or qualifications may not have the same importance in all cultures. More than credentials are needed to establish a relationship between patient and health professional in which open discussion can take place. Building a trusting and open relationship in which such discussion can take place in the interaction is crucial to the patient education process. Health professionals must be perceived as sincere and genuinely interested in helping patients to obtain their maximal health status. They must also be perceived as trustworthy and accepting rather than condemning, criticizing, or making light of the patients' beliefs or cultural practices.

Patient education is often conducted with the assumption that the patient shares the same values, attitudes, and philosophy as health professionals presenting the information. This may not be the case, especially with patients from other cultures. Unless this is recognized, it is likely that attempts at effective patient education will fail. Lack of knowledge or understanding of cultural differences or unwillingness to accept patients' alternative beliefs, values, or attitudes can lead to the inability to empathize or to see the patient's point of view. These factors can prevent health professionals from being able to construct the patient education interaction to meet patients' needs and to devise solutions to potential barriers to patient compliance that would be acceptable to all involved. Before trying to change patients' attitudes, beliefs, or health practices, health professionals should first try to understand them, respecting patients' cultural identity. Health professionals who demonstrate a critical attitude toward patients' behaviors, attitudes, or customs will only alienate patients and discourage opportunity for further patient education encounters.

In some instances, health professionals may avoid conducting patient education with patients from other cultures altogether, feeling the situation to be unmanageable. Such a defeatist attitude makes health professionals seem abrupt and distant, further diminishing the opportunity for effective patient education in the future. In other instances, health professionals may conduct patient education with no alteration or consideration of cultural factors, ignoring, denying, or minimizing differences that do exist.

Even when health professionals are sensitive to cultural differences, they still may not feel they have the knowledge or skills for effective patient education with patients from other cultures. In some instances, health professionals may be overly sensitive, so that they are not as direct in the patient education interaction as they would be with other patients. Because of their fear of offending the patient in some way, health professionals may not address certain issues or may fail to obtain information that could make the patient education interaction more effective. In the same vein, health professionals may not attempt compromises or negotiation, feeling that such efforts may be misinterpreted by patients. At times, health professionals may deny that there are any differences in values or priorities. By acknowledging and understanding differences, health professionals may be able to use them to help patients follow recommendations.

In some instances, health professionals may merely expect that patients will follow directives without examining patients' feelings about the recommendations or assessing whether or not they can be carried out. For example, the concept of prevention may be totally foreign to individuals in some cultures. In addition, when recommendations involve a procedure such as mammography or Pap smear, patients may consider the suggestion a lack of respect or violation of privacy. To make patient education interactions most effective, it is crucial that health professionals consider specific experiences, beliefs, and values related to the patient's cultural background.

Effective patient education demands an understanding of the norms and shared values of patients' culture as well as an understanding that individual differences are present in every culture. Patient behavior should be evaluated within the patient's cultural frame of reference. Knowledge of patients' culture gives health professionals a more complete picture of patients' perspectives of their condition and helps health professionals determine what type of patient education is best suited to patients' needs. Health professionals' understanding of the norms of patients' cultures and the extent of patients' immersion in those cultures can be critical to understanding patients' responses to medical advice.

An understanding of cultural backgrounds of patients enables health professionals to appreciate attitudes of individuals of different cultures to hospitalization, dietary restrictions, or other treatment regimens. In addition, health professionals can become more sensitive to difficulties and fears patients in a new country may have, the frustration those with language difficulty may feel, and the importance and significance of spiritual and religious rituals. Health professionals must show respect for patients' cultural beliefs about illness and provide patient education that enhances patients' understanding within their own cultural framework. At the same time, health professionals must make some determinations regarding which behaviors are culturally based and which are unique to the individual.

Cultural differences are too complex and diverse for simple approaches. Cultural patterns are only rough approximations and do not consider individual differences within the culture. There are broad variations of individual behavior within each culture. Although some generalizations may be true for the majority of individuals within a culture, they certainly are not true universally. Likewise, no culture is static. Therefore, culturally sensitive patient education requires ongoing work and modification to reflect changes within the patient's culture. There will always be exceptions. Although there is not a standard way to work with patients of different cultures, it does require a comprehensive approach that raises the awareness and sensitivity of health professionals to cultural issues to be incorporated into patient education. Health professionals cannot know specific customs, values, and beliefs of every ethnic group. Health professionals should, however, develop an openness to cultural differences and not impose their values on patients from a different ethnic background.

Patients may find proposed treatments unacceptable because they clash with group norms and, before accepting the treatment, may discuss the recommendations with other members of their culture, seeking group acceptance before modifying behavior. In different ethnic communities, the reputation of the health professional frequently travels by word of mouth. Consequently, if the health professional is viewed as one who works within the cultural framework of the patient, credibility will be gained.

At times, patient education involves problem solving and negotiation, identifying barriers that may prevent patients from following through with advice and recommendations given. The same is true with patients from different cultures. Health professionals must be aware of and sensitive to cultural differences, not making assumptions and generalizations based on stereotypes but, rather, attempting to understand the patient as an individual.

COMMUNICATION ISSUES IN CROSS-CULTURAL PATIENT EDUCATION

Patient education is a process of interpersonal interaction and communication as well as a process of transfer of health information. Presenting patient education information to any patient is directed toward helping the patient to:

- understand his or her diagnosis and treatment
- understand aspects of prevention
- incorporate the information into daily life, and
- make truly informed choices about the extent to which he or she will follow treatment recommendations

Before effective patient education can occur, however, health professionals and patients must accurately send and receive both verbal and nonverbal messages. In conducting patient education across cultures, it is important to adapt not only the content of the health information but also the methods by which the content is conveyed. Communication styles may be different and may be a source of misunderstanding. There should be a concerted effort to make information fit the patient rather than insisting that patients fit information. Barriers to effective communication in the patient education process can occur at any time, even when both patient and health professional are from the same culture. When health professionals and patients are from different cultural backgrounds, however, the barriers to effective communication become greater, and a greater opportunity for misunderstanding exists. In addition to such misunderstandings impeding the accurate transfer of information in the patient education process, misunderstandings can also lead to alienation and disintegration of the relationship between patient and health professional.

Patients from different cultures may not use the standard language spoken by health professionals or may not speak the language at all. Often, in an attempt to speak the language of the health professional, patients may use simple phrases because of their limited vocabulary in the language. It is at times easy for health professionals to assume, because of a patient's difficulty in using the language, that he or she has limited intelligence. The health professional may begin to think of the patient as a child and begin treating him or her in that way, which only serves to build further barriers to effective patient education. In most instances, patients' inability to use a new language adequately is not a reflection of level of intelligence or education but, rather, merely unfamiliarity and inexperience with the new language.

Even if the language of the health professional is the primary language of the patient, regional differences may exist within the same language. Language variations related to words and expressions may be as important as recognition of differences of values and customs. Subcultures within the same country may also use nonstandard language as the norm, with their own phrases and words to express concepts. Language of the subculture may be a way the patient has found to adapt and function in his or her own world. Although foreign sounding to the health professional, the language of the subculture may be highly developed and structured and quite adequate for conveying ideas. If health professionals cannot relate to patients' language systems, then they probably will have difficulty building rapport.

Likewise, health professionals may, because of their own lack of understanding of the patient's language, attribute inaccurate characteristics or motives to the patient. Misunderstandings that arise from cultural variations in communication may lead to alienation and/or inability to develop trust and rapport, which may result in termination of the patient education intervention. Although breakdown in communication can and does occur at times between health professionals and patients from the same culture, the problem can be exacerbated between people from different racial or ethnic backgrounds. Health professionals from one social class may assume that patients are using the same class rules when communicating and that the words and phrases have the same meaning, whereas this may not be true.

Meanings of language are communicated in many ways. In addition to verbal expression, nonverbal communication is often as meaningful or more meaningful than words expressed. Lack of understanding of the nuances or the importance of nonverbal behaviors in different cultures can also cause misunderstanding and consequently serve as a barrier to effective patient education. In addition, the ways words are communicated—such as rate, inflections, loudness, hesitations, and silences—are all used to communicate a variety of different meanings. A gesture, tone, inflection, posture, or eye contact may enhance or negate a message.

For example, people from some cultures may feel uncomfortable with stretches of silence, whereas those from other cultures may give silence specific meaning. Some cultures may use silence as a sign of respect or as a sign of politeness. In other cultures, silence may be used to signify agreement or to emphasize a point. If the health professional is from a culture in which silence is not part of regular communication, a patient education interaction in which the patient remains silent may be interpreted as lack of understanding or disinterest on the part of the patient. If the health professional is uncomfortable with silence, he or she may keep talking to fill in the silence or believe that the patient education session has failed.

Health professionals may expect patients to be inquisitive and open, approaching the patient education interaction with a certain degree of sophistication. Persons not fitting into this framework may be considered resistant or defensive. Take the case of Ms. Bobnon, an international student who was receiving routine prenatal care from Dr. Tate. At each visit, Dr. Tate attempted to talk with Ms. Bobnon about diet and activity during pregnancy, what to expect at different stages of pregnancy, and how to prepare for the baby. Throughout each visit, Ms. Bobnon remained silent, never asking questions and offering no comment. Dr. Tate became increasingly frustrated and shared with the nurse that he had concern about Ms. Bobnon's ability to care adequately for the baby given that she seemed to have so little interest in the patient education information. Dr. Tate did not understand that, whereas in some countries, patients are expected to ask questions or state their opinions about their treatment, some cultures may view this as rude and disrespectful, and consequently patients do not ask questions during the patient education interaction, which was true in Ms. Bobnon's case. Health professionals unaware of such differences may also interpret this reticence of asking questions as a sign of ignorance, a lack of motivation, or an ineffective patient education interaction when, in fact, patients may believe they are merely being respectful.

For the most part, health professionals may believe that being frank, open, and direct when conveying patient education information about health and health care is most desirable. Many cultures, however, have norms that value indirectness or the use of euphemisms in conversation. People from different cultures may vary in their information orientation. Whereas some cultures may value facts and directness, others may place more importance in having their own questions and concerns answered. In some cultures, indirectness in speech is considered an art. Directness may be considered forceful, or the patient may view the health professional who is direct as being rude and pushy. Such actions may alienate the patient. Under these circumstances, openness and directness, especially if the information is perceived to be a particularly sensitive topic, may be viewed as too blunt or as a source of embarrassment, thus alienating the patient. Take the following example of Mr. Delano.

Mr. Delano, a nurse, had recently begun working in an adolescent health center where most of the patients were of the same ethnic background, a background different from his own. Having worked with adolescents of his own background for a number of years, Mr. Delano prided himself on being able to build rapport quickly and to conduct patient education effectively. One program he had been particularly proud of was the acquired immunodeficiency syndrome (AIDS) prevention program he had established at another health clinic. He became increasingly disillusioned and discouraged at the neighborhood health center, however, when it became obvious that not only were the adolescents at this center unreceptive to this information, but they seemed to be avoiding talking with him about other issues as well. Although Mr. Delano interpreted this behavior as the patients' lack of ability to confront the issue, in fact, the patients were offended by what they perceived as Mr. Delano's brashness and insensitivity in being so direct in his discussions.

Volume of speech may also be interpreted differently in other cultures. Speaking in a soft voice may not indicate shyness but rather politeness, and speaking in a loud, brash manner may not indicate anger or hostility. Likewise, the speech patterns or tone of voice of the health professional may be interpreted by the patient as indicating that the health professional is upset, embarrassed, rude, or sarcastic.

Nonverbal behavior also has an important impact on interpersonal communication. Nonverbal behavior is culture bound, and consequently the health professional cannot make universal generalizations about different nonverbal behaviors and their meanings. These behaviors operate primarily without the awareness of the individual exhibiting them and often may be a more accurate reflection of feelings than are words. Nonverbal behaviors may be used as a way to exhibit social control, such as getting up and moving to the door as a signal that it is time to end the conversation. Nonverbal behavior is also a way of demonstrating warmth or friendliness. The extent to which these concepts are acceptable to display among strangers or acquaintances, however, varies from culture to culture. For example, in some cultures, a handshake may be a traditional form of greeting, whereas in other cultures, body contact is avoided, but gestures such as bowing are considered polite. In other cultures, more intimate forms of greeting, such as hugging, are considered appropriate in most social situations.

Eye contact is another nonverbal behavior that has different meanings in different cultures. In some cultures, eye contact is considered important, demonstrating attention and interest, whereas in other cultures, eye contact may be considered confrontive, aggressive, or hostile. In the patient education interaction, eye contact may be interpreted by health professionals as a sign that patients are interested or listening. Aversion of the eyes may be interpreted as a sign of discomfort, guilt, indifference, depression, or disregard. Some cultures, however, assume that merely being there and sitting quietly indicate interest. Styles of communication with the eyes may be different between cultures and may lead to misinterpretations.

Health professionals use patients' nonverbal behavior as cues to discomfort, fatigue, disinterest, embarrassment, or a variety of other factors that can impede effective patient education. However, when conducting cross-cultural patient education, the same rules of interpretation of nonverbal behavior may not be applicable. Being aware of differences in the meaning of nonverbal behavior can help the health professional avoid misinterpretations.

Likewise, health professionals should be aware that their own nonverbal behavior may also be a help or a barrier to effective patient education. Individuals from different cultures may be very sensitive to behaviors exhibited by health professionals. In some cultures, greater sensitivity and awareness of the nonverbal behavior of others, especially those in power, may have been learned as a matter of survival. In some instances, the health professional may be unaware that certain nonverbal behaviors are offensive to the patient. In other instances, however, the nonverbal behavior may be the unconscious reflection of the health professional's bias.

Take the case of Dr. Frankel, who had asked Mr. Su, a patient from a cultural background different from her own, to return for blood pressure checks due to an elevation of blood pressure on several visits. When Dr. Frankel diagnosed Mr. Su as having hypertension, she took Mr. Su into her office to talk about the condition and its treatment. Rather than sitting beside Mr. Su as she usually did when conducting patient education, however, she sat at her desk with Mr. Su placed on the other side. She used less eye contact, and after presenting the information arose from her desk, walked to the door and asked Mr. Su to call her if he had any questions. Although the content of the information was the same as that Dr. Frankel routinely presented, her nonverbal behavior communicated feelings of indifference and disinterest. Attitudes, beliefs, and feelings are deeply ingrained into our total being. No matter how unbiased health professionals believe they have been verbally, if they have not recognized and adequately dealt with their own biases, they may still communicate bias through nonverbal cues.

Use of space as an aspect of culture is an important factor in communication. Reactions and behaviors in interaction with others are to some extent a reflection of the spatial dimension to which we are all culturally conditioned. Conversational distance, or the amount of space between two people talking, varies considerably from culture to culture. Some cultures dictate a much closer stance than normally comfortable for people from other cultures. If the patient's conversational distance according to his or her culture is closer than that of the health professional's, and the health professional backs away from the patient, the patient may interpret such behavior as aloofness or the desire not to communicate. On the other hand, health professional may interpret the close proximity as patients' attempt to become intimate. Personal space may also be interpreted as a sign of dominance and status. The higher the status of the individual, the more space he or she is allowed to occupy.

Even the setting in which patient education takes place is important. The placement of furniture where both health professional and patient sit may have implications that could have an impact on the effectiveness of the interaction and can enhance or retard the patient education process.

Bodily movement may also lead to misunderstanding because the same movement can have contrasting meanings. For instance, whereas in some cultures a raised thumb is given to show approval, in some cultures, the same movement may be considered an insult. In some cultures, nodding the head up and down while the other individual is speaking demonstrates listening and understanding of what is being said. However, not all cultures use this movement. Its absence, therefore, could be interpreted by health professionals as lack of interest or understanding on the part of patients, when in fact it is merely not a behavior commonly used in the patient's culture.

Communication styles may either enhance or negate the effectiveness of patient education. When the communication style of health professionals is different from that of patients from another culture, patient education may not be effective, and several problems may arise. The health professional may not seem credible to the patient, and the patient may not incorporate the information or may not attend subsequent sessions. The health professional may terminate patient education early due to what he or she considers poor motivation or lack of interest on the part of the patient, or the patient and health professional may be unable to establish rapport, which is crucial to effective patient education.

It is important for health professionals working with culturally diverse populations to be aware of differences in communication practices and differential meanings of nonverbal behavior. Health professionals should guard against possible misinterpretation by patients of actions and/or information and should be aware of how their own nonverbal behaviors may reflect stereotypes or bias about various cultural groups. Health professionals should be able to shift their communication styles and delivery of information to suit the needs of the culturally different patient.

Likewise, it is important to recognize that health professionals cannot understand all variations and nuances of all cultures. When there are personal limits to the extent to which health professionals' communication style can be altered, they may need to seek other alternatives, such as learning more about the specific culture, seeking information from others from the patient's cultural background who can provide insight, or anticipating their own limitations and the impact on the patient. In most instances, however, the most effective means of helping patients appears to be communicating acceptance and understanding of the patient's world view and acknowledging to patients that health professionals understand that the material they are presenting is from a different cultural perspective. This alone may be enough to bridge the communication gap between patient and health professional.

USE OF AN INTERPRETER

When patients and health professionals do not speak the same language, an interpreter, if available, may be used to assist in the patient education interaction. Use of an interpreter alone, however, does not always ensure that patient education interactions will be successful. Just because an individual speaks the same language as the patient does not mean that all communication conveyed between parties will be effective. Whereas normally the information exchange in patient education interaction takes place between two people, the health professional and the patient, use of an interpreter adds one more dimension, which can increase the complexity of the interaction.

Interpreters, even though able to communicate in the patient's language, may or may not also be familiar with the patient's culture. Even if the interpreter is familiar with the patient's culture, he or she may consciously or unconsciously insert personal bias into the interpretation from patient to health professional or health professional to patient. In addition, issues of confidentiality may occur if the patient is being given or has asked for information of a particularly sensitive nature.

Although in larger cities professional interpreters may be available, this is not always the case. In instances where a neighbor, family member, or sometimes the patient's child is asked to interpret, health professionals should be aware that the educational and social background of the interpreter is just as important to consider as that of the patient. In order to interpret accurately, the interpreter must understand both the content and the context of the message. The interpreter must also be able to convey information from health professional to patient and from patient to health professional in as unbiased a way as possible. If the interpreter's own values and beliefs are in conflict with the patient's or the health professional's, the information may be slanted toward a particular view of the interpreter rather than given as the information was originally presented.

Patient teaching using an interpreter takes longer. Each message must be repeated twice. The health professional should attempt to present information with as little technical jargon as possible and attempt to keep explanations simple and unambiguous. The health professional should not forget the patient's presence and should avoid talking only to the interpreter as if the patient were absent. As the information is translated by the interpreter and given to the patient, the health professional should be attendant to the patient's response, reactions, and expressions, and if they indicate that the patient is anxious, upset, or has any other negative response, the interpreter should be asked to identify what specifically made the patient respond in that way. At times, it may be important for the health professional to obtain a word-for-word translation of what was said. Obtaining this type of feedback provides the health professional a chance to clarify or amplify any points that were unclear or misunderstood, as well as providing the opportunity to make sure the message was interpreted accurately.

Although it is helpful in many patient education situations to have written materials that can reinforce information health professionals have given the patient verbally, this may be even more important in the case of individuals who speak a different language. If written materials are used, however, it is just as important to make sure the translation is correct in writing as it is to make sure the verbal translation is correct. Having the interpreter back-translate the information can help identify problems or inaccuracy of the original translation so that they may be corrected.

SOCIAL-CULTURAL VARIATIONS

Patient education is greatly influenced by the social-cultural framework from which it arises. Identification with the cultural group norm may affect not only patients' health behavior but also the degree to which they adhere to patient education instructions. As a result, individuals from different cultures may respond quite differently to the same type of patient education information.

Cultural responses to patient education on a variety of topics are illustrated by the following examples. For instance, prenatal patient education, which is accepted as a routine part of good prenatal care in some cultures, may in other cultures be viewed as unnecessary or even a violation of privacy. Some cultures may believe that this type of information is best shared between females in the culture or that such information should be passed from mother to daughter rather than given from a health professional who is a stranger. As another example, patient education about tobacco and alcohol use may be viewed differently by patients from different cultures. Although in some cultures, both are taboo, in others, both are used as part of ceremonial ritual. While in some cultures, the use of one or both is considered socially appropriate, in other cultures, the use of one or both may be considered socially irresponsible. Patient response to patient education about either will be determined to some extent by the cultural view and tradition from which they come. Diet is often important to ethnic identity, having religious as well as nutritional connotations, often including not only what foods are eaten but how they are prepared. Patient education about nutrition or diet changes alone may be ineffective, unless the cultural meaning of food and tradition of preparation are understood.

In some cultures, individualization and independence are highly valued. For example, in the United States, patient education traditionally emphasizes assisting patients in self-direction through the presentation of information regarding their condition and/or treatment or means of prevention of illness. In the United States, patient education practice arises out of the belief that patients should be given information from which to make their own decisions and out of the belief that information regarding health and health care will help the individual follow medical advice, which will in turn enhance their well-being. Given this philosophy, helping patients to engage in necessary behavior change is the ultimate goal of patient education. Although health professionals may emphasize self-determination and self-direction, other cultures may value the mystique of health professionals, believing they have healing powers, or they may expect a more authoritarian approach.

The information health professionals believe to be necessary may not be the same information believed by the patient to be necessary. Consequently, patients may not value information and also may not ascribe to the self-reliance and self-determination with regard to health care and treatment that health care professionals hold to be important. When the views between patient and health professional become too diverse, patients may choose to abandon the setting, seeking help and advice from those whose beliefs and practices more closely resemble his or her own.

Information given may also be in conflict with the patient's traditional beliefs or superstitions regarding cause and/or treatment of disease. Patients in a new culture may be living a dualistic life in which they are attempting to retain their traditional values while still trying to live and function in a dominant culture different from their own. This conflict can be the source of considerable stress. Patients may fear retribution if they disagree or allow health professionals to know their true feelings. Consequently, they may take great efforts to hide their true thoughts or their behavior for fear of offending or threatening the health professional. Instead, while appearing to accept the information, they may quietly discount all of it, not following through on medical advice. Public acceptances of information do not necessarily guarantee follow-through with the advice given.

Health professionals may assume that the major goal of patients in health care settings is to "get better." In some cultures, however, patients may have a stoic acceptance of poor health with little effort to change. Such patients may accept life, illness, and death as a destiny of nature, not under individual control and not to be interfered with. In other instances, illness may be viewed as a human weakness, and, consequently, admitting illness by receiving treatment or learning more about the illness or treatment may also be viewed in a negative light. Some cultures ascribe a spiritual nature to illness, believing that illness is the will of another who wishes the illness upon them. Such attitudes may be difficult for health professionals to accept unless they understand the cultural context.

Social class and economic status can also contribute to patients' reactions to patient education interactions and their ability to follow through with recommendations. Individuals of lower socioeconomic class or those living in poverty may have yet another layer of values and priorities from those of middle or upper class individuals from their same culture. Whereas some patients from culturally different backgrounds may be well educated and financially solvent, this certainly is not true for all patients.

Patients with poor socioeconomic status may in turn have less education and have received poorer health care because of limited access to health care or to good health care practices. These individuals may, for instance, view such recommendations as "regular exercise, plenty of rest, and a diet of fresh fruits and vegetables" as a luxury rather than a legitimate recommendation they can follow. Not taking into account patients' economic backgrounds and the role this plays in their current health status is a mistake that can interfere with the total patient education process.

Coming from a lower class background often compounds cultural variations. The gap between a health professional from a middle-class environment that is predictable and a patient from a lower socioeconomic class environment that is unpredictable may be immense. Individuals from a lower class or socioeconomic background have different access to resources, which may affect the extent to which they are willing or able to follow treatment recommendations. For instance, follow-up visits may be difficult if the patient has no access to transportation. Walking in order to obtain more exercise may be unreasonable if the neighborhood in which the patient lives is unsafe. Other directives may be those that the patient cannot afford.

Health professionals may be future oriented, thinking ahead to issues of prevention, whereas some patients may be past or present oriented, with the satisfaction of basic needs of the moment being the most important. Health professionals may view some patients as unable to plan and become frustrated at what they perceive to be lack of motivation. However, in a cross-cultural context, the patients' views and behavior are understandable and appropriate for their environment. Individuals who are unemployed, underemployed, or for other reasons live in a state of poverty may feel in day-to-day jeopardy because of their struggle to meet the daily needs of food and shelter—factors that health professionals may take for granted. The patient may only be able to concentrate on immediate, short-term goals rather than long-term goals or prevention. The health professional may attribute the attitudes displayed by the patient to cultural or individual characteristics rather than to adversity of the patient's circumstances. In these instances, the patient education intervention may be more effective if the health professional first attends to the patient's perceived immediate needs and focuses on short-term, one-day-at-a-time goals rather than emphasizing long-term outcomes.

Because of patients' environments, and/or inexperience with patient education, their expectations may be quite different from those of the health professional. Many patients may expect merely to be given some tangible treatment and may see no reason for additional information. If this is the case, health professionals may perceive patients as hostile and even resistant. Under these circumstances, the result may be premature termination of the patient education interaction.

Just as health professionals may hold myths and stereotypes about different cultural groups, they may also hold myths and stereotypes about patients from lower socioeconomic backgrounds. Stereotypes that these patients are unreliable, irresponsible, and impulsive may be based on other aspects of behavior, such as arriving late for appointments or missing the appointment altogether. Rather than making assumptions or basing opinions on these stereotypical images, health professionals should attempt to ascertain the reason for the missed appointment. In many instances, for example, the reason for the missed appointment may be related to not owning a car and thus being dependent on others for their transportation or owning a car in serious disrepair. Even if public transportation is available, it is at times costly and at times undependable. Patients may also have difficulty arranging child care and may not find it manageable to bring children with them, especially small children. Health professionals must appreciate and be prepared to respond to the needs of the individual, especially if the situation is confounded by economic hardship, discrimination, or other stressors within the environment.

FAMILY ISSUES AND CULTURAL DIVERSITY

The role and influence of family on patients' willingness and ability to carry out treatment recommendations are important in any patient education interaction. However, specific roles and expectations of family members are not the same across all cultures. Health professionals must define and respect family members' roles, enlist family support for continuing treatment, and increase their confidence in the proposed intervention. It may be important to incorporate the family into the patient education intervention and to praise the family for its efforts that have helped the patient adhere to the medical advice.

Cultural beliefs affect family roles and relationships and can have an impact on patient education in a number of areas. Child-rearing practices and gender role are two examples. Discipline—how it is administered and by whom—may have strong cultural overlays that may influence the patient's receptivity to patient education information about the topic. In addition, gender roles and expectations may make a difference in how, when, and to whom patient education information is given and how willing the patient is to follow the recommendations.

In some cultures, men and elders are viewed as having higher status and are regarded as the major decision makers in families, with little input from others. Gender roles, perceptions, and expectations may also be different. Some cultures place major emphasis on the male of the household being independent and the caretaker of his family. If this is the case, it may be difficult if the treatment recommendation puts the patient in a position where he must be in a dependent role, whether in the hospital or at home. An older patient who does not speak the language of the health professional may feel threatened by having to depend on his or her children to translate information given. It may be difficult for the patient under these circumstances to maintain dignity and respect in a dependent role that may be required because of the condition. In some cultures, the husband, even though not the patient, is expected to be given the information and make decisions about the recommendations for his wife. The husband may be resentful if a male presents information directly to his wife or may resent his wife having more knowledge about her condition or treatment than he has. If the husband is the patient, he may feel resentful of having to be dependent on his wife for part of his care.

In some instances, when one family member has become acculturated, strain may be experienced between family members for accepting advice that appears to go beyond the values of the culture. For instance, in cultures where celibacy before marriage is expected, any discussion about contraception prior to marriage may be viewed as offensive.

In some instances, a family member may inherit two different cultural traditions. Reluctance to accept certain treatments should not be viewed as a sign of disinterest or irresponsibility but rather may reflect a conflict between duality of membership in two groups. The health professional may undermine the patient's cultural concept of extended family by asking to talk with the patient alone without the presence of relatives. Health professionals' persistence in encouraging patients to be self-reliant in their treatment may violate cultural views of appropriate role behaviors.

APPROACHES

To conduct patient education effectively with people from different cultures, health professionals must be willing to alter their own behavior, attitudes, and communication styles and to examine their own biases and stereotypes. Patient education interventions that are culturally appropriate are dependent not only on knowledge about different cultures but sensitivity as well. Health professionals must have the ability to demonstrate tolerance of others' frames of reference and points of view This does not mean that there must be all over, blanket acceptance of beliefs or practices that could be harmful. Abusive practices are not acceptable regardless of tradition. When cultural practices are not harmful, they can be incorporated with medical recommendations. Although there is no cookbook formula for working with patients from different cultures and ethnic backgrounds, there are some general guidelines.

Health professionals should not discredit patients' cultural beliefs and practices and should treat beliefs, practices, and traditions with respect. Health professionals should attempt to reflect back their interpretation of the patients' perspectives for clarification and to demonstrate to the patient that they have both heard and respect the patient's point of view.

Health professionals should assess patients' beliefs and maintain openness and flexibility. For example, if to the question, "What do you think is causing your cold?" the patient responds, "The bad wishes of my neighbor," the health professional, rather than criticizing or discounting the belief, should attempt to learn more about the belief. Accepting patients' beliefs and feelings is not the same as validating their beliefs.

As much as possible, health professionals should attempt to incorporate the patients' beliefs and practices into the treatment recommendations. If some of the patient's cultural beliefs or practices have the potential for harm, the health professional should consult others who have more insight into the culture so that alternatives may be identified. Depending on the immediacy of the threat and the extent of danger, the health professional may need to obtain more immediate consultation from a supervisor or from other outside agencies. Before this step is taken, however, health professionals must be certain that the perception of harm is accurate and not simply a result of their own bias or lack of understanding of what the belief or practice actually encompasses. For instance, in some cultures, babies are carefully swaddled and kept in the swaddling for hours at a time. Although from a perspective that infants need to have full freedom of movement, the practice may seem appalling, if no harm has been shown from this practice, the health professional would hardly be justified in reporting the family for child abuse. The case would be different, of course, if a prenatal patient confided to the health professional that if the baby were not the right gender, it would be drowned at birth.

Health professionals should assess who the patient looks to for social support and advice. Again, rather than attempting to discredit these sources, the health professional should demonstrate understanding of their importance to the patient and include them when appropriate. If, for example, the person of authority and respect is an elder in the group, whether related or not, that person may have more influence on the degree to which the patient is willing to accept and follow treatment recommendations than has the health professional.

Although health professionals, especially if working predominately with one ethnic group, should strive to learn as much as possible about that group, each patient from the culture should be approached as an individual. Health professionals should avoid stereotyping and making assumptions about patients based on the norms of the group without first assessing the individual patient's values and beliefs. Individual variation within cultures exists. Health professionals should also remember that the term *normal* means average. It is a statistical phenomenon that may vary in different cultures. Normal is relative.

When communicating with patients from different cultures, health professionals should take into consideration the interaction of class, language, and cultural factors and their impact on verbal and nonverbal behavior. Health professionals should take care not to misinterpret patients' behaviors and to be aware of their own behavior and how patients respond. If, for example, every time the health professional moves close to the patient, the patient moves away, before making the assumption that the patient is unfriendly, the health professional should consider other reasons for the behavior, such as cultural definition of socially appropriate distance. Likewise, the health professional should avoid moving close if he or she observes that the patient's response is one of discomfort.

Health professionals should convey patient education instructions in a culturally appropriate manner. Some cultures may consider directives offensive. Other cultures may expect a more direct approach to health advice. Health professionals should be aware of the possible misinterpretation of examples or analogies and should use these with care. Abstract examples may be taken literally. Health professionals should also be aware that some words may not have correlates in all languages or may have a different meaning from the one intended. As much as possible, health professionals should attempt to be clear and concrete in instruction to avoid misunderstanding.

Health professionals should know when to be action oriented and when to work with patients toward achieving goals at a slower pace. Patients may not care about long-term effects but rather may have different priorities of what is important to them immediately. Helping patients from different cultures through situational problems and dealing with their priorities demonstrates respect, builds greater trust and rapport, and helps to ensure additional patient education interaction.

Above all, health professionals should be genuine. Health professionals should not be afraid to acknowledge unfamiliarity with a culture and should not be afraid to apologize for any *faux pas*. Statements such as "I have had little experience with people of your culture, but I would like it if you could help me learn," or "I didn't mean to offend you. Please allow me to try again," convey caring and concern and will be accepted by most people as such. Health professionals should not pretend to know about a culture unless they really do. A brief visit to a country is hardly sufficient for anyone to understand fully the traditions and nuances of that culture. The understanding is most likely at best superficial and prone to subjective interpretation of the experience. In addition, it negates the differences of different regions of the country, different subcultures, and education and economic variations. Statements such as, "I'm well aware of your customs in Mexico; I spent a week in Tijuana last summer," not only serve to discredit the health professional but may also be offensive.

Conducting patient education with patients from another culture can be challenging but also enriching for health professionals. The interaction offers not only the opportunity to help patients but an opportunity for health professionals to expand their own knowledge of other cultures.

8

Effective Communication of Health Advice to Enhance Patient Compliance

EXCHANGING INFORMATION

Effective patient education requires more than giving patients factual information or having them recite facts. To be effective, patient education must be based on patients' individual needs and given in a manner that facilitates their ability to carry out recommendations. This requires a degree of interpersonal skill and sensitivity from the health professional. Health professionals must be able to listen to, observe, and understand what patients are saying before they can give them information that will be most meaningful and best meet their individual needs.

Communication in patient education is a two-way process involving interchange between patient and health professional. It is a complex process that is essential to identifying patients' needs. It alters patient teaching to best meet those needs and help patients follow recommendations. Although it is vital to communicate information clearly in a way patients are most likely to comprehend and remember, health professionals' skills in patient interviewing are just as important. These include the ability to recognize patients' verbal and nonverbal cues, respond accurately and appropriately to patients' cues, and provide support and feedback. All are critical components in the patient education process. Such skills promote a sense of trust, which in turn promotes an open and honest relationship. Such a relationship is crucial if health professionals are to elicit accurate information from patients, encourage them to express concerns, and identify any misconceptions or misunderstandings they may have.

RELATIONSHIP SKILLS: BUILDING RAPPORT

The object of patient education is not only to help patients comprehend information but also to help them put the information to use in their daily

148

lives. This is most readily accomplished in the context of the relationship between patient and health professional. The quality of this relationship can have a significant impact on the outcome of treatment and on patients' ability and willingness to carry out recommendations. Although evidence suggests that one important factor in the relationship may be the professional's ability to communicate information effectively to patients about their condition and treatment, findings also indicate that the health professional's ability to establish rapport with patients may also be a factor.

Rapport, although difficult to define, is essential to establishing a good relationship between patients and health professionals. A part of rapport is health professionals' ability to make patients feel cared for and respected as individuals. The degree to which patients feel comfortable in sharing information about themselves, as well as their feelings and concerns, is determined to a great extent by health professionals' ability to communicate a caring, respectful attitude. Basic aspects of a relationship that facilitate open communication and rapport are acceptance, understanding, empathy, and trust. Although these terms have become platitudes for some, they are essential in building a relationship that can influence the effectiveness of patient education.

Acceptance and Understanding

Acceptance demonstrates respect for people regardless of their circumstances and placement of value on individuals simply because they are human. Acceptance of a person does not mean blind acceptance of all their behavior. For example, showing acceptance of a patient who has emphysema but continues to smoke heavily does not mean condoning the smoking behavior. It does mean continuing to respect and value the patient as a person.

Everyone appreciates being treated in a respectful way. Feeling that one is respected is an integral part of relationship building. Demonstration of respect facilitates communication and trust and is the first step in building rapport. When patients detect an attitude of indifference or disinterest displayed by health professionals they are less likely to engage in open communication.

Health professionals who show acceptance of patients are able to accept patients' views, although they may be different from their own, and exhibit a nonjudgmental attitude. A tolerant attitude by health professionals establishes open communication and enables patients to change. Consider the differences in the following remarks made by health professionals while conducting patient education. The patient in the example has liver damage and has been instructed to give up consumption of alcohol:

> *Patient:* I don't think I can function without being able to have a drink every now and then. Whenever I'm tense or depressed, alcohol has been the only thing that can help me keep going.
>
> *Health Professional A:* Alcohol isn't a way to solve problems. In your case, it'll only make your problems worse.

Health Professional B: So coping with some of your feelings is at times difficult for you.

The remark of Health Professional A is judgmental and demonstrates little empathy for the patient's feelings. Such a remark, rather than helping to establish a relationship for an effective educational encounter, will probably alienate the patient, making further successful educational interventions unlikely. The remark of Health Professional B, however, neither judges nor condones. The remark communicates that the health professional recognizes the patient's feelings and accepts them as such. Acceptance is not synonymous with approval; it does, however, establish an atmosphere in which patients can openly share their feelings and concerns. Lack of acceptance may cause patients to withhold information that could be of value to the health professional in developing the most effective education plan. Without a feeling of acceptance, patients may be reluctant to return for further patient education.

Health professionals must be able to communicate to patients not only acceptance but also understanding of them, their feelings, and their concerns. Understanding means the ability to grasp patients' perspectives and to interpret the meaning of their words and behavior accurately.

Before acceptance and understanding can be demonstrated, health professionals must first be attentive to what the patient is saying. Flipping through a chart or looking at other material while the patient is trying to describe their situation or express their concerns does little to build rapport. Likewise, even though health professionals may be able to repeat verbatim what the patient has said, such attention is superficial listening at best. Many patient cues may have been missed. Patients who sense a lack of genuine concern may also be reluctant to ask questions or express feelings. Patients want to know they have been given the health professional's full attention. This means listening to words and ideas as well as being aware of what patients may be expressing through their behavior. Not only the content of what is being said but also the feelings expressed along with it must be considered. Giving patients full attention during education activities helps demonstrate concern and caring for them as unique individuals. This alone can be helpful in communicating that the information given is important and can be of help.

Communicating Empathy

Failure to establish empathy can be a serious barrier to effective patient education. Empathy is the ability to view feelings from patients' perspectives and to communicate acceptance and understanding to patients. Health professionals communicate empathy by putting aside their own feelings and values, putting themselves in the patient's shoes, and seeing feelings and attitudes from the patient's point of view. Before beginning teaching, it may be helpful for professionals to pause and ask themselves: "How would I feel if I were in the patient's situation? If I were given these recommendations under the circumstances the patient is in, how might I feel? How might this affect my reaction to the recommendations?" Empathy must be an accurate understanding of the patient's perspective. The following example illustrates empathetic and nonempathetic responses.

Mrs. Vicker had just had a mastectomy. In preparation for Mrs. Vicker's discharge from the hospital, the nurse had begun to teach her exercises that had been prescribed to increase her range of motion, as well as how to change her own dressings. During a teaching session, Mrs. Vicker became tearful.

> *Mrs. Vicker:* I'm so ugly now. I'll never be the same. I'll never be able to function again as I did before, either as a wife or just in general. Sometimes I think it would have been better if I never would have consulted the doctor when I found the lump in my breast.
>
> *Nurse A:* Don't be silly. The mastectomy saved your life. Lots of women who have had mastectomies lead full, happy lives. There are so many things left for you to enjoy in this world. I think you're just feeling sorry for yourself. You should appreciate what you have.
>
> *Nurse B:* I know this isn't easy for you. You're pretty discouraged now, aren't you?

Nurse A's response not only shows rejection of Mrs. Vicker's feelings but shuts off further expression of concerns that may be important to effective patient education. Nurse B's response is empathetic. It demonstrates acceptance and understanding of Mrs. Vicker and encourages her to express her feelings more directly. It is important for health professionals to realize that an empathetic response does not involve giving advice or coming up with solutions. It merely communicates to patients that the health professional recognizes their feelings and accepts their expression of them.

The creation of a nonjudgmental atmosphere in the educational interaction is important in building rapport and, consequently, in creating effectiveness in patient education. A positive, noncritical attitude establishes a relationship that increases the probability that patients will be more honest in their responses to health professionals. If patients feel that acceptance is dependent on repeating what they feel the health professional wants to hear, rather than what is actually true, much valuable information is lost that could contribute significantly to the effectiveness of patient education.

Through exploration and discussion, health professionals can identify patients' needs and concerns. This step is crucial if health professionals are to work with patients to accomplish educational goals later. Before this point can be reached, a relationship built on understanding, acceptance, and honesty and communicated through accurate empathetic responses must be established.

Building Trust

Developing trust facilitates rapport as well as establishes credibility. Patients are less likely to follow instructions that they feel were not given with their best interests in mind or that they believe are inaccurate or inappropriate.

Part of trust comes from health professionals' ability to communicate genuine concern for patients. Part also comes from patients' beliefs that health professionals are competent in their skills and that they are approaching patients in a truthful, honest manner. Before patients can trust health professionals' recommendations, they must have some trust and confidence in health professionals themselves.

To some degree, trust is built into the relationship between patient and health professional by virtue of the health professional's expertise. This is communicated to patients by the health professionals' role, title, and academic and/or scientific degrees. Patients already have some expectations about health professionals' knowledge base by knowing, for example, the professional role they fill, such as physician, nurse, dietitian, or pharmacist. Although this can be an asset from some vantage points, health professionals cannot rely solely on their professional role to create trust in patient education interactions. Health professionals should be comfortable with patients and not hide behind learned roles and words. Although a professional demeanor must be maintained to establish credibility, the approach to patients should also be personal to establish trust.

The manner in which health professionals present information is critical in developing a sense of trust and confidence. If information is presented in an abrupt, matter-of-fact way without demonstrating sensitivity to patients' reactions, patients may be less likely to be convinced that the health professional has any knowledge of or concern for them as individuals. Health professionals who drone on with facts without considering the emotional impact of their statements stand to lose patients' cooperation as well as their trust no matter how well the information is organized.

Health professionals who seem unsure of the information they are presenting also risk losing credibility and trust. Consider the following statement: "I think this is the way Dr. Jacobs wanted you to take your medicine—or maybe it was two times a day rather than three—that's probably right, take it two times a day." The statement does little to instill confidence. The patient may doubt (and rightfully so) the accuracy of the instructions and consequently be reluctant to follow any of the instructions given. Chances are good that the patient will not be eager to seek further advice from the health professional or to seek answers to possible questions. In instances when health professionals do not know the answer or have information readily available, they should acknowledge to the patient that they do not know and offer to try to find the answer or the additional information requested.

To be effective in communicating information, health professionals must be confident that the information they are presenting is accurate. Professionals must also have a good understanding of the information they want the patient to learn. This, of course, necessitates health professionals' willingness to stay abreast of changes in health literature and to review and update their own knowledge base as needed.

Consistency of information given in patient education is also important to developing trust. Health professionals who contradict themselves in the presentation of information or who contradict information given by other health professionals also cause the patient to doubt which information is factual and which recommendations they should follow. Consistency of information given by one health professional or by several health professionals working with the same patient is important in building trust. The case of Mrs. Kramer, who had been given diet instructions from both the dietitian and the physician for her diabetes, is an example.

> *Dietitian:* I note from your chart that you enjoy having a glass of wine before dinner. I've incorporated that into your diet plan by taking away one of the other exchanges, so now you can still enjoy a glass of wine.

> *Mrs. Kramer:* But Dr. Gephardt said I was to avoid alcohol totally in any form because it could be very harmful to me because of my diabetes.

Mrs. Kramer is put in the position of not knowing who to believe and which instructions are correct. Communication between health professionals conducting patient education is crucial to provide consistency. Likewise, the health professional must make sure that information is consistent from one teaching session to another if credibility is to be maintained. The preceding situation might have been avoided had there been better communication between the dietitian and the physician. Neither appeared to have an understanding of what the other would tell the patient. Of course, patients can at times misinterpret information. Under the circumstances, the dietitian should clarify what the patient was actually told by the physician without disrupting the credibility of either of them. The dietitian may respond with a statement such as. "Certainly using alcohol in excess and without appropriate planning can be harmful. Although alcohol in small amounts can be incorporated into the diet plan, all patients are individuals and respond differently. Let me check with your physician and see what is best in your case."

In addition to credibility and consistency, one of the major variables in developing trust is honesty. Honesty is more than merely being truthful. It conveys a sense of openness between health professional and patient, and promotes confidence that the health professional is being genuine in the interaction with the patient.

In the case of Mrs. Squires, newly diagnosed as having diabetes, the nurse had spent several teaching sessions explaining the importance of controlling diabetes with accurate administration of insulin, as well as following the prescribed diet. Consider the effects of each of the following statements made by the nurse:

> *Mrs. Squires:* It sounds so easy when you talk about it all, but diabetes will still make a big difference in my life. We've always gone to a lot of parties and dinners, and I love sinfully rich desserts. We've lived that kind of life for so long. It's all going to be very difficult. Sometimes I wonder if it's all going to be worth it. I've known people who followed their diet and insulin instructions faithfully and still developed complications. I'll bet you wouldn't think all of this was so easy if you were going to have to do it.

Nurse A: The people you've mentioned were probably cheating on their diet and insulin all along and you just didn't know. If you value your life and your health, you'll follow the instructions. You'll just have to get your priorities right. If I were you, I wouldn't think twice about following the instructions to the line.

Nurse B: I know following these instructions won't be easy for you. I, too, would find it very difficult. And you're right, there are no guarantees that following all the instructions will mean you'll remain 100% complication-free. However, we do know that the better control maintained, the greater your chances of having fewer complications. Tell me a little more about what you feel will be the most difficult for you.

In her response, Nurse A lost credibility by denying the accuracy of the patient's observations without further exploration and was critical of Mrs. Squire's feelings. This response lessened the possibility that Mrs. Squires would express her feelings honestly with the nurse again. The blanket statement that the nurse would have no difficulty deciding what to do conveyed a sense of superiority over Mrs. Squires. This lessens the probability that Mrs. Squires will respond honestly or trust the nurse with her feelings in the future.

Nurse B's response was open and honest not only in acknowledging personal feelings that indeed the task of administering insulin and following a special diet was difficult but also by showing a willingness to explore Mrs. Squires' feelings further. The nurse demonstrated acceptance of the patient's concerns and reinforced her for expressing them. This increased the possibility that Mrs. Squires would feel comfortable expressing concerns in the future. Encouraging the patient to be honest in expressing her concerns created the opportunity to provide support for Mrs. Squires and to identify alternatives and compromises that may be possible to increase her compliance with the recommendations given.

Honesty must always be used with sensitivity and discretion. Truth dumping, which consists of the indiscriminate disclosure of facts without regard for a patient's feelings or the impact the information will have, is just as detrimental to the development of trust as being dishonest. Forming a social unit with the patient in which there is mutual caring and respect helps patients come to trust health professionals. This component may be one of the key elements in helping motivate patients to follow health advice.

NONVERBAL BEHAVIOR

Communication is the key component in effective patient education. Communication, however, consists of more than verbal exchange. Many messages are also conveyed by body movements, facial expressions, touch, eye contact, and tone of voice. Such nonverbal behaviors communicate the attitudes, beliefs, and emotions of both patient and health professional in subtle ways. Awareness of nonverbal cues can help the health professional to communicate more effectively so that both patient and health professional receive and interpret messages the way they were intended.

Patient Cues

Much information can be gained from patients' nonverbal cues during a teaching interaction. Cues may indicate the patient's emotional state, a lack of understanding, possible discomfort, or just that further information is needed.

Nonverbal cues help health professionals obtain a more accurate interpretation of patients' statements by linking their behavior to the words they speak. Noting patients' facial expressions as well as their words increases understanding of the meaning of their message. Nonverbal behavior also helps health professionals determine the most appropriate way of responding to a patient at a given time. For example, a different response would be required for a patient who appeared angry than for one who appeared sad.

Nonverbal cues from patients are available to health professionals throughout teaching interactions. How does the patient appear as the health professional enters the room? Is the patient's body posture relaxed or tense? Does the patient appear nervous or at ease? Does the patient's body posture or position change during the teaching session? Does the patient maintain eye contact with the health professional or look around the room or at the floor? Does the person avoid eye contact only when certain issues are discussed? Does the patient's facial expression appear pleasant or worried? Angry or bland? What changes occur in the patient's facial expression when various topics are discussed? Does the patient appear attentive or distracted? Does his or her facial expression indicate understanding or confusion? Disagreement or acceptance?

For observation of nonverbal behavior to be useful in the teaching interaction, the behavior must be interpreted correctly; however, no communication, verbal or nonverbal, has meaning out of context. For example, if the health professional notes that the patient has begun to fidget during a teaching session, it is difficult to know the meaning of the behavior without gathering further information about it. Fidgeting could mean that the patient is uncomfortable physically or uncomfortable with the content of the information being presented. Fidgeting might also mean that the patient is anxious to end the session because of time constraints.

Nonverbal cues alert health professionals only to the fact that some message is being delivered. Health professionals must then gather sufficient additional information to interpret the message correctly. Interpreting nonverbal cues without clarification may lead to ineffective patient education. If, for example, the health professional observes the patient fidgeting throughout the interaction and interprets the behavior as disinterest when the patient is actually physically uncomfortable, further teaching efforts may be abandoned rather than rescheduled for a time when the patient is more comfortable and, thus, more receptive. Such misinterpretation of cues might communicate to patients that the health professional is insensitive to their needs and thus interfere with building the rapport that can be crucial to future teaching interactions.

Noting how closely patients' nonverbal communication parallels their verbal responses can also give health professionals valuable information to facilitate effective patient education. If patients' nonverbal behavior appears to conflict with their verbal responses, health professionals have an indication that further clarification of the message is needed. For example, if a patient states that he or she will have no difficulty following the treatment regimen but frowns while making the statement, additional information about the response is needed before its meaning and that of the nonverbal behavior can be interpreted correctly. The frown may indicate a lack of understanding of the instructions. It may indicate that the patient disagrees with the treatment prescribed or that the patient will have some difficulty carrying out the recommendations. Without further clarification, the health professional cannot respond in a way that will contribute the most to effective patient education, either by giving additional information, negotiating aspects of the regimen, or helping the patient resolve problems that might interfere with following the instructions. A statement such as, "I notice you were frowning when you said you would have no difficulty following treatment," provides the opportunity for opening additional dialogue and, consequently, clarification of the meaning of the observed behavior.

Observation of nonverbal behavior is, of course, only one part of making communication effective. When nonverbal cues are observed, health professionals need to decide whether behavior should be clarified at the time or merely noted and added to the data already obtained.

Whether patients are confronted with health professionals' observations of cues immediately or observations are noted for future investigation depends on several things. To some extent, the timing of the confrontation depends on the relationship between the health professional and the patient. How and when the patient is approached also depend on the health professional's clinical judgment concerning the particular teaching situation.

In some instances, it may be better merely to note nonverbal behavior as a part of information to be followed up with additional observations. In others, failure to clarify the meaning of the nonverbal behavior when it occurs may be a substantial barrier to effective patient education.

At times, failure to clarify the meaning of nonverbal behavior is due to the health professionals' lack of knowledge of how to approach the patient. Clarification of nonverbal behavior should be done in a nonthreatening, nonaccusing way that communicates that the health professional has made an observation and is only trying to understand the patient and the meaning of the behavior. For example, when a patient is noted to fidget during the teaching interaction, the health professional may say, "You seem to be somewhat uncomfortable. Is there anything I can get for you, or would it be better to stop for today and to continue this teaching at a later time?" At this point the patient has the option either to deny discomfort or to go on to explain the behavior. If the patient chooses to deny discomfort and offers no explanation for the restlessness, the health professional may want to note the observation and look for cues that may give additional insight into the behavior. If the patient offers an explanation, such as, "I just can't sit in one spot too long because of my back. Could I just stand up and walk around a little before we go on?" or "My neighbor brought me to the clinic today, and she's been waiting for a long time. I hate to have her wait much longer," the health professional can then take appropriate action based on the additional information received.

Any communication has two frames of reference. In this case, the two belong to the patient and the health professional. Continuing the teaching interaction without noting or clarifying nonverbal messages, or interpreting nonverbal behavior without checking for its accuracy, can have a great impact on the extent to which patient teaching is effective.

Cues from the Health Professional

It is important for health professionals not only to understand patients and the meaning of their nonverbal behavior but also to understand themselves, their usual patterns of communication, and how these factors can influence the teaching interaction. Health professionals need to be aware of unintentional cues and messages they may be conveying to the patient through nonverbal communication.

Nonverbal behaviors of health professionals can be interpreted by patients in a variety of ways. Patients can interpret a hurried approach or poor eye contact as a lack of interest in them as people. Health professionals' projection of approachability may not only have an impact on patients' receptivity to information presented but may also be a factor in patients' willingness to express views honestly or to give the health professional the information needed to construct the most effective teaching plan.

The manner in which health professionals present information may also influence the degree to which patients carry out the recommendations given. If the health professional fidgets, appears tense or nervous, or seems to lack confidence while presenting information, patients may not take the information seriously or may question its credibility. Presenting information in a disinterested, routine way can also have negative effects. Patients may interpret the manner of presentation to mean that the health professional is not interested in them as individuals or has not considered their special problems and concerns. Patients may therefore not be willing to follow the recommendations and may take it upon themselves to modify the instructions as they feel best meets their needs.

Nonverbal cues such as eye contact, a relaxed body posture with no excess gesturing, and a warm and friendly manner communicate that the health professional is accepting of and interested in patients as persons and is considerate of their special needs. Showing attentiveness and a nonhurried approach also indicates a willingness to answer patients' questions. Asking patients whether they have any questions when their nonverbal behavior contradicts the stated willingness to answer them is unlikely to receive an honest response. Effective patient education is dependent on patients' ability to follow the regimen accurately. If they are unsure of how or why it is to be carried out, the possibility of their following the regimen accurately is decreased. If patients feel an openness to questions and a willingness by health professionals to answer them, however, doubts, a lack of understanding, or misunderstanding of the information presented can be identified. This type of information exchange affords health professionals an opportunity to correct any problems that may interfere with patients' willingness or ability to carry out the regimen.

Touch can also be of help in the patient teaching interaction. It can be used to convey acceptance, support, and caring to the patient. Touch can, of course, be overused. If health professionals use touch appropriately and with discretion, however, it can increase rapport and influence the success of patient teaching.

Touching takes many forms—from a simple handshake to a touch of the arm to an arm around the shoulder. How and when touch is used in patient education depends on the clinical judgment of health professionals as well as a number of other variables. It stands to reason that explaining why an antibiotic is prescribed for strep throat may not require touching to communicate reassurance, support, or acceptance to the extent that teaching a patient with a terminal illness may make use of it.

Beginning a teaching session by putting an arm around an individual is obviously not as appropriate as a handshake, especially if this is the first interaction between patient and health professional. In other instances, putting an arm around an individual after the patient has shared a particularly emotional bit of information does more to convey reassurance and acceptance than a handshake.

Other variables to be considered in the use of touch during patient education include the age difference between patient and health professional, the gender of each, and cultural differences that may exist between the two. Touch is perceived in different ways by people of different ages, gender, and cultures. From an awareness of variables mentioned in previous chapters, health professionals can increase their skill in determining the degree to which touch should be used in individual teaching encounters. It is important for health professionals to remember that touch, although at times helpful in effective patient education, can also be misinterpreted. Good judgment in the use of touch appropriate to the circumstances can be of great help in enhancing rapport between patient and health professional, thus facilitating the effectiveness of patient education.

RESPONDING TO PATIENTS' VERBAL CUES

Throughout the teaching interaction, whether during the initial stages of rapport building and data gathering, information transfer, or evaluation of teaching effectiveness, health professionals' responses to patients' verbal statements can facilitate or hinder the degree to which teaching goals are reached. Knowledge of a variety of available responses can be of value in making the teaching session as productive as possible.

Probing Responses

A probing response is an open-ended statement that attempts to obtain additional information from the patient. Although such responses may be used most frequently in the initial data-gathering stages of teaching, such responses are helpful whenever health professionals want to obtain additional information. In the initial stages of teaching, when health professionals want to assess patients' understandings or feelings about their conditions, examples of probing statements may be, "Tell me your understanding of your condition," or "I'm wondering if you've known anyone else with this condition and, if so, what your impressions have been."

Such statements encourage patients to express their views and are more productive than closed statements requiring a yes or no response, such as, "Do you understand your condition?" or "Have you known anyone else with this condition?" Such closed statements give health professionals very little additional information regardless of patient response and may discourage patients from elaborating. Probing statements may be especially valuable in the closing portion of teaching, when health professionals are attempting to evaluate the extent to which patients understand the information given. Closed statements such as, "Do you understand what you're supposed to do?" or "Are the instructions clear?" are likely to elicit an affirmative response regardless of patients' level of understanding. Patients may not wish to reveal that they do not understand and therefore may answer yes regardless of their understanding of the material presented.

In some instances, patients may feel that they do understand the material presented and what they are supposed to do when they actually have misinterpreted or misunderstood the advice given. A probing statement such as, "Just so I know that I've been clear in my instructions, could you tell me how you're to take your medicine," or "Could you briefly summarize for me what we've talked about today," gives health professionals far more information and provides the opportunity to correct misinformation or misunderstanding before the patient leaves the health facility.

Clarifying Responses

A clarifying statement facilitates correct understanding. Statements of clarification help health professionals make sure they are interpreting patients' verbal statements the way they were intended. Accurate perception of patients' verbal statements is important throughout the teaching interaction. Clarification of patients' statements can help determine, to a great extent, the direction teaching takes. If, for example, after receiving diet instructions, the patient says, "This diet will be almost impossible for me to follow," the health professional may clarify the patient's response with a statement such as, "Do you mean that you will have difficulty because of willpower or because of the life style and schedule you have?"

In assuming that the statement in the preceding example means that the patient has no willpower, the focus of teaching may be misdirected. The actual problem may be that the patient's schedule is such as to render it difficult to have three scheduled meals a day in the amounts specified. If this is the case, the focus of teaching should be directed toward suggestions that could help the patient follow the recommendations.

Reflecting Responses

A reflecting statement facilitates further communication by encouraging patients to elaborate on a statement already made. Reflecting statements can help health professionals gain more understanding of patients' concerns and perspectives, which can in turn facilitate the effectiveness of patient education.

For example, Mr. Abernathy was scheduled to be admitted to the hospital for an angiogram as well as other diagnostic procedures. A few days before admission, Mr. Abernathy visited the clinic, at which time the physician explained the procedure to him, helping him understand what to expect. As the visit with the physician was drawing to a close, Mr. Abernathy said, "I sure hope whoever does this test knows what they're doing. I'd sure hate to end up worse than I am now."

In response to Mr. Abernathy's statement, the physician may have made a reflecting statement, such as, "You're feeling anxious about this test," or "You're nervous about having the test performed." Such a statement would not only facilitate further communication but would also help identify additional information that may indicate the cause for Mr. Abernathy's concern. Was Mr. Abernathy's anxiety partly based on misunderstanding or lack of understanding of what had been said? Had he had previous negative experiences or known others who had negative experiences related to an angiogram? Identifying the patient's concerns and perspectives through reflecting statements helped the physician assess whether Mr. Abernathy needed additional information, clarification of information, or additional reassurance and support.

Statements that close the door on identification of the patient's additional teaching needs produce less than satisfactory results. Such a nonproductive response to Mr. Abernathy's statement might be the following:

> "Oh, hundreds of patients have this done every week with no problems. The persons doing the test are highly trained and well qualified for the job. It's a highly valuable technique for understanding just what exactly is causing your symptoms. You'll do fine."

It is unlikely that such a statement would elicit further insight into Mr. Abernathy's concerns. While at first glance the statement may appear to give further information and support, it may in actuality only indicate to Mr. Abernathy that the physician has little concern for his feelings. In addition, the statement produces a barrier to further communication and, consequently, to identification of further teaching needs.

Unless health professionals identify and perceive patients' true concerns, it is difficult to meet their needs. Unless patients' fears, concerns, and/or misunderstandings are accurately identified and addressed, there is a chance that these will take priority with the patient. The end result will be noncompliance.

Confronting Responses

A confronting response describes an observation of people's verbal or nonverbal behavior of which they may or may not be aware. Confrontation does not imply that health professionals take on an adversary role with patients. Rather, it implies that a statement is made that gives honest feedback about what health professionals perceive to be happening with the patient.

Confrontation should not make inferences about patients' motives for the observed behavior. It merely gives patients an opportunity to elaborate on or deny observations brought to their attention. For example, if a patient has canceled several appointments for teaching about hypertension at the last minute, a statement such as, "I see you've been canceling your appointments at the last minute. Obviously you're having difficulty accepting your condition," may not only be untrue but may actually serve to alienate the patient. A more positive use of confrontation in this situation may be a simple observation of fact, such as, "I see you've canceled several of your appointments."

Confrontation should not take the form of a formulated question such as, "Why are you uncomfortable?" Such a question also assumes that the health professional's interpretation of the observed behavior is correct and can put the patient on the defensive. Confrontation should not communicate hostility but should reflect sympathetic interest. An example of the use of confrontation is illustrated by the following case.

Mrs. James had been scheduled for a hysterectomy. She was seen at the physician's office before admission to the hospital for preoperative teaching and a history and physical. The physician began discussing the surgical procedure but noticed that Mrs. James appeared more quiet than usual, her eyes tearing at several points. Several times, the physician asked Mrs. James if she was all right or if anything was bothering her. Each time she responded that nothing was wrong. Toward the end of the teaching session, the physician decided to confront Mrs. James with his observations with the statement: "Although you say nothing is wrong, I see tears in your eyes." Mrs. James began to cry, stating that she feared that she would no longer be perceived as a woman by her husband.

By confronting Mrs. James with his observations, the physician gained information that could then be pursued. The confrontational statement made by the physician consisted of observations, rather than accusations such as, "You aren't telling me the truth. If nothing is wrong, why are you crying?"

If used excessively and inappropriately, confrontation—like other responses—loses its value. Used correctly, however, confrontation can facilitate patient responses that might give the health professional new insights to be used in patient teaching.

INITIATING PATIENT TEACHING

Patient education can take place in informal interactions or during more formal interactions in which patient education is the major purpose of the meeting. The initial approach to patient teaching may differ depending on the circumstances.

In situations in which teaching is a routine part of an interaction between patient and health professional, such as during a clinic visit or medical procedure, there is no reason to delimit the teaching portion of the interaction. Patient teaching under these circumstances becomes a normal part of the communication between patient and health professional.

In cases where patient education is the only purpose of the interaction, the approach to patient teaching may be different. If the health professional is unfamiliar with the patient, before initiating teaching, the health professional should offer an introduction defining his or her professional role and the purpose of the interaction.

When meeting new patients, health professionals should not make the assumption that patients prefer to be called by their first names. More appropriately, the health professional may give the patient the choice with a statement such as, "Would you prefer I call you Mrs. Smith or Jane?" Such a statement conveys regard for the patient as an individual, helping to build rapport.

When initiating the teaching interaction, health professionals may also put patients at ease through touch, asking how they feel or briefly engaging in some other pleasant form of conversation that communicates a personal interest. The following example illustrates the preceding points. The patient has been referred by a physician to a dietitian for special diet instruction. The greeting by the dietitian in initiating patient teaching follows:

> *Dietitian:* Hello, Mr. Jones (smiling and extending hand for handshake). I'm Miss Smith, the dietitian. Dr. Johnson has asked me to talk with you a little about your diet. (Miss Smith sits down.) Would you rather be called Mr. Jones or Don? (Patient responds.) I see from your chart that you have a little girl who is six. I have a niece her age. They sure have a lot of energy at that age, don't they?

In the statement, the dietitian has introduced herself and defined her professional role and why she is interacting with the patient. She has also offered a statement that communicates that she knows something about the patient as an individual and that serves to put the patient at ease before moving directly into the teaching to be conducted.

Communication is also enhanced if, when initiating patient teaching, health professionals establish comfort in the environment, such as providing adequate ventilation or a quiet area where there will be a minimum of distractions. In a physician's office, for example, the physician may say something like, "I wanted to talk with you in a little more detail about your blood pressure, but it's really stuffy in this examining room. Why don't we go to my office where it's a little more comfortable?"

The main thrust of the initial interaction in patient teaching is to gather data, make an educational diagnosis, and build rapport. Part of this time can also be used to identify patients' current knowledge and/or attitudes about their condition or treatment by encouraging them to express their views or knowledge. This step, whether teaching about acute or chronic disease, is important to efficiency and effectiveness in patient education. The following statements are examples of types of approaches health professionals might use to elicit this type of information:

> From our test results, it appears you have a urinary tract infection. Can you tell me a little bit about what you know about urinary tract infections?

> As you know, your diagnosis of emphysema has been confirmed. I want to talk with you about emphysema in more detail, but first would you tell me a little about what you already know about emphysema?

Both statements give health professionals an opportunity to determine the patient's level of understanding about the condition, avoiding possible redundancy in teaching. Such statements help health professionals discover any misinformation or misperceptions patients may have, so that those may be addressed. This approach also helps build rapport by letting patients know that the health professional is concerned about what they think about their condition.

ESTABLISHING GOALS FOR COMMUNICATION

The content of patient education depends on the needs and interests of the particular patient, the circumstances under which the teaching is taking place, and the goals to be accomplished. Although health professionals may feel that patients should be as well informed as possible in all areas of their health and health care, it is important to establish realistic goals and to assess the feasibility of meeting those goals.

For example, it is doubtful that health professionals could expect to be successful in patient education if the goal is to eliminate smoking in a 25-year-old patient who smokes two packs of cigarettes a day, has no symptoms, and has no desire to quit smoking. Considering the lack of insight into the patient's reasons for smoking and knowledge of how difficult it is to change such behaviors, a more realistic goal under these circumstances might be to increase the patient's awareness of the hazards of smoking and to work toward motivating the patient to cut down the number of cigarettes smoked each day.

Determining goals for patient education does not have to be difficult if health professionals take the time to ask themselves, "What do I want the patient to be able to do as a result of this instruction?" From this question, the content of patient teaching can also be determined if health professionals ask themselves, "What information does the patient need to carry out the instructions?" These two questions will yield different answers for different patients with various disease conditions. Different goals and content obviously are required for teaching patients with acute conditions or chronic conditions or for teaching people about health promotion. In any teaching situation, short-term or long-term goals may be established.

For example, when teaching a patient about medication prescribed for a urinary tract infection, short-term goals might be the following:

• The prescription will be filled.
• The patient will take the medication as prescribed.

Once these goals have been identified, the health professional might ask, "What information does the patient need to know to accomplish these goals?" Answers might be

• the name and type of medication
• the length of time the medication is to be taken
• why it is important to take the medication as directed
• what the patient should expect from the medication (such as discoloration of urine or potential side effects of the medication)
• any special action the patient should take (stop the medication and call the physician if rash occurs, etc.)

Without the information the health professional has identified by asking the question, "What does the patient need to know to accomplish the goals?" the patient may not get the prescription filled because he or she doesn't understand why the medication is important. The patient may not take the medication for its full course or may discontinue it as soon as symptoms subside. He or she may discontinue taking the medication without consulting the physician if side effects occur.

The same teaching interaction could also identify long-term goals. One long-term goal that the health professional may establish in the example of urinary tract infection might be, "The patient will decrease the frequency of reoccurrence of urinary tract infections." To accomplish this goal, the health professional may determine that the patient needs to know ways to prevent urinary tract infection from occurring, such as good hygiene or increasing fluid intake.

Short- and long-term goals may also be established for teaching about chronic conditions or health promotion. Because teaching about chronic disease may involve much more complex information, as well as being affected by patient reactions to the condition, short-term goals may be thought of as building blocks for each teaching session, on which the accomplishment of long-term goals can be based. In teaching patients with diabetes how to inject insulin, short-term goals might be directed toward teaching them to draw up the correct insulin dose and then inject it. The long-term goal may be to render them independently able to manage their own insulin injection accurately at home on a daily basis.

Patient teaching for health promotion may also have long- and short-term goals. In the previous example of the 25-year-old patient who smokes two packs of cigarettes a day, the short-term goal may be to increase the patient's awareness of the hazards of smoking. However, the long-term goal may be to motivate the patient to cut down smoking.

When communicating health advice and determining goals for patient education, health professionals should recognize that although some goals can be accomplished in the immediate teaching session, others require days, weeks, or months of teaching before they can be reached. This is especially true when patient teaching involves the development of specific skills or a change of attitude on the part of the patient.

In setting goals for patient education, health professionals should establish priorities for the sequence of information. Information that is necessary to enable patients to function safely and adequately should be covered first. Goals that are dependent on the accomplishment of prior goals can be included at a later time. Goals should go from simple to complex, with complex goals being built on those that are less difficult.

When establishing goals for patient instruction, health professionals should be explicit. A goal such as, "For the patient to know about his condition," says little about the specific outcomes to be expected. Evaluation of the extent to which the goal is reached is consequently more difficult.

The more explicit health professionals can be in determining behavior patients are to demonstrate as a result of patient teaching, the more efficient and effective can be the teaching directed toward accomplishing that behavior.

COMMUNICATING INFORMATION

Although effective patient education is greatly dependent on the interpersonal skills of health professionals and their ability to ascertain patient needs, health professionals' ability to relay information in a clear, concise manner is also of major importance. Information alone is not sufficient for patient education to be effective, but obviously patients must have the facts before they are able to follow the recommendations given. Organizing and presenting the information in a clear way that patients can understand also requires skill by health professionals.

Approaches to Information Giving

Giving health advice to patients may be done on a formal or informal basis and may be direct or indirect. Varying approaches to patient education are appropriate at different times. The approach used is dependent on the circumstances.

Informal patient education, for example, may be done when patients' need for information is identified unexpectedly. For example, a preteenager being seen at an office visit for a sore throat asks, in passing, about menstruation. A need for information has been identified and may best be met when the need arises, rather than requiring the patient to return at a later time for a formal teaching session.

Informal patient education may also be done when health professionals observe an additional need for information. For example, this may be the case if, in observing a young mother at an office visit in which her 2-year-old is being seen for otitis media, the health professional notes that the child has not had a needed immunization. Although not directly related to the condition or treatment for which the child is being seen, a need for patient education regarding the importance of immunization is identified. The need can be addressed informally during the office visit. Other examples of informal patient education are giving patients explanations of what is being found during a physical examination, recommendations for treatment of a condition for which they have sought advice, or any other explanation that is part of their regular clinical encounter.

Informal patient education takes place during a regular clinical encounter when the sole purpose of the interaction between patient and health professional is not patient education. Although informal patient education is done spontaneously rather than at a predetermined time, the need for presentation of information in a clear, organized manner based on the patient's level of need should not be minimized.

Formal approaches to patient education consist of specific times set aside for the major purpose of communicating information to patients, or when the sole purpose of the interaction is patient education. Formal approaches may be used, for example, during preoperative teaching, when giving patients with chronic disease specific instructions about their condition or care, or when giving specific instructions to a hospitalized patient about home care.

A formal approach does not mean that health professionals lecture patients or that patients remain passive listeners. Even in formal approaches, patient education may take the form of discussion and information exchange between the two parties. Patient education should remain as much as possible a two-way process of communication, keeping patients actively involved.

Although presenting information to patients at a time they are ready to receive it and in amounts they are able to comprehend is desirable in most situations, a more direct approach may be necessary in certain situations. If, for example, a child is examined in the emergency room for a head injury, and the decision is made to send the child home for continued observation, a more direct approach to patient education may be desirable. Teaching parents signs and symptoms they should be aware of that may indicate complications of the head injury or teaching them what they should do if such symptoms are observed cannot be postponed. Information given to the parents in these circumstances is crucial. Even more critical is the health professional's assurance that the information has been understood.

An indirect approach to patient education may be used when time is not of the essence. In this case, information may be given in an easy, give-and-take method that combines information giving with discussion. This approach assists the health professional in involving patients and identifying their feelings. This approach might be used with a prenatal patient who can receive some patient teaching about infant care over several prenatal visits.

Avoiding Jargon

Health professionals must remember that they have special medical knowledge and a special medical vocabulary that the patient may not have. Medical jargon should be avoided. For instance, teaching patients with emphysema about their condition with an explanation such as, "Emphysema means basically that there is dilatation of the alveoli with inherent loss of elasticity," probably will have little meaning to many of them. Time spent giving patients information they cannot understand is not only an inefficient use of time but is also unlikely to reach the anticipated goal of patient education. A better explanation might be, "In the lung, there are tiny air sacs in which outside air and air that is inside your body, which is a waste product, are exchanged. In emphysema, these little air sacs become bigger and lose their ability to stretch."

Patient education can involve teaching patients medical terms as well. In this case, the lay term may be used with the medical term. Such might be the case in explaining a gastroscopy to a patient. The health professional may say, "During the procedure, we'll place a hollow tube down your food pipe or esophagus." This technique serves to acquaint patients with the medical terminology while still conveying the content of the message. It also helps health professionals avoid the feeling that by using simpler language they are talking down to patients.

The level of language used when explaining things is determined to some degree by the assessment of patient variables discussed in preceding chapters. It is also important for health professionals to recognize that patients' ability to form concepts may often be related to their level of language acquisition. Not only the words used but the content, too, may be determined by patients' use of language. Patients with relatively low levels of sophistication may not want or be able to conceptualize the same educational content as those with a greater level of sophistication.

The use of analogies can be helpful in explaining medical terms and concepts to patients. For instance, the heart may be described in terms of a pump; an aneurysm, in terms of a hose with a weakened area susceptible to different water pressures. Such analogies may help patients conceptualize information in a way that is more meaningful to them.

Health professionals should not make assumptions about patients' level of language and ability to conceptualize without further data gathering. Patients should not automatically be placed at a particular level of ability to understand without being considered as an individual. Just as it is faulty for health professionals to assume that patients of lower educational levels are unable to understand various explanations, so is it faulty to assume that those with a higher educational level or apparent levels of sophistication necessarily understand medical terminology. An example illustrating this point is the case of Mrs. Lindquist.

Mrs. Lindquist was working on a doctoral degree and had consulted her physician because of excessive uterine bleeding. Upon examination of Mrs. Lindquist, the physician reported that she had a fibroid tumor and that he felt surgery would be necessary. Assuming the patient understood the diagnosis, no further explanation of the condition was given other than routine preoperative teaching. The patient suffered a miserable week until surgery, thinking that any kind of tumor meant cancer.

This type of misunderstanding can be avoided by clarifying medical terms that may be misconstrued. Just as some patients may think that the word *tumor* is synonymous with the word *cancer*, numerous other terms may be misunderstood, such as *vaginal infection* and *gonorrhea*. When giving explanations, health professionals should clarify each term, saying something such as, "The tumor is benign, which means it isn't cancer," or "You have a vaginal infection, which should not be confused with a venereal disease like gonorrhea." In doing so, health professionals prevent misunderstanding by taking a few additional seconds of time.

Clarifying Perceptions

Health professionals should keep in mind that they and the patient may be from significantly different social backgrounds. Differences in social status or background may mean discrepancies in life experiences, values, attitudes, and perceptions. Health professionals and patients may perceive illness differently and may perceive information differently as well. The thought patterns of health professionals may be so different from those of the patient that there may be total unawareness of patients' faulty interpretation of information given. Such is the case of the patient in the following example.

Mr. Castillo was given a prescription for medication for hypertension. He received instructions about hypertension as well as instructions to take his medication once a day. At a follow-up visit, the physician discovered that Mr. Castillo had taken hardly any of the medication. When Mr. Castillo was asked why he had failed to follow the instructions, he stated that he thought he had been following them. He continued that he thought *hypertension*, although realizing that the term meant high blood pressure, also meant that he would feel extremely tense, which he interpreted to be the cause of his elevated blood pressure. Because he had not felt tense since his last appointment, he had seen no reason to take the medication.

Health professionals should, throughout teaching interactions, periodically check for understanding and interpretation of information presented. Patients should be encouraged to ask questions. Asking simple questions, such as, "Does this make sense to you?" or "Are there points I haven't made clear or that you would like to talk about some more?" give patients the opportunity to clarify any information of which they may be uncertain. Asking patients to summarize information is another means by which their understanding of the information presented can be assessed.

If health professionals keep in mind that the main goal of patient education is to communicate information in such a way that patients understand and are able to put it to use, the process becomes easier. This means that if slang terms are needed to get a point across, then they should be used. If the patient does not understand the term *urinate*, but rather uses the phrase *make water*, then using the patient's terminology is the most efficient way to communicate. Health professionals working in an area where slang terminology prevails may save themselves considerable time and create more effective and efficient communication in patient education if they take the time to learn some key slang words and phrases and the conceptualizations they denote. It obviously is just as important for the health professional to perceive accurately words that have meaning to the patient as it is for the patient to perceive accurately what is meant by medical terms used.

Being Specific

It is important to be as specific as possible when giving patients instructions. Vague instructions are not likely to be followed as accurately as those that are to the point. Comments such as, "When you go home after surgery, take it easy for a few weeks," can mean different things to different people. To the man who is used to heavy labor, mowing the lawn may seem like taking it easy, even though he uses a push mower. A housewife who has help with the laundry and cooking may believe that lifting her 20-pound child can also be a strain.

Several studies illustrate the importance of being specific with instructions. In one study, a diuretic was prescribed for water retention. More than half the patients for whom the medication was prescribed thought that its purpose was to help them retain water rather than eliminate it (Mazzullo et al. 1974). In the same study, an antibiotic was ordered every 6 hours. Only a small number of patients interpreted the instructions to mean every 6 hours around the clock. Patients interpreted the instructions to mean that they should take the pill every 6 hours while they were awake. Consequently, a number of patients for whom the medication was prescribed received only three-quarters of the amount of medication prescribed in a day's time.

The more specific health professionals are about directions, the more likely patients will be to carry them out accurately. Instead of saying, "Take it easy after surgery," health professionals may specify exactly what is meant by "take it easy." Specific instructions, such as, "Avoid lifting over 10 pounds," or "Avoid going up and down stairs," are more explicit in helping patients know exactly what is meant. With medication, health professionals may specify exact times the medication is to be taken, such as (in the case of every 6 hours) 8 A.M., 2 P.M., 8 P.M., and 2 A.M.; or health professionals may work with the patient in arranging times to suit their individual schedule, such as 6 A.M., 12 noon, 6 P.M., and 12 midnight.

Being specific also means that health professionals emphasize which instructions are most important to follow and elaborate on why recommendations are important. If, for example, a patient is being given two medications—one of which is to be taken as needed but the other to be taken in the treatment of a specific disease—vague instructions about the two medications may be confusing. As a result, the patient may take neither medication accurately. For example, if the physician prescribes an analgesic and an antibiotic for a 3-year-old patient with otitis media, it might be important to give specific instructions to the parents, such as the following:

> I am giving your child a prescription for two medications. One is to help relieve the symptoms, but the other is to treat the cause of the symptoms and fight the infection that is causing them. The first medication is for the symptoms. It's a local anesthetic that will reduce the pain. Fill the ear canal with the drops, and place a cotton plug in the ear canal. Repeat every 2 to 4 hours as necessary to relieve the pain. Usually after 2 days the symptoms will be gone, and you won't need to continue using this medication. The other medication is amoxicillin, an antibiotic that will fight the infection. Give your child one and a half measuring teaspoons by mouth every 8 hours around the clock so the organisms causing the symptoms are killed. You should continue using this medication even though your child may have no further symptoms, otherwise the organism causing the infection may not be killed, and the infection could become full-blown again.

The more specific health professionals can be in giving patients information, the more likely patients will be to have a clear understanding of what they are to do. Consequently, they will more likely be able to carry out the instructions accurately. Being specific takes little extra time if the health professional is aware of the variety of ways in which information may be misinterpreted by the patient. Time spent in making the instructions as specific as possible is time well spent.

HELPING PATIENTS REMEMBER INSTRUCTIONS

It is not enough for patients to understand instructions. They must also be able to remember them. Studies indicate that patient recall of information received during physician visits is generally no more than 50% (Ley 1972, McGrath 1999). The reason for such low rates of retention is thought to be linked to large amounts of information given to the patient at one time, the patient's high anxiety, the small amount of medical knowledge held by the patient, and the intellectual level of the patient.

In conducting patient education, health professionals should use simple but accurate words and should provide enough information so the patient can put it into perspective. Explanations should be limited in accord with the emotional and intellectual capacity of the patient. Health professionals should be aware that patients may suffer from information overload if they receive too much information at one time. Quantity of information is not always linked with patients' understanding. At times, an abundance of information can fatigue patients and interfere with their remembering.

Specific techniques can be used to help increase patients' ability to recall information. Patients may not remember all the information given, especially if it is complex. Discussion of the information under a topical outline may help them organize the information in their minds, thus providing a structure that can be more easily remembered. For example, the health professional may say, "I am first going to explain to you the treatment prescribed for your condition. Then I'll discuss what we expect the treatment to do, and finally I'll discuss how you are to carry out the treatment." If the information is complex, it may be divided into several sessions. For example, "Today I'm going to explain what diabetes is. Tomorrow we'll talk about your diet, and the next day we'll begin to talk about insulin injections." Specific instructions, such as teaching patients to administer their own insulin, may have to be broken down into smaller steps.

When patients are given a large amount of information at one time, they may have difficulty detecting which information is most crucial. Repetition of important instructions facilitates their ability to decipher what is most important as well as helping them to remember the information given. Important instructions may be repeated in a slightly different way, not only to increase retention but to clarify the instructions as well.

Another way to help patients remember instructions is by writing them down or using simple handouts. Although never meant to replace one-to-one communication between patient and health professional, written instructions may help patients remember instructions after they return home or may clarify instructions they cannot remember clearly. Pictures of simply drawn diagrams can also be used in patient teaching to illustrate points. The phrase, "A picture is worth a thousand words," is important to remember when teaching patients.

In all instances, verbal and written communications should complement each other. Health professionals should remember that the overuse of handouts can be detrimental to effective patient education. Although use of handouts alone may appear to be a way to save time, it can also be impersonal. Handouts are of little value if the patient does not understand them or does not read them. Further discussion of the use of handouts and other visual aids in patient education appears in Chapter 16.

Helping patients remember instructions should not be a difficult task if the health professional remembers

- organization of material
- clarity and specificity of instructions
- repetition of important points

- illustration or demonstration of points
- reinforcement through written instructions.

REFERENCES

Ley, P. 1972. Comprehension, memory and the success of communications with the patient. *Journal of Instructional Health Education* 10:23–29.

Mazzullo, J.M., 3rd, Lasagna, L., Griner, P.F. 1974. Variations in interpretation of prescription instructions. The need for improved prescribing habits. *Journal of the American Medical Association.* 227(8):929–931.

McGrath, J.M. 1999. Physicians' prescriptives on communicating prescription drug information. *Qualitative Health Research* 9(6):731–745.

Making the Patient a Partner in Patient Education

9

THE ART OF NEGOTIATION

Webster's New World Dictionary defines *negotiation* as "the process in which there is conferring, discussing, or bargaining to reach an agreement" (Guralnik 1978). In terms of patient interaction, negotiation is a somewhat foreign term to many health professionals who believe that patients who come for help or advice should and will automatically follow the recommendations given merely because they were offered. In such interactions, health professionals and patients are too often at odds, with health professionals making invalid assumptions about the patient's ability or willingness to follow the regimen. Patients, on the other hand, may withhold important information about their inability or unwillingness to follow the recommendations given or may never be given the opportunity to disclose such information.

The concept of negotiation in patient education may be met with varying degrees of acceptance by health professionals. Some may feel that negotiation interferes with what they consider to be the major goal of patient education: to offer information that will help patients improve or maintain health. If negotiation is included, some health professionals may fear that patients may not choose what is best for them. Given this point of view, then, it would seem that negotiation could make patient education less effective. The problem with this view, of course, is that it assumes health professionals know what is best for patients and their health. This may not be the case.

To make recommendations that patients are unable or unwilling to follow is inefficient and ineffective for both patient and health professional. Conflict exists if health professionals blindly advise patients, expecting them to follow the directions without understanding their feelings or identifying barriers to patient compliance. Negotiation identifies areas of agreement and disagreement and provides a forum for discussion of solutions. Although some health professionals may find the concept of negotiation alien, and not within the framework of health care to which they have grown accustomed, patient education can be only as effective as patients' ability to carry out recommendations. Negotiation can increase the likelihood that patients will be helped to find solutions to problems that may interfere with their following health advice.

CHANGE IN PATIENT STATUS

In the past, patients were viewed as passive recipients of health care (Ong et al. 1995). Generally, neither patients nor health professionals expected patients to play any active role in their health care, much less negotiate with the health professional about the recommendations given. It was expected by both patients and health professionals that health professionals were the ultimate authority by virtue of their expertise and would therefore make the final decision about what was best for patients (Stone 1979).

Often, information about their health and health care tended to be kept from patients by well-meaning health professionals, who rationalized this information deprivation with statements such as the following:

Patients don't have the ability to understand.

If patients had all the information, they would worry needlessly.

Patients really don't want to know all the information. That's why they're seeking advice from a health professional.

Some health professionals felt that their professional role would be diminished by sharing too much information with the patient. Other health professionals felt that keeping some mystery in their role was in itself therapeutic. Some felt that if patients were given too much information, they would lose respect for the health professional. Still other excuses for failing to give information ranged from, "Patients wouldn't remember anyway," to "Giving the patient information takes too much time."

When patients did challenge the lack of information given them by health professionals, they were frequently looked upon as "troublesome patients." The "good" patient was thought of as the one who sat passively, offering no criticism and asking few questions. Patients were frequently treated in a paternalistic way, with a benevolent attitude being displayed by health professionals connoting, "What you don't know won't hurt you." When occasionally patients did challenge a recommendation or ask a question, they were frequently met with comments such as, "Oh, don't worry about that. I have everything under control," or "I'm not able to disclose that information. You'll have to ask your physician."

As patients became more sophisticated and aware through the media and other information sources, faith in health professionals as the final authority diminished. The advent of self-help and patient information groups increased patients' desires for increased involvement in their care. Media publicity also decreased patients' view of health professionals as omnipotent guardians of their health; in some instances, it increased distrust of health professionals themselves.

At the same time, studies being conducted in patient compliance indicated that many formerly held beliefs about patients and about giving patients information about their condition and treatment were in error. Health professionals began to realize that if information were conveyed properly, patients could understand explanations and that, through various strategies, their recall of information could be increased. Contrary to previously held beliefs, patients did want more information about their condition and treatment (Beisecker and Beisecker 1990); rather than having more problems as a result of knowing what to expect, patients who were better informed had fewer problems (Stewart 1995). Also in contrast to earlier beliefs, patients—instead of losing respect for the health professional as a result of being given more information—actually were more satisfied with the care they received if adequate information was given (Dansky et al. 1996).

Patient teaching, if conducted efficiently, can save health professionals time by decreasing unnecessary phone calls and return visits. Withholding information can increase patients' anxiety rather than decrease it. Patients frequently misinterpret a lack of information as meaning that the truth is so negative that it cannot be shared with them. In addition, patients are much more anxious if they do not know what to expect, even if by being informed they know they can expect pain or discomfort.

Although increased information has many positive results, information alone is not associated with patient compliance (Blessing-Moore 1996). Although health professionals now tend to agree that patients should be informed, it has also become increasingly evident that health professionals—if they are to effect positive outcomes in patient compliance—must take another step. Patients need to feel they are not only recipients of information but also that they play an active part in their own health. Even though patients now receive more information, they still are often not actively engaged in the teaching process. It becomes increasingly obvious that effective patient teaching is a shared responsibility between patient and health professional.

MODELS OF PROFESSIONAL RELATIONSHIPS AND NEGOTIATION

Szasz and Hollender (1956) described three types of relationships that embrace models of interaction in the physician–patient relationship. These conceptual models are (1) activity–passivity, (2) guidance–cooperation, and (3) mutual participation. Although described a half a century ago, examples of these relationships can still be found in interactions between health professionals and patients today. These conceptual models can also be applied to patient teaching between patients and health professionals. The success of patient teaching may be determined to a great extent by the model of interaction health professionals use when conducting patient teaching.

Perhaps the oldest of the three models and the one most used in the past was the activity–passivity model. In this model, health professionals took an active role, assuming full responsibility for determining goals. Patients assumed a passive role, being recipients of care and having little input into the treatment or care being received. This model, if applied to patient education, might be reflected in the one-sided communication of information given by the health professional to the patient in which there is little or no consideration for the patient's feelings or his or her ability to follow the advice given. The teaching method would probably resemble a lecture approach, and the patient would have little opportunity to respond to the information presented. Although this model is the least desirable for effective patient education, under special circumstances it may be necessary, such as during an emergency when the patient or family must be given instructions quickly, and there is little opportunity or necessity for negotiation. Use of this model under less stressful circumstances is likely to achieve less than the desired results.

The second model, that of guidance–cooperation, is probably more familiar to health professionals. In this model, although patients are more active than in the previous model, most of the responsibility for goal setting still belongs to the health professional. This model implies that by virtue of health professionals' training, they have special knowledge and expertise that patients seek to receive help for their perceived needs. The model assumes that because patients are seeking help, they are also willing to cooperate with health professionals. Using this model, it may be assumed that the major goal for patient education is to help patients gain information so they will be able to follow recommendations given by health professionals. Because patients are in the position of seeking help, it may be assumed by health professionals that they are also willing to "cooperate" and "comply" with the recommendations given. Carried to a further extreme, the model may be one in which the major goal of patient education is to enforce patient compliance by trying to shape or mold patients' behavior into what health professionals believe will be best for the patient in the current situation.

The guidance–cooperation model places health professionals in a paternalistic role. Patients are *expected* to comply with the recommendations. There is little opportunity for patient input or disagreement with the recommendations made. Even though characteristics of patients may be taken into consideration when determining the manner in which instructions are given, and even though patients may be encouraged to be actively involved in the teaching process by asking questions or offering feedback about their level of comprehension, the possibility that health professionals might actually negotiate the recommendations with patients is not recognized. This model removes the patient from the decision-making process and from assuming responsibility for participating in decisions about recommendations. Although this model may at first glance seem more efficient, it probably results in less effective patient education by lessening the mutual participation between patient and health professional in the teaching relationship.

The last of the three models, the mutual participation model, might also be called the model of negotiation. This model assumes both patient and health professional to be equal members of the interaction. Patients and health professionals work together, sharing information and reaching a common goal of agreement in treatment. In patient education, patients become active participants in the process, forming a partnership with health professionals in decision making. The patient's own experiences provide clues for the most effective plan. Health professionals essentially are facilitators as well as educators, helping patients to help themselves. Such an approach does not mean that health professionals abandon what is medically sound advice, nor does it mean that persuasion in patient education in this model has no place. It does mean that health professionals base patient education on the information they gain from the patient and work with the patient in problem solving to best suit the patient's needs.

Each model of interaction between patient and health professional may be appropriate at different times. It would obviously be inappropriate to engage in a mutual participation model with a small child or under emergency circumstances, just as it would be inappropriate to engage in an activity–passivity model when discussing elective cosmetic surgery with a patient. The health professional's judgment and awareness of the use of different models in various teaching situations are of crucial importance. In most teaching situations, however, respecting the patients' needs and rights, working with patients in defining goals, and problem solving with patients will most likely result in effective patient education.

In the first two models, agreement between patient and health professional is taken for granted. Both models assume that patients do not know enough to dispute the word of health professionals. In both the first two models, it is assumed that health professionals know what is right and best for patients and that the major goal in teaching is to get patients to accept the professionals' views or plan with little alteration.

The model of mutual participation is characterized by high degrees of empathy and recognition of patients' individual needs. In this model, health professionals do not profess to know what is best for patients or all the variables patients must face in following recommendations. The model is based on negotiation—two-way communication of information and equality between patients and health professionals. Although health professionals and patients have different levels of knowledge (i.e., medical knowledge of health professionals and knowledge by patients of their own psychosocial needs), it is a combination of both that best enable the patients to follow the recommendations. If patients have no knowledge of what they are to do, recommendations cannot be followed. On the other hand, if health professionals have no knowledge of the problems and barriers patients experience in following recommendations, it is unlikely that the recommendations will be followed.

Even when a point of disagreement is reached, it is far better for health professionals to recognize areas of dissension and seek alterations that may still be within the framework of a therapeutic end than to be unaware of alterations in treatment the patient may establish independently, without the health professional's knowledge. Focusing on points on which patients and health professionals do agree and continuing to search for alternatives and solutions in areas where they disagree may result in increased compliance as well.

SHARED RESPONSIBILITY IN PATIENT EDUCATION

The mutual participation model, if used in patient education—although assigning the patient more responsibility in the patient–professional interaction—does not lessen the responsibility of health professionals; it merely alters the focus of the responsibility.

Patients' personal responsibility is the central theme of negotiation. The responsibility of health professionals, however, is to identify concerns, values, or problems that may interfere with patients' success in following recommendations. To do this, health professionals must build an atmosphere of trust in which patients feel comfortable.

Health professionals have the responsibility not only to communicate instructions in a way patients can understand but also to assess whether patients can follow the regimen. In patient education, therefore, health professionals must address issues relevant to the patients' situations that may be a barrier to carrying out recommendations. The mark of success in patient education is not patients' ability to regurgitate information but their ability to incorporate instructions into their daily lives, away from the direct supervision of health professionals. During patient education interactions, health professionals should identify patients' feelings about the information and recommendations being given and assess problems or limitations they may have in carrying out instructions. Only in this way can health professionals help patients discover alternatives and solutions that may increase the likelihood that they will be able to follow through with the plan. This is best accomplished when patients have had a part in formulating the plan.

Passive patients who have little to do with formulating the plan for treatment are also likely to feel less responsibility and commitment for carrying it out. If, as in the activity–passivity model, health professionals accept full responsibility for decisions about the recommendations patients are to follow, patients may also delegate full responsibility to the health professional for treatment failure, rather than examining the possibility that their own actions or lack of action contributed to the problem. In assigning major responsibility for positive treatment outcomes to health professionals, rather than accepting their role in carrying out recommendations, patients may place unrealistic demands and expectations on health professionals. If patients' expectations are then not met, the result may be anger and hostility toward health professionals. The point can be illustrated with the case of Mr. Morris.

At 32, Mr. Morris was obese and hypertensive. His physician, concerned about the elevated blood pressure, talked with him about hypertension. The physician used an active-passive model of interaction, being directive and parental in giving instructions. The physician's statement was as follows:

> I want to get your blood pressure down. In order to do this, I'm ordering this medication and a low-salt/low-calorie diet. The diet I'm prescribing will help you lose weight as well as help lower your blood pressure. I'm referring you to the dietitian for further explanation of the diet. I'll monitor how effective my plan for lowering your blood pressure has been by having you return for follow-up visits.

After several follow-up visits, it was noted that Mr. Morris had not lost weight, nor was his blood pressure any lower. Upon leaving the physician's office. Mr. Morris, exasperated, remarked to a friend the following:

> I've been spending all this money going to that doctor for my blood pressure, and still it's no better and I haven't lost an ounce. I don't think she knows what she's talking about. She just wants my money. I'm not going back if she can't seem to help me.

Mr. Morris did not accept responsibility for his role in contributing to the treatment failure. Even though he was placed on a low-salt/low-calorie diet, he frequently ate snack foods filled with salt and calories. Likewise, he sometimes forgot to take his medication and had neglected to have the prescription filled immediately because of its expense. Because the physician had accepted most of the responsibility for Mr. Morris's treatment, Mr. Morris placed most of the blame for treatment failure on her, expecting her to "heal" him. Had the physician taken a less dominant role, including Mr. Morris as an active participant in his own health care, the outcome might have been quite different.

Motivating patients to accept responsibility for their health and treatment begins by engaging them as active participants in the patient education interaction from the start. Whereas some patients may find it difficult to assume responsibility for their actions, health professionals may work toward this goal. With Mr. Morris, more active participation could have been solicited with a statement from the physician such as this:

> We're going to have to work together to get your blood pressure down. There are two things we need to do in order for that to happen. One is to work on helping you to reduce your weight and to decrease your salt intake, and the other is to have you take a medication to reduce your blood pressure. We'll talk together about how we can best work that out for you. I can prescribe these things, but obviously most of it will have to be up to you to follow the instructions at home. Let's talk about any problems you feel you may have in doing these things.

Such an approach assigns a portion of the responsibility to Mr. Morris and communicates to him that the physician feels that he is a responsible adult who has an active part in his health care and treatment.

Through patient education, health professionals not only communicate information but offer help and support to patients so that they may come to terms with problems and feelings they have in carrying out the instructions.

Health professionals can provide much help by exploring patients' feelings and concerns and by working with them in finding solutions. If patients say they are unable to follow the instructions, health professionals may focus on alternatives that can assist them. In the case of Mr. Morris, the dietitian and/or the physician might have reached some compromises on the diet, or perhaps a less expensive medication for hypertension could have been ordered. As it stood, Mr. Morris felt little commitment for carrying out the regimen and, consequently, did not do so.

Just as it is important for health professionals to include patients in the patient education process and to help them assume shared responsibility for outcomes, it is also important that the health professional realize that patient responsibility can be overemphasized and can have effects opposite from what is desired. If patients are made to feel that they have sole responsibility and control of their health, they may feel that the health professional has no expertise of value to them and may neglect further medical treatment totally. Secondly, if this view is held too strongly by the health professional, little will be done to help the patient overcome barriers in the way of following the regimen. The end result, of course, still is patient noncompliance.

In the previous example, an overwhelming amount of the burden would have been placed on Mr. Morris had he been told, "Whether you have a stroke or not because of your blood pressure is up to you." Such a statement would most likely decrease rapport between the physician and Mr. Morris. Another nonproductive attitude by the physician might be expressed, "I gave the advice and he didn't follow it, so there's nothing I can do." This approach leaves Mr. Morris with no alternatives. It also damages the relationship between the patient and the physician, which may be crucial in working out solutions so Mr. Morris can follow the advice given. A more productive statement might be, "Despite the diet and medication we talked about last time, there still is no weight loss. Can we try to figure out why? Can we talk about any problems you might have been having in following the regimen?"

Health professionals who are committed to effective patient education must also accept some of the responsibility for its outcome. Health professionals, of course, have the responsibility to communicate the information necessary to enable patients to understand the recommendations that are to be carried out. Just as important, however, is the health professional's responsibility to determine any obstacles or barriers that could hinder successful communication or prevent patients from following recommendations. This means that health professionals must also be aware of patients' limitations in accepting health advice or in following the regimen.

THE BOUNDARIES OF PATIENT EDUCATION

Just as patients' perspectives on illness might differ from the perspective of health professionals, so may there be differences in the way recommendations are perceived. Although health professionals may not perceive recommendations as being difficult or unreasonable to carry out, patients may view them in quite a different light.

As mentioned in previous chapters, patients' beliefs, values, and social influences may have significant impact on the extent to which they follow any given regimen. To conduct patient education without considering the impact of the recommendations on patients' lives is to discount their point of view. Values held by health professionals may not be the same as those held by patients. Recommendations that seem simple to health professionals may be overwhelming to patients when trying to implement them. Patient education outcomes held as ideal by health professionals may not be the outcomes that patients value.

It is not surprising that the degree to which patients are willing to follow recommended regimens is related somewhat to their perceptions of the cost associated with following instructions. Although cost in terms of financial considerations may certainly be an issue, cost may be measured in a variety of other ways as well. To patients, cost may also be measured in terms of pain and discomfort, lack of function, risk, or perceived loss of self-esteem. Cost is, of course, evaluated subjectively by patients and assessed in terms of their own lives and the impact that following or not following recommendations will have on them. This concept has relevance whether it is used in teaching patients about acute illness, chronic disease, or preventive practices. Not only must patients believe that treatment will be effective; they must also believe that the treatment or change in life style will be worth the cost.

Mr. Ueda's case illustrates this point. Mr. Ueda was a 58-year-old pharmacist who owned and operated two pharmacies in the small city in which he lived. He had had angina for several years, although he continued his work at full pace as much as possible until the condition became so incapacitating that bypass surgery was recommended. Mr. Ueda had an uneventful postoperative course and, before leaving the hospital, received a series of patient education sessions concerning recommendations for him upon returning home.

One of the recommendations given Mr. Ueda was that he cut down on his hours of work and, preferably, that he relinquish some of his responsibility at both pharmacies, taking on more of a supervisory role. Reasons for a slower pace were given, and Mr. Ueda appeared to understand the possible consequences of not cutting down his workload. Only a week after his discharge from the hospital, however, the physician received a worried call from Mr. Ueda's wife, stating that he had returned to nearly a full workload at both pharmacies. Obviously upset, she asked that at Mr. Ueda's next visit, the physician make a special effort to "talk some sense into him" so that he would be encouraged to follow recommendations. At the next visit, the physician began to talk with Mr. Ueda about his obvious noncompliance. Mr. Ueda replied that he had spent much time and effort developing the pharmacies and took much pride in being actively involved in their management. Although he fully understood what the additional strain of maintaining his current level of activity might mean, he was also aware of the personal loss he would experience if he would cut back on his involvement.

Although he was willing to follow the other recommendations given, the personal cost of decreasing his involvement with the pharmacies was, to him, not worth the benefits that the physician and Mr. Ueda's wife believed the decreased workload would bring. Mr. Ueda stated, "What would extra years of life mean to me if I were miserable sitting at home? If as a result of my work I have a shorter life, at least the time I have had will be well spent. I can only hope that if I die early as a result, that it will happen at work where I have invested so much of myself."

The physician, realizing that additional lecturing or informing Mr. Ueda of the reasons why the recommendations should be followed would be to no avail, began to think of ways that alterations could be reached. The physician negotiated with Mr. Ueda, arranging some rest periods during the day as well as talking with him about the possibility of working 6 days with shorter hours instead of 10 hours for 5 days. Through this process of negotiation, the physician and Mr. Ueda were able to reach a satisfactory plan that more closely approximated the goals of both. Without such negotiation, the additional time and effort spent in patient education would have been less than effective. The value that the physician and Mr. Ueda's wife placed on the possibility of longer life as a result of decreased activity was not shared by Mr. Ueda. Negotiating recommendations within the framework of Mr. Ueda's values increased the likelihood that Mr. Ueda would more closely adhere to the new recommendations.

WHEN NEGOTIATION FAILS

It appears that effective patient education is most likely the result of mutual participation, respect, and shared decision making between patients and health professionals. Patients' personality, values, attitudes, and life situation are all key components of the process. Likewise, the personality, attitudes, and values, as well as the skill, of health professionals in communicating health advice also affect the success of patient education.

The concept of negotiation is not to assure patients that they receive only what they want in terms of treatment recommendations. It is rather a process by which both patient and health professional engage in discussion to determine goals that can be acceptable to both and to establish what each is willing to compromise to reach the mutually established goals. Health professionals seek to offer advice they feel is professionally appropriate, whereas patients seek to reach goals that are consistent with their own expectations and priorities. Compromises in patient education are acceptable as long as both patient and health professional are able to maintain their own particular standards.

Although the concept of negotiation would seem the ideal solution in ensuring that patient education goals are reached, the reality of all human encounters is that conflict is bound to occur at some point. Obviously, the nature of the condition for which patient education is being conducted is also a major factor in the degree to which negotiated goals can be established. For instance, insulin-dependent diabetics who object to injecting themselves with insulin may have few alternatives that can be negotiated. Under emergency situations, time or circumstances will probably preclude negotiation.

There are times, however, when patients and health professionals may be unable to reach an acceptable compromise even when negotiation of alternatives would be possible. What happens when there appears to be a stalemate between patient and health professional? Several courses of action can be taken.

One course of action may be coercion, in which either the patient or the health professional or both be used to coerce the other into accepting each other's point of view. Coercion may be used to punish the other with the threat of rejection. The health professional may try to coerce the patient with a statement such as, "Miss Lorig, if you won't make a commitment to losing weight as we discussed, then it's useless to go on with these teaching sessions, and I won't see you anymore."

The patient's use of coercion of the health professional may also be an attempt to punish by rejection with such a statement as, "I really don't see why I can't be given more Valium for my symptoms. The relaxation exercises you've talked with me about will never work. If you won't see that I get more Valium, then I'll just go to someone else who will."

Coercion by health professionals alienates patients. If punishment in the form of rejection is also used, then health professionals lose the opportunity not only to supply future patient education but also to provide support in other aspects of recommendations of the treatment regimen that patients may be willing to follow.

A more productive means of handling the problem may be for the health professional to accept the fact that the patient is not following the regimen as recommended. The health professional can then work with the patient in areas of the regimen in which he or she is cooperating. The health professional can monitor the patient's progress and remain available to answer questions, offering alternatives when and if the patient is ready to accept them.

Such an approach does not mean that health professionals show approval of patients' noncompliant behavior. Health professionals may still be honest with patients about views of why the recommendations should be followed. By demonstrating acceptance of the patient as a person despite the noncompliance, however, and by keeping channels of communication open, the possibility for further patient education and negotiation is also kept open.

When patients demonstrate coercion and attempt rejection of the health professional as a way to get what they want, especially when the request goes against the health professional's judgments and standards, such demands need not necessarily be met. The health professional may explain why the demands cannot be met and continue to demonstrate a willingness to work with the patient despite areas of disagreement. Health professionals obviously cannot control patients' behavior or whether or not they will return. Health professionals can, however, continue to show respect and acceptance of patients as individuals with differing opinions. This approach may increase the probability that additional patient education can be accomplished in the future.

Another course of action that may be adopted by either patient or health professional when negotiation fails to reach a compromise is to ignore the problem. Patients, realizing that a stalemate has been reached, may merely resign themselves to agreeing outwardly with the health professional when in actuality they disagree with the recommendations and have little intention of following them. The health professional, uncomfortable with a situation in which there is conflict, may pretend that the conflict is resolved and discontinue further discussion. In additional encounters between patient and health professional, the charade may be maintained. The patient may not admit to not following advice. The health professional, to avoid further confrontation, may avoid asking the extent to which the patient is following the instructions given.

Avoidance of confrontation over conflicts in negotiation does not appear to be the most effective solution to the problem. When disagreements are reached and cannot be resolved, it is more effective for both patient and health professional to be open and honest about areas of disagreement, focusing on areas in which agreement can be reached. In so doing, health professionals are able to obtain an accurate picture of patients and their progress. Patients then have the option of returning to the health professional at a later time for advice and information without losing face.

The case of Mr. Perkins illustrates productive outcomes of the appropriate handling of occasions when negotiation between patient and health professional fails. Mr. Perkins had arteriosclerosis and subsequently was diagnosed as having an aortic aneurysm, which was repaired. The nurse practitioner working with Mr. Perkins' family doctor visited him while he still was in the hospital to begin discharge planning and to conduct patient teaching. Mr. Perkins had been a heavy smoker for many years, a behavior that was definitely contraindicated, especially because of the arteriosclerosis and the surgery he had experienced.

In addition to other instructions for discharge, the nurse discussed techniques that might be helpful to Mr. Perkins in stopping smoking. The nurse's approach was open and warm, and feedback from Mr. Perkins regarding his perceptions and feelings about the recommendations were frequently elicited by the nurse. With regard to the instructions to quit smoking, Mr. Perkins said, "I've been smoking for over 30 years. That isn't a habit that would be easy to break even if I wanted to."

The nurse responded with various attempts at negotiation—ranging from having Mr. Perkins cut down on the number of cigarettes smoked to, at the very least, switching to cigarettes that contained less tar and nicotine. Mr. Perkins, out of exasperation, finally said, "I enjoy smoking. I like the cigarettes I've smoked for 30 years, and I don't intend to stop."

The nurse, recognizing the futility of continuing to negotiate further, stated the following:

> Mr. Perkins, you know from our discussion why the advice to stop smoking is crucial. I can't, however, force you to stop and I can't tell you that it's okay if you don't. I'll continue to help you with other aspects of your treatment, though, and if you do change your mind about smoking, please contact me and we'll go over ways that that might be accomplished.

The nurse's attitude toward Mr. Perkins was one of cooperation and respect for his decision while still communicating that his choice was not within the standards of what was therapeutically thought best. At subsequent visits to the physician's office, the nurse practitioner continued to ask Mr. Perkins about his smoking as well as other aspects of his regimen, offering him support and encouragement for following the other instructions well while still leaving open the option to work with him to stop smoking.

Although Mr. Perkins may never stop smoking, because of the nurse's attitude many other goals for patient education were accomplished. Failure at negotiation does not mean that nothing more is to be accomplished. It means the health professional remains alert and aware of other issues in which positive outcomes might be effected for the patient.

FACILITATING PATIENT DECISION MAKING

A variety of factors determine how patients make decisions about the extent to which they follow health instructions. As with other decision-making processes, there may be conflict invoked in the patients' decisions of which instructions they are willing or able to follow. Following instructions may mean that the patient accepts some short-term losses or inconvenience in order to reach the long-term goals that compliance proposes to attain. In some instances, the short-term effects of following the treatment may not seem worth the effort taken to reach the long-term goals. Such might be the case of patients following recommendations for preventive health practices. The time and effort spent in exercising, dieting, or quitting smoking may not have immediate results that are reinforcing enough to motivate patients to continue, especially when the long-term goals seem nebulous at best. In terms of treatment regimens for various conditions, the "cure" may seem worse than the treatment itself, causing patients to discontinue treatment despite their knowledge of the consequences. This may be true in the instance of medications that have side effects or treatments that involve discomfort, it may also be true when treatment interferes with patients' other priorities. Such was the case of Mrs. O'Fallin.

Mrs. O'Fallin was pregnant with her fourth child and had suffered kidney damage in the past. She continued to have recurrent urinary tract infections, which were watched closely by the physician and treated aggressively to prevent the infection from affecting her kidneys. She had returned to her physician for a prenatal visit after having been seen by the physician for a urinary tract infection a week previously. At that time, she had been given a prescription for antibiotics along with instructions on how to take the medication and why taking the medication as directed was crucial. At the prenatal visit, the physician was shocked to learn that Mrs. O'Fallin had not had the prescription filled despite knowing the risk involved if recommendations were not followed.

Mrs. O'Fallin's explanation of how she reached her decision seemed to her quite simple. Her husband was temporarily laid off from his job. Their youngest child had been quite ill and required medication. Money was not available to fill both the prescriptions for Mrs. O'Fallin and their child. Mrs. O'Fallin, therefore, chose to risk her own health rather than risking the health of her child. The physician saw the situation in quite a different light. From the physician's standpoint, Mrs. O'Fallin's health was crucial to her unborn child as well as to the continuing care of her other children. Mrs. O'Fallin's decision not to follow recommendations was, however, based on her beliefs and priorities despite knowledge and explanation of the risk involved.

In making decisions about the extent to which instructions will be followed, patients can react in a variety of ways depending on how they balance the consequences of following or not following instructions.

- Patients may totally ignore the information given and continue in their current pattern of action or inaction despite the consequences to their health and well-being. Such might be the case with persons who continue to smoke heavily even though evidence links such activity to a variety of diseases, and warnings of the consequences of smoking are highly publicized.

- Patients may totally adopt the recommendations given without question, being complacent and passive in the process. In this situation, patients place the decision of what is best solely in the hands of the health professional giving them the advice and instruction, basing their strict adherence to the instructions on the faith that the health professional's advice is sound.

- Patients may appear to have decided to follow instructions but actually choose to follow only selected aspects of the recommendations, procrastinating about the rest or blaming others for their inability to follow all of them. Excuses such as, "My wife forgot to remind me to take my medication on vacation," or "I was waiting until I tie up a few loose ends at work to begin the treatment," may be examples of this process of decision making.

- Instructions given may seem so threatening or so impossible that patients, discounting the instructions, frantically search for what they consider easier solutions to their problems. Such may be the case of patients who, after receiving instructions, elect to seek more "natural" means in the form of health foods and other folk remedies instead.

- Patients weigh the pros and cons of the instructions given, ask questions, seek additional information, and make a decision of whether or not to follow the instructions based on their investigation and assimilation of the information gained. An example of this type of decision-making pattern may be determined by patients who, before deciding whether or not to have elective surgery, research the risks versus the gains, seek a second opinion, and base their decision on facts gathered.

The last pattern of decision making, except in emergencies when there is no time to gather additional facts, probably leads to the best decisions. Although health professionals cannot coerce patients into this form of decision making, they can do various things to facilitate the process.

First, when involved in patient education, health professionals should be realistic in relaying the consequences of following or not following the instructions. Reasons for following instructions should be based on facts regarding the probability that the outcome of following them will be positive, rather than making promises based on personal bias or conjecture. Such statements as, "If you'd quit smoking you'll live to be a hundred," are unrealistic in terms of the outcomes patients can expect if they follow instructions. A better statement, based on fact, may be, "There is considerable evidence supporting the view that smoking is linked to a variety of diseases and that, as a whole, persons who smoke less tend to have increased longevity." The second statement, based on fact, is more likely to be taken seriously by the patient than one that appears to have no supporting evidence.

When following or not following instructions seems critical to a patient's well-being, health professionals may be tempted to use threat and fear arousal in an attempt to motivate the patient to make the decision to adhere. Studies indicate, however, that as the degree of fear is increased, adherence to recommendations decreases (Leventhal 1971). If the consequences of not following instructions are blown out of proportion or are based more on emotionality than fact, the patient maybe less apt to take the instructions seriously. If, for example, the health professional says, "If you don't take your medication for your hypertension as directed, you're going to have a stroke and die," the patient only has to know of one other individual who has not complied with the same regimen and has had no serious consequences to discount the credibility of the statement.

Fear arousal can also raise patients' anxiety levels to a degree that they deny that the threat exists to protect themselves from increased anxiety. Under these circumstances, patients may react to the preceding statement by ignoring the health advice totally rather than admitting the seriousness of their condition.

Before patients can be motivated to action or before they can make an adequate decision about the extent to which they will follow the regimen, they must be given a realistic view of what following or not following the instructions will mean. A statement by the health professional, such as, "Just take these medications for your hypertension as directed," will do little to help patients in decision making. By receiving information based on fact, however, patients are better able to weigh the risks and benefits of following the instructions realistically and make a more rational decision on how closely they will adhere to them. Consider a statement such as, "Hypertension if uncontrolled by medication could lead to stroke. The purpose of the medication that has been prescribed is to help you to keep your blood pressure at a safe level." The statement communicates the seriousness of the condition and the importance of following the regimen without being unnecessarily alarmist in the warning.

The second way health professionals can help patients in decision making is by helping increase their awareness of their use of excuses and rationalizations and how these are interfering with following recommendations. In confronting patients with their excuses or rationalizations, health professionals should not actively accuse patients of making excuses but rather refute the excuses or rationalization with factual information.

As an example, a patient may say. "If I have a Pap smear and they find cancer, there is nothing they can do, anyway." Rather than telling the patient she is wrong or that she is being unreasonable, it is more productive for the health professional to counter with facts, such as the cure rate for cervical cancer when it is detected early.

Rather than attacking patients' excuses or rationalizations, through raising patients' awareness of their use health professionals can assist patients in acknowledging their tendency to rationalize. This technique helps patients explore excuses they are making so that more effective decision making may result.

Another way health professionals can help patients to make decisions effectively about following recommendations is to prepare them realistically for what they might expect from following or not following the regimen. The information should address both positive and negative effects that may result if recommendations are followed. Health professionals frequently refrain from sharing possible side effects of treatment or medication for fear that patients will be less likely to follow recommendations or that patients' knowledge of potential side effects will increase their chances of developing them.

Withholding such information often has effects opposite those intended. Patients who have not been forewarned about what to expect may be more likely to discontinue treatment if negative effects are experienced. If patients know what to anticipate, are reassured, and are told what to do if negative side effects occur, however, the likelihood that they will continue treatment is increased.

There is also little evidence to support the belief that patients who are informed about possible side effects are more likely to develop them. Realistic expectations can help patients cope more effectively with negative effects of following instructions as well as help them experience a more active sense of control.

Patients' verbal commitment to following negotiated instructions can be helpful in increasing the effectiveness of patient education. Many people feel uncomfortable going back on their word, especially when the commitment made to a particular action is made verbally in the presence of a respected and esteemed person. Such might be the case of a patient making a commitment to follow instructions in the presence of the health professional who has delivered them.

Such a commitment may be obtained by the health professional, saying something like, "Now that we've reached an agreement and appear to have worked out most of the problems that there seemed to be with regard to the instructions, tell me what exactly you are going to do when you go home." Commitment may also be more formalized in terms of establishing a contract between patient and health professional that outlines specifically what is expected.

Facilitation of decision making is helpful to health professionals in effective negotiation in patient education. Although patients have final control over whether or not instructions will be followed, guiding patients in effective decision making is an important aspect in patient education.

PATIENT CONTRACTING

Patient contracting is one method that can be used to help patients follow through with the recommendations given and to help them reach mutually accepted goals that have been decided upon through negotiation. Negotiation was previously described as discussing or bargaining to reach an agreement. Contracting is an active process in which patients and health professionals work together to establish specific measurable goals. Whereas negotiation establishes a general framework for the partnership, contracting specifies the particulars. Responsibility to reach the goal is shared rather than being one-sided. Both patient and health professional clearly know and agree on what can be realistically expected from each other.

The process of contracting is based on a theory of learning that specifies that behavior can be increased when there are positive consequences that closely follow performance of that behavior. Through contracting, patient education goals are made in measurable and observable terms. Through specific identification of what the patient is to do, the patient knows what to expect, the health professional is able to facilitate the meeting of specific goals by reinforcing behavior that contributes to meeting the goals, and there is an observable process through which patient progress can be monitored.

Contracting focuses on increasing patients' skills in carrying out recommendations, emphasizing patients' strengths rather than weaknesses. If certain instructions seem unmanageable or overwhelming, rather than dwelling on patients' inability to carry out recommendations or on the mammoth nature of the task, emphasis is placed on small parts of the task that the patient can accomplish. Breaking recommendations into small, attainable steps makes the plan more realistic for the patient to follow. Through feedback and monitoring of progress, health professionals are able to reinforce patients at each level of attainment, as well as noting problems patients may have with various aspects of the regimen. If problems occur at different points, the contract can be negotiated, and additional strategies that might help the patient attain the goal can be used. Rather than emphasizing patients' failures to comply with recommendations, contracting emphasizes what has been accomplished and continually searches for additional methods to help patients follow the recommendations that have been decided upon.

Just as with other approaches to effective patient education, contracting, in order to be effective, must be based on patient needs. This means that assessment of the patient and the current situation is essential if contracting is to be optimal. Establishing background data regarding the patient's current life style and activities enables health professionals to be aware of patient strengths that can be used to facilitate following instructions. In addition, health professionals are able to identify potential barriers that may need to be altered if the goals are to be reached. Gathering these types of background data with patients builds a framework from which they can make their own decisions. After mutual goals have been established, health professionals are then able to supply information patients want and need to reach the goals.

Helping Patients Identify Goals

Instructions that appear simple to implement to the health professional may seem overwhelming to the patient. Recommendations may seem unrealistic to patients, and thus many of them may be abandoned. The goal of health professionals may be to help patients carry out all the recommendations at once, without realizing that such an ambitious goal may actually sabotage the possibility of carrying out any of them. Patients, discouraged at what appears to be impossible goals, may selectively choose recommendations to follow or may give up the treatment regimen completely. A more realistic approach may be to identify with patients' short-term goals and strategies that can help them eventually reach the long-term goals. The case of Mr. Gunter is an example.

Mr. Gunter had rheumatoid arthritis. The physician had talked with him about the importance of energy conservation in treating the condition and specified the importance of alternating periods of work, activity, therapeutic exercise, and rest in order to avoid fatigue. The physician had asked that the nurse conduct more in-depth patient education with Mr. Gunter about his condition and treatment.

The nurse spent considerable time talking with Mr. Gunter about energy conservation, in addition to other aspects of treatment. The nurse began by helping Mr. Gunter establish some goals and priorities. The first step was to obtain background data concerning his daily activities and to help him to decide which of those activities were the most critical to him.

At first Mr. Gunter became frustrated at establishing any priorities of activity. He stated, "I can't change my job, and I don't want to be the only inactive one when I'm home with my family. All my activity is important. I just don't see how I'm ever going to be able to get these rest periods in." In talking with Mr. Gunter, the nurse discussed the possibility that everyone engages in a certain amount of activity because it is expected rather than actually examining whether or not the task is worth doing. In helping Mr. Gunter establish some priorities about activity, the nurse asked him to ask himself the following questions about his activities; "Does this task really need to be done? Why does it have to be done? What would happen if it were eliminated? What makes it so hard to think of giving up this task? Is this something that has to be done by me or could someone else help to do it?"

In establishing priorities, the nurse was careful to help Mr. Gunter not exclude tasks for his own enjoyment. Having energy left over to enjoy activities with his family because of rest periods established during the day became reward-ing in itself and reinforced Mr. Gunter to continue the regimen. By working with Mr. Gunter to establish how these rest periods could be accomplished at work, the physician's recommendations for energy conservation were broken down into small, manageable steps with strategies that allowed Mr. Gunter to reach the goals established.

At several points during the establishment of priorities, Mr. Gunter appeared reluctant to make the commitment to rest at specified periods. The nurse contin-ued negotiating and continued further exploration of Mr. Gunter's resistance by saying, "We don't seem to be able to agree on time throughout the day when you could rest. What do you think might make it easier for you to rest?" The statement prompted Mr. Gunter to relay his concerns about what fellow workers would think about his taking frequent rest periods. The nurse and Mr. Gunter were then able to talk about potential problems and to establish strategies for coping with them.

Goals in patient education may be numerous. Health professionals may not have the time or opportunity to address all the issues of complicated regimens at one time. It might be important to remember, however, that accomplishing short-term goals is a step toward accomplishing long-term goals. Those teaching situa-tions in which there will not be ongoing contact with the patient are better geared toward establishment of short-term, prioritized goals that can be reached. In cases where there will be ongoing, continued contact with the patient over time, such as in a clinic setting, short-term goals can be building blocks toward the end goal.

Recommendations that require complex life-style changes may be more dif-ficult for patients to accomplish than those requiring only simple, short-term changes. For example, following a strict, long-term diet regimen will probably be more difficult for patients to accomplish than taking one pill a day for 1 week. If health professionals are unaware of the differences in the level of difficulty and expect patients to have complete success with each of the recommendations, both patient and health professional may become disillusioned and disappointed if the patient fails. Establishing less complicated, short-term goals with which patients will have a better chance of success can enhance motivation as well as create additional opportunities for patient teaching. For instance, if a goal is to have a patient stop smoking cigarettes completely, a more realistic goal and point of negotiation might be to establish a maximum number of cigarettes he or she will smoke during the day rather than setting the goal of complete cessation too quickly—a goal that will probably be met with failure. Although both health pro-fessional and patient may agree on an ultimate end, the goal is more easily reached if it is tackled with small steps along the way.

Making Goals Observable

One of the difficulties in determining the effectiveness of patient teaching is often establishing what outcomes are expected and how those outcomes may actually be measured. Joint establishment of goals between patient and health professional is important, but making the goals specific is just as crucial. Contracting helps establish outcomes that are less vague, more observable, and consequently more easily measured by patient and health professional.

For example, in the previous case, one of the goals that Mr. Gunter and the nurse agreed on was that he would lie down in the lounge at work during coffee breaks in the morning and afternoon, as well as for 30 minutes during his lunch hour. Mr. Gunter was asked to keep a record of how often the goal was reached. Upon returning to the clinic, the nurse noted that Mr. Gunter frequently missed lying down during the lunch break. The nurse helped Mr. Gunter examine factors that interfered with his accomplishing that part of the regimen. The main problem appeared to be that another employee frequently rested in the lounge, leaving no space available for Mr. Gunter during his lunch hour. Rest periods during the coffee breaks appeared to present no problem.

The nurse discussed the possibility of staggering lunch times or of finding another place to rest, but neither of these approaches was feasible. The nurse was able to negotiate with Mr. Gunter, however, that on days when he was unable to rest at noon, he would lie down for 30 minutes upon returning home. At subsequent visits, it was found that this solution tended to be more satisfactory for Mr. Gunter, thus increasing his amount of rest time during the day. If the goal for education outcomes had only been based on Mr. Gunter's knowledge of the importance of rest, or had the goal only been that he have frequent rest periods during the day, neither patient nor health professional would have been able to determine efficiently the extent to which the instructions facilitated the outcome, nor would barriers that impeded reaching the goals have easily been identified and overcome.

Unless goals are clearly specified, health professionals cannot assume that terms mean the same thing to the patient as they do to them. In Mr. Gunter's case, instructions such as, "Take frequent rest periods throughout the day," may have meant sitting down once or twice during the day, whereas the nurse's concept of the instructions was something quite different.

If patients have difficulty attaining a goal, they may be encouraged to keep a diary in which they record events that occur in relation to their following instructions. In this way, the patient and health professional may be able to examine more closely the factors that interfere with the patient's progress and therefore discuss alternatives that would help the patient to attain the goal.

An example is the case of Mr. Henry, who was given dietary instructions in which specific recommendations were, "Avoid caffeinated beverages such as coffee, tea, and cola drinks," By keeping a diary of his activities during the day and the extent to which instructions were followed, Mr. Henry discovered that the major time for noncompliance occurred in the morning shortly after arriving at work. In more fully investigating the circumstances, he discovered that every morning when walking past the lounge to his office, he smelled the aroma of coffee that was served there. The aroma was sufficient stimulus for him to be tempted to have a cup of coffee. By identifying specific situations contributing to his noncompliance, Mr. Henry and the health professional were able to establish ways in which the problem could be dealt with. As one solution, Mr. Henry agreed to try walking to his office another way to avoid walking past the coffee room.

By making instructions specific and observable, goals can be counted, measured, and recorded. By keeping a diary, situations that may interfere with compliance can be described. Contracting can be used to establish a procedure in which both health professionals and patients know what the expectations are and to provide a mechanism for continual evaluation and feedback that can be useful in modifying instructions as need indicates.

Reinforcing Patient Behavior

A reinforcer is anything that is a positive consequence of behavior and increases the likelihood that the behavior will occur. In the case of patient education, it may seem that behavior that maintains or enhances patients' health or sense of well-being should in and of itself be positive enough in consequence to ensure that they will follow recommendations given. It is obvious, of course, that this is not the case. Not all patients place the same value on health itself. Likewise, some treatments, although having positive consequences on long-term health, may cause short-term discomfort and inconvenience, which decrease patient motivation to follow the regimen before the long-term reinforcement is reached.

Contracting uses reinforcement as a way to increase the likelihood that patients will follow instructions to reach agreed-upon goals. Because all persons do not come from the same environment or background, what is reinforcing for one individual may not be reinforcing for another. A significant part of successful contracting is to identify factors that can be used as reinforcement to help patients reach their goals. It is important that health professionals be aware of their own value judgments so as not to impose on patients those things the health professionals consider reinforcing. To work effectively, reinforcers have to be meaningful to patients. The issue is not to identify acceptable reinforcers but to find effective reinforcers unique to the individual that will help him or her reach a specified goal.

Reinforcers for patients may change over time as people's circumstances change. Health professionals using contracting in patient education therefore must be aware of the changes that occur and the consequences those changes have on patient behavior.

Reinforcers may involve praise and recognition, attention, or, in some instances, more tangible factors. The health professional and patient together may discuss what potential reinforcers are available. Some reinforcers may be a natural part of patients' daily lives. These can be used and capitalized on. For instance, a patient who is trying to lose weight and is praised by her husband every time another pound is lost probably has a more powerful reinforcer in her immediate environment than any number of tangible reinforcers the patient and health professional could come up with. In this instance, the contract between patient and health professional would consist of a specified number of pounds to be lost by the patient, perhaps weekly. Although the health professional might continue to reinforce the patient through praise for progress at each visit, the health professional, also aware of the potency of the husband's praise, might reinforce him as well for his positive contribution to the patient's success. Just as a spouse, friends, or other individuals in the patient's life can be positive reinforcers, they also have the potential to sabotage the patient's success. Health professionals who are aware of the importance of social reinforcers can consider these variables and include them as factors in the patient education plan.

In other situations, praise of the patient by the health professional may be reinforcing. In some instances, helping patients to determine ways they can reinforce their own behavior may be important. In the case of the patient on a diet, a reinforcer might be to buy a new article of clothing every time a specified number of pounds has been lost.

Reinforcement is most effective if applied in a consistent, systematic way. If, for example, the health professional praises a patient at one visit for losing weight but then neglects to give him or her praise on subsequent visits, the effect of the initial reinforcement may be lost.

It is also important for health professionals to recognize that removing unpleasant factors associated with certain behavior may also be reinforcing and therefore increase the likelihood that the patient will follow directions. If, for example, a patient experiences negative side effects from antihypertensive medication and an alternative medication is not feasible, the professional may be able to tell the patient that with sufficient weight loss, the medication could be discontinued. The potential of having the medication removed may in itself be reinforcing and increase the likelihood of the patient's losing weight.

Nearly anything can be a reinforcer. When negotiating a contract, it is important for the health professional to remember that, to be effective, reinforcers must be important to the patient. Reinforcers must also be accessible and consistently applied if they are to increase patients' ability to follow instructions. The best way to find reinforcers is to talk to and listen to the patient. Because the reinforcer must be important to the patient, the unilateral selection of reinforcers by health professionals is of little value.

Decreasing Patient Behavior

Although many instructions in patient education focus on helping patients do something, such as follow a diet or take their medication at regular intervals, sometimes instructions are directed toward helping them decrease behavior, such as smoking. It is important for health professionals to remember that it is easier to increase a behavior than to change a behavior that has become a daily part of the patient's life style.

To decrease behavior through contracting, it is again important that patients and health professionals establish baseline records of the frequency with which the behavior is being performed. Situations that surround the behavior when it occurs should also be identified. For many such activities, the behavior patients want to decrease may be so much a part of their daily routine that they are unaware that it is occurring. They may also be unaware of what stimulates the behavior to occur.

In smoking, for example, by record keeping patients may note that every time they have a cup of coffee, they also smoke a cigarette. They may find that even though they frequently do not drink the coffee, merely getting it is the stimulus to smoke a cigarette. One way to help the patient cut down on smoking, then, may be for the patient to avoid having coffee. By avoiding getting the coffee, the stimulus for a cigarette is decreased. Although in most cases, asking the patient to make two major changes in life style at one time may make the likelihood of success more difficult, in this case the behaviors are linked so closely, one serving as a cue for the other, that change of one necessitates change in the other. Without such record keeping, the patient may have been totally unaware of the correlation between the two behaviors or the frequency of having a cigarette. In recording the baseline data, it is also important that patients be aware of events that may be reinforcing them to continue the behavior. In the same example, although getting the coffee served as the stimulus to smoke, the reinforcer might be that a coworker, when seeing the patient light a cigarette, would come over to join him. Thus, a pleasant social encounter resulted from the patient lighting a cigarette. Removing the coffee as a cue for cigarette smoking as well as removing the pleasant consequences of smoking may help decrease the smoking behavior of the patient. Further help may be offered by helping the patient to find ways of having the same pleasant social interaction without smoking.

Obviously, the more complex the behavior the patient is trying to decrease, the more complicated are events surrounding the behavior; consequently, they are more difficult for the patient to record. To obtain a more complete pattern of behavior, it may be helpful to include family members in recording behaviors. Family members may observe circumstances surrounding the behavior of which the patient may be totally unaware. Including the family in contracting can help members understand how to provide reinforcers for the patient's success at decreasing behavior. Working with family members can also help them to realize what they may be doing unknowingly that makes it more difficult for the patient to decrease behavior.

An example of including family to assist patients to reach their goals may be illustrated by the same example of smoking used before. If a family member consistently offered the patient coffee at home without realizing that the gesture offered a cue to smoke, one step in helping the patient to decrease smoking would be to help that family member understand how he or she was contributing to the patient's behavior. On the other hand, again if the family member joined the patient upon noting him light a cigarette, the attention may serve as a reinforcer for smoking. The family member then may be encouraged to seek other situations in which to give the patient time and attention, thus avoiding reinforcing the patient upon smoking. It is important for the health professional to know that including the family in contracting should also be a patient's decision. A secret coalition between health professional and family is not the optimal way to help patients reach their goals or to build an atmosphere of mutual trust and respect.

One of the major difficulties in decreasing behavior is, of course, identifying all the reinforcers that encourage various behaviors to continue. In many instances, if reinforcers are identified, they may not all be controlled. Many reinforcers are subtle. It is important for health professionals to recognize that a variety of techniques may be needed to decrease behavior effectively. By keeping records, the patient and health professional can keep track of the degree to which behavior is decreased. If behavior is not decreased as a result of the current techniques being utilized, this is a clue that another strategy should be tried.

Helping Patients Remember with Contracting

Contracting helps patients and health professionals identify problems the patient may be having in following the instructions given in patient education. Although there may be many variables attached to patients' inability to follow instructions, one factor may simply be that they have difficulty remembering what they are to do. Health professionals can help patients find ways to help them remember what they are to do by providing cues for the desired behavior.

For example, there may be many reasons for patients not to keep a follow-up appointment. If the health professional finds that a major reason for the patient's consistent failure to keep appointments is the inability to remember the time, a series of strategies may be implemented. Examples of such strategies may be making a phone call to the patient the day before the appointment as a reminder, having the patient write the appointment on a calendar immediately upon returning home, or asking a family member to remind the patient of the appointment. No matter what the technique decided on, the strategy is designed to provide cues to the patient that will initiate the desired behavior.

The same strategy may be used to help patients remember to take medication or to follow a variety of other instructions, if, for example, the patient is to take a medication before meals but has difficulty remembering to take the medication before lunch at work, the health professional may help the patient to identify reminder cues. Cues might consist of attaching a reminder note to the money to be used to buy lunch or placing a cue elsewhere in the patient's environment to stimulate the desired action of taking the medication.

Family or friends can also help patients to remember what they are to do. Both patient and significant others must, however, express a willingness and interest in having this type of involvement. Before enlisting the help of family or friends, it is important for the health professional to be aware of the relationship between the significant others and the patient. Health professionals should avoid placing patients in a situation in which reminders become nagging rather than a positive stimulus to carry out the desired behavior. Health professionals must also recognize that although enlisting the help of family or friends can be beneficial, under other circumstances, it could foster a dependent relationship in which patients assume increasingly less responsibility for their own care. A careful evaluation of a patient's family circumstances is critical if the desired outcome is to be reached.

Considerations in the Use of Contracting

A variety of issues should be considered when using contracting to increase patient compliance. There are definite advantages to contracting. First, it is a positive approach that focuses on future actions that can be taken rather than dwelling on past failures or difficulties the patient had in following recommendations. Second, in contracting, problems or instructions are translated into specific behavior, which prevents inaccurate perceptions of what is to be done. Both health professionals and patients have the same perceptions of goals and behaviors. Expectations are clearly outlined. Because goals and behaviors are explicit, there is a system for monitoring the extent to which the desired behaviors are reached. There is also a means for identification of specific problems that may interfere with carrying out the instructions. Contracting requires health professionals to focus on patients' environments and ways in which the environment influences their ability to carry out instructions. The patient and health professional work together to determine goals and strategies by which goals can be reached.

Despite its many advantages in patient education, contracting also has some pitfalls. For contracting to work effectively, health professionals should have ongoing contact with patients during which progress may be monitored and problems, if they arise, identified and dealt with. In many health care settings, this is not feasible. Health professionals may have only one contact with the patient, limiting the extent to which ongoing monitoring, reinforcement, and negotiating can be conducted. This, however, does not eliminate the possibility that ongoing follow-up can be done.

Health professionals frequently neglect to recognize that contracting, like other forms of patient education, is a highly complex process involving detailed assessment of the patient and the environment. The process requires a commitment by the health professional to work with patients in reaching their goals. The application of contracting in a haphazard way can be more detrimental than helpful and can be perceived by patients as a cold and technical way of approaching their problem. To be effective, the health professional must work closely and consistently with the patient in establishing goals and reinforcing and monitoring their attainment.

Contracting may also be viewed by some as dealing so specifically with observable behavior that the feelings and emotions of the patient are ignored. To be effective, contracting must consider these aspects and how they are reflected in the patient behavior observed. Contracting must be specific to the individual and his or her particular circumstances rather than a series of the same strategies applied to all individuals in the same condition. The plan must remain flexible and must accommodate individual patient needs.

Contracting is not a means to coerce patients into compliance with recommendations. It is a technique by which health professionals work with patients to find ways that may help them follow instructions most effectively. Ideally, contracting gradually enhances the individual's own self-control and self-regulation, consequently increasing each person's responsibility for personal health.

Contracting alone may not be sufficient to reach all goals of patient education. It is a tool that can be used for some patients in a variety of teaching situations. Not all patients may be comfortable with this approach, nor will all health professionals be willing to adopt it. Constraints on both patient and health professional must be considered. If applied appropriately, with good judgment, and in the right circumstances, contracting and continued negotiation can be one means to increase the effectiveness of patient education.

REFERENCES

Beisecker, A., Beisecker, T. 1990. Patient information-seeking behaviors when communicating with doctors. *Medical Care* 28:19–28.

Blessing-Moore, J. 1996. Does asthma education change behavior? To know is not to do. *Chest* 109:9–19.

Dansky, K.H., Colbert, C.J., Irwin, P. 1996. Developing and using a patient satisfaction survey: a case study. *College Health* 45:83–88.

Guralnik, D.B. (Ed.). 1978. Webster's new world dictionary of the American language, 2nd college edition. Cleveland: William Collins and World Publishing Co., 952.

Leventhal, H. 1971. Fear appeals and persuasion: the differentiation of a motivational construct. *American Journal of Public Health* 61(6):1208–1224.

Ong, L.M., deHaes, J.C., Hoos, A.M., Lammes, E.B. 1995. Doctor-patient communication: a review of the literature. *Social Science Medicine* 40:903–918.

Stewart, M.A. 1995. Effective physician-patient communication and health outcomes: a review. *Canadian Medical Association Journal* 152:1423–33.

Stone, G.C. 1979. Patient compliance and the role of the expert. *Journal of Social Issues* 35(1):34–59.

Szasz, T.S. and Hollender, M.H. 1956. A contribution to the philosophy of medicine: the basic models of the doctor–patient relationship. *Archives of Internal Medicine* 97:585–592.

Illiteracy in Patient Education and Patient Compliance

10

TYPES OF ILLITERACY

Literacy, as defined in the United States, is described as "an individual's ability to read, write, and speak English, and compute and solve problems at levels of proficiency necessary to function on the job and in society, to achieve one's goals, and develop one's knowledge and potential" (National Literacy Act 1991). Literacy, by definition, is obviously more than knowing how to read. It is a complex concept, including a constellation of skills that, in addition to reading, impacts on patients' vocabulary development (Doak et al. 1996) and, consequently, their ability to think, organize, interpret, and analyze information (Lasater and Mehler 1998). Even though a patient possesses adequate reading skills, they may still be unable to grasp the meaning of words or to comprehend the concepts the words are meant to convey.

Reasons for illiteracy are numerous. Illiteracy may be related to a learning disability. *Learning disability* is a broadly defined term, consisting of many types. A learning disability may be related to genetic factors, or it may be caused by an injury to the central nervous system, such as with traumatic brain injury, stroke, meningitis, or dementia. Causes other than biologic factors may also be responsible for illiteracy. Individuals with inadequate educational preparation may also have inadequate vocabulary skills development with the resultant inability to read, comprehend, conceptualize, synthesize, or adequately formulate questions. Cultural factors may also be a cause for illiteracy. Individuals who do not speak the language of the country in which they are living are at a functional disadvantage. Whether they are recent immigrants or have lived in a country for many years, unless the language of the new country has been learned and mastered, individuals are functionally illiterate even though they may be literate in their native language.

ILLITERACY AS A DISABILITY

In a world of technologic advances and greater college attendance than ever before, it is difficult to believe that a high number of individuals lack the literacy skills needed to function effectively in society. Educational attainment is not, however, always an indication of an individual's literacy. This functional disability has impact on the person's ability to work and to enjoy many leisure activities that are taken for granted, such as reading a newspaper, a book, or a magazine, or reading to children or grandchildren. Illiteracy also interferes with the ability to read signs, directions, or other written material that is necessary for convenience and in some instances well-being.

This disability is often not identified in everyday life. People may go to great lengths to hide their inability to read or to understand the written word. Surprisingly, many of these individuals may be high school graduates and, in some instances, college graduates. Unfortunately, educational levels may not mean that individuals have attained a level of literacy competence.

The impact of illiteracy on the individual's health and health care has only recently been realized. Patients' ability to understand health information is a prerequisite to patient compliance (Lasater and Mehler 1998, Mayeaux et al. 1996). To maximize positive outcomes in health care, patients need to be able to read and understand instructions, prescriptions, informed consent, and other written documents to optimize their potential for following recommendations through their own informed choice. Too often, however, patients are given written materials, including informed consent forms, without consideration of whether or not they can read and/or comprehend them.

Ability or inability to read and understand health information also can affect the degree to which patients follow preventive health practices. With the increasing amount of health information available in magazines and newspapers, as well as brochures, pamphlets, books, and other written materials designed to help individuals be better informed about health and health care, it is easy to assume that everyone has the opportunity to be well informed. For those unable to read these materials, however, this is not the case.

Take the example of Mrs. Peterson, a concerned mother who wanted to do the best for her children but had not had them immunized. A single parent with no family, Mrs. Peterson had decided to move to a large city several hundred miles from her home. Before moving, she asked a friend who previously had lived in the city for the name of a clinic where she could receive health care for her children. Several months after moving to the city, Mrs. Peterson brought her children to the clinic recommended by her friend for a routine checkup. The nurses at the clinic discussed the importance of childhood immunizations with

Mrs. Peterson, and she seemed genuinely interested and concerned. They also told her of the availability of free immunizations at the local health department and advised her that she could call there for further information. When Mrs. Peterson returned to the clinic a few months later, the nurses discovered that she still had not obtained the immunizations for her children. They were shocked at what they perceived as Mrs. Peterson's lack of motivation to obtain the immunizations despite their encouragement to do so.

"I know Mrs. Peterson is having financial difficulty," one nurse exclaimed, "but it's not as if she has to pay for the immunizations. The announcement of their cost-free availability at the health department is posted all over the clinic waiting room and every examining room. She couldn't have helped but see them. Besides, we also included the notice along with the financial statement for her last visit, and she came in personally to pay that bill, so I know she saw the notice. I become so angry when parents are irresponsible."

The nurse's assumption, of course, was that Mrs. Peterson was able to read the notices. What the nurse did not know was that Mrs. Peterson was unable to read. Although she had asked several of her neighbors about the health department, its location, and the days immunizations may be available, they had said they were unsure. They suggested that she look up the number in the telephone book and call the Health Department directly. Not knowing her neighbors, she was embarrassed to tell them that she could not look up the number because she could not read. She was equally embarrassed to admit this to the nurses at the clinic, fearing that they may consider her unfit to care for her children. Obviously, she was also unable to read the announcements that had been posted.

Mrs. Peterson's example is only one of many similar situations that occur only too frequently in health care facilities everywhere. The extent of illiteracy in the general population is unknown. It is estimated that nearly 20% of the adult population in America has reading skills below the fifth-grade level (Davidhizar and Brownson 1999). Many more individuals are only marginally competent (Doak et al. 1996). This means many of the patient education materials available for patients about prevention or explanation of disease or illness and directions regarding treatment regimens are all of little benefit for this group. The impact of this fact on health and health care of individuals is immense.

Health professionals should always take the time to thoroughly explain aspects of illness and prescribed treatment to patients and should never depend on patient education materials alone. When information is complex, however, written patient education materials are used as supplemental material that patients can take home to read, review, and synthesize at their leisure. For those unable to read, of course, these materials are of little benefit. Too often, health professionals do not take the time to assess the degree to which patients can read and comprehend materials they are given.

Unless the problem is identified and adequately compensated for by the health professional, it can have potentially serious consequences. Take, for example, Mr. Kelly, who had been diagnosed as having diabetes. He had collapsed at work, was admitted to the hospital, and at that time had received his diagnosis. During his hospital stay as well as a few weeks after his discharge, he received patient education about diabetes and its management from the diabetes education team. He appeared to comprehend the information they presented and took home all the material they provided for review and more thorough study, as they suggested. Two months after his hospital discharge, he was admitted to the hospital emergency department in a diabetic coma. During the course of his hospitalization, a member of the diabetic education team approached Mr. Kelly to assess his understanding of the regimen and to provide any additional instruction that might be needed.

"Did the materials I gave you before provide enough information?" the diabetic educator asked. "Oh yes," replied Mr. Kelly. "There were pages and pages. There's a lot of information there."

The diabetic educator continued, "I was wondering what we might be able to do to help you to avoid going into a coma again. Do you have any idea of how this might have happened?"

"Well," said Mr. Kelly, "everything you told me when we talked before was so clear. I understood everything, really, but then after I got home I couldn't remember exactly what you said about everything so I did the best I could, but I guess that wasn't enough."

"We give people the materials you took home for that reason," said the diabetic educator. "Didn't they help?"

"I know they would have if I could have read them." replied Mr. Kelly. "The pictures are all real helpful, but you see, I never learned to read."

No one had thought to check Mr. Kelly's ability to read, understand, and use the materials he was given. As a result, the use of materials as a backup was futile.

Use of patient education materials as a substitute for direct information given by the health professional is always an ineffective way to teach patients. When patients have low literacy skills, the materials are even more ineffective. The key to effective patient education is to provide information to patients in a way that will best increase their understanding. Before that can be done, health professionals must be able to assess patient's strengths and weaknesses. Assessing patients' literacy skills is no exception.

MYTHS ABOUT ILLITERACY

Many myths and stereotypes surround beliefs about illiteracy. Just as myths and stereotypes interfere with adequate appraisal in social situations, so can they become a barrier to the health professional finding the best way to help patients learn. Because of preconceived views of illiteracy, health professionals may not even assess this important factor in interacting with patients.

The stereotypical view often held about people with low literacy skills is that they are from a lower socioeconomic level, use poor grammar, often are unemployed, and are uneducated. Although this may be the case in some instances, it is not true in many. The problem of illiteracy can be found in many types of individuals and is not limited to a specific group or educational or socioeconomic stratum (Lasater and Mehler 1998).

Another misconception about illiteracy held by health professionals at least until recently is that while it exists in many parts of the world, it does not exist in the United States, where education for children is mandated by law. As more research is conducted, this too has been demonstrated to be a myth with no basis in reality. Results from the 1993 National Adult Literacy Survey revealed the magnitude of the problem in this country (National Center for Education Statistics 1993). Almost half of the United States adult population has deficiencies in reading or computational skills (Ad Hoc Committee on Health Literacy for the Council on Scientific Affairs, American Medical Association 1999). Although some individuals drop out of the educational system because of frustration, illiteracy can be found in people from many educational levels.

A common belief among health professionals is that patients unable to read will let the health professional know. This most often is not the case (Weiss and Coyne 1997, Williams et al. 1995). If patients are unwilling to admit that they do not understand everything the health professional has said for fear that the health professional will see them as stupid, admitting that they are unable to understand or read the written word is even more difficult. There is considerable social stigma attached to the inability to read, particularly in a situation where the health professional may be viewed as educationally elite. Patients may go to great extremes to hide their illiteracy. Such statements as "I can't read this now, I forgot my glasses," or "I'd like to take this home to read it more thoroughly when I have the time and am not so preoccupied," can easily be overlooked as possible cues for further assessment of level of literacy.

Perhaps an even more destructive view by health professionals of illiteracy is that it is directly related to intelligence. This, of course, is also a myth with no basis in fact (Doak et al. 1996). Although some individuals with low literacy skills may have additional problems related to cognitive function, in many instances, individuals may have high intellectual skills in certain areas but are nonfunctional in reading.

ASSESSING PATIENTS' LITERACY SKILLS

Recognizing that illiteracy is a potential problem is the first step to assessment of literacy skills of patients. Because patients are not forthcoming about their inability to read or understand information, health professionals should assess the reading ability and understanding level of patients before conducting patient education. Health professionals should not assume that they will be able to recognize patients with poor literacy skills. Even when they suspect that patients may have difficulty reading or understanding, health professionals may feel uncomfortable or not know how to address the issue with the patient. As a result, the problem goes unresolved, and the patient does not receive the assistance needed to fully incorporate information provided in the patient education interaction.

Direct questioning of patients about their reading ability has been shown to be highly ineffective. Patients go to great lengths to hide their reading difficulties or when they do admit having difficulty reading, they often underreport the extent (Parikh et al. 1996). Merely asking patients whether they are able to understand the material is insufficient because most patients with limited literacy skills will most probably attempt to hide this deficiency (Weiss and Coyne 1997).

Screening for patient literacy can contribute to the effectiveness of patient education. Several instruments have been developed that can be used to assess patients' literacy. The Rapid Estimate of Adult Literacy in Medicine (REALM) is a word recognition test and was designed to be used with patients in health care settings (Davis et al. 1993). It is designed to assess adult patients' ability to read common medical words and can be administered in about 3 minutes. A second instrument, the Wide-Range Achievement Test–Revised (Jastak and Wilkinson 1993) is also a word recognition test and provides an approximate grade level of reading ability.

As in most areas of assessment of patients' strengths and weaknesses, the best method of assessment of degree of literacy involves observing, being alert to cues, and conducting sensitive and timely direct questioning. The task is made easier in an atmosphere of genuine concern, trust, and conveyance of a sincere desire to help. Take the example of John. John had been a patient of Dr. Marshall for almost a year after being referred to her for treatment of ulcerative colitis.

Dr. Marshall had taken considerable time teaching John about his condition and treatment and had given him a number of books and patient education materials to increase his understanding. John always gratefully took the materials and when returning the books Dr. Marshall had lent him, always made a point of telling her how much he appreciated her lending the books to him. Dr. Marshall never questioned John's ability to read until one day at a visit. She gave John information on a new treatment alternative, saying, "I'm still tied up with another patient, but I'd like you to read this while you're waiting so we can discuss it today before you leave."

Upon returning later to discuss the material with John, Dr. Marshall said, "Well, John, what do you think?"

"I'm not interested," John replied.

"Really, I'm surprised," Dr. Marshall said with astonishment. "What were your major objections?"

John refused to give any specifics saying only that he would take the material home to think about it. The next day, Dr. Marshall received an enthusiastic call from John saying that he would like an appointment with her as soon as possible to discuss beginning the new treatment. When he returned to Dr. Marshall's office, she asked John why he had suddenly changed his mind. John shrugged, dismissing the question; however, when Dr. Marshall gave John the questionnaire that was required to be filled out by all patients beginning the new treatment protocol, John threw it down saying, "I don't know why I have to do this."

Dr. Marshall proceeded to talk with John and finally said, "John, you know a lot of people in our country have difficulty reading. I wondered if maybe that applies to you. If it does, please let me help." John began to cry, telling Dr. Marshall of the complex ways he had learned to cover up his disability. Dr. Marshall made the appropriate referrals, and John not only began the new treatment but learned to read as well.

Patients' illiteracy can have profound effects on their health and health care. Given that the purpose of patient education is to communicate information to patients that they can use to promote their own health and well-being, it is important that health professionals spend time assessing patient skills in this area, make appropriate alterations when necessary, and, in some instances, as in the case of John, make referrals as necessary.

ASSESSING READABILITY OF MATERIALS

Patients read at different levels. Therefore, it is important for the health professional, before giving materials to a patient, to assess the grade reading level of written materials and make sure the readability level matches the patient's ability. Materials that are appropriate for someone reading at the tenth-grade level may not be appropriate for someone reading at the fifth-grade level or below. Both vocabulary and sentence structure influence readability of materials. To know which level may be best for a particular patient, the health professional should have some understanding of how to assess readability of materials to be used for patient education. Although there is no universally accepted way to assess the degree of difficulty of reading materials, there are a number of different formulas and tools that can be used. The range of rating may vary with the procedure used, but these formulas can provide at least cursory information related to readability. Perhaps one of the simplest and easiest formulas to use is the SMOG formula. The SMOG formula is one of a number of formulas used to establish readability. It is quick, easy to use, and predicts grade level difficulty within 1.5 grades 68% of the time. The procedure for using the SMOG is as follows (Doak et al. 1996):

1. Choose ten consecutive sentences near the beginning of the material to be reviewed.

2. Choose ten consecutive sentences from the middle and ten consecutive sentences from the end of the material.

3. In these 30 sentences, count the number of words containing three or more syllables, including repetitions.

4. Consider hyphenated words as one word. Proper nouns are also counted. Numerals and abbreviations should be counted as they would if the words

were written out. For instance, the numeral 25 consists of three syllables, *twenty* having two syllables and *five* having one syllable. The abbreviation *Dec.* for *December* consists of three syllables. When sentences are divided by a colon, each portion of the sentence is considered a separate sentence.

5. Compare the total number of words containing three or more syllables with the SMOG Conversion Table (Table 10-1).

The SMOG formula is only one of a number of tools available to measure readability. The SMOG is generally most useful when used for shorter materials. There are also a variety of computer software programs available to measure readability. It is important, however, that health professionals remember that, although patients' ability to read written material is important, even more important is their ability to comprehend the content and concepts contained within.

TEACHING PATIENTS WITH LOW LITERACY SKILLS

Some people have never learned to read. Other people may be able to read but may be unable to comprehend fully what is written. In the latter instance, the person may be able to read the words but unable to grasp the meaning of the words. How health professionals alter patient education depends on the specific situation at hand.

TABLE 10-1	SMOG Conversion Table
Word Count	**Grade Level**
0–2	4
3–6	5
7–12	6
13–20	7
21–30	8
31–42	9
43–56	10
57–72	11
73–90	12
91–110	13
111–132	14
133–156	15
157–182	16
183–210	17
211–240	18

Although a number of written patient education materials are available, patients with low literacy skills may not have the skills necessary to utilize the materials. Some patients are able to read simple material but not able to read more complex information. A brief pamphlet or instruction sheet outlining information may be easier for patients to assimilate than material that contains comprehensive explanations. Health professionals should assess written materials for readability in all instances and match the reading level with patients' needs. Organization of material is also important. Material should contain only essential information—that which is most important for the patient to know. For instance, although it may be helpful for a patient with diabetes to know the exact mechanism of the disease, it may be most important for them to know signs of diabetic coma and insulin shock and steps to take if either of them should occur. Those items most important for the patient to know should be listed first. The use of headings also helps patients to focus on key concepts of the message contained within the handout and presents patients with the opportunity to retrieve specific information easily for review. Underlining or highlighting in color may help draw patients' attention to important points they are to remember. Material should be arranged in logical, sequential steps of presentation.

Health professionals can select a number of commercially prepared patient education materials that are written at a level compatible with patients' ability. In some instances, it may be more practical for health professionals to develop their own materials. If this is the case, health professionals should remember to avoid jargon, use simple terms with few syllables, and use short sentences. The use of words should be consistent and the material contained within the pamphlet directly related to what the health professional wants the patient to be able to do after receiving the information. Low-literacy materials used for patient teaching should be written with large print for ease of reading.

In some instances, patients with limited literacy skills may need more time to read or to absorb material presented. Providing patient education materials to the patient before the teaching session so they may become familiar with the handouts may be helpful. In other instances, it may be helpful for the health professional to read the material aloud while the patient follows along.

Visual presentation of concepts can add to patients' ability to comprehend and remember material presented. The adage "a picture is worth a thousand words" is particularly true for patients with low literacy skills. Handouts with graphic representations to illustrate points should be used as much as possible. If pictures are used to convey patient education information, the health professional should ensure that the visual aids are not demeaning to the patient or that they do not treat the patient in a childlike manner. Visual aids are meant to enhance the patients' ability to learn, not to create an emotional barrier because of embarrassment.

When most patient education information must be communicated verbally, organization of information and presentation of information in a logical sequence is especially important. Health professionals should be sensitive to the patient's need to remember the material without benefit of written materials for review. Health professionals should attempt to avoid proceeding too rapidly and should present the most important information first, repeating it throughout the interaction. As much as possible, focus should be on what patients are expected to do rather than overloading patients with peripheral information. It may be beneficial to present smaller amounts of information over several sessions rather than overloading the patient with information in one setting. Information should be presented in logical segments using terms with which the patient is familiar. Analogies should be simple with familiar themes. When patient education involves a task, such as reading a thermometer or giving an injection, demonstrations may help patients achieve understanding. Likewise, having patients do a repeat demonstration enables health professionals to check patients' understanding of the procedure they are to perform.

Audiovisual aids can be used to supplement patient education information presented. Patients might be encouraged to return to review the materials as often as they like, or if practical, audiovisual materials may be loaned to the patient so they are able to review the material at home.

In all instances, the health professional should review and restate information presented, but when patients have low literacy skills, reviewing material is essential. Health professionals should verify patients' understanding of the information by having them confirm their understanding in their own words. Because of the patient's potential sensitivity to the problem of illiteracy, health professionals should take care that the patient is not treated in a condescending manner. Patients' understanding of information can be obtained with a simple statement such as: "Just so I can be sure I have been clear in my explanation, could you briefly summarize the information we've just discussed?" (or "How are you to take your medication?" or "What foods are you to avoid?" etc.).

The patient's response to the previous statement gives the health professional the opportunity to identify any misunderstanding and then to fill in or correct any information that was missed or misunderstood. Interaction and feedback from the patient should be encouraged frequently. When the patient has not understood or has misunderstood information, the health professional should attempt to present the information in a slightly different way, using the patient's frame of reference as much as possible.

Patients with low literacy skills are capable of learning and understanding patient education information if health professionals take time to present information in a way that best meets the patient's needs. Although these inter ventions may at first seem time consuming, the results in terms of increased effectiveness in patient education for patients with low literacy skills can well be worth the extra effort.

If the patient's literacy problem involves fluency and vocabulary, the health professional should be especially cautious not to use jargon and should make sure that the words used are actually conveying the intended message. For example, Ms. Wayne, the patient educator at the outpatient health facility, had been asked to give a presentation on cancer to a group of senior citizens. She said, "Any change in color of your stool is an important sign that you should report to your doctor." One participating in the group raised his hand and asked, "I haven't talked with my doctor yet, but I am remodeling my bathroom. Is one color better than the other?" Terms that are common to health professionals are not always familiar to patients. Health professionals should, as much as possible, use whatever terms best convey the message to the patient.

REFERENCES

Ad Hoc Committee on Health Literacy for the Council on Scientific Affairs, American Medical Association. 1999. Health literacy: report of the council on scientific affairs. *Journal of the American Medical Association* 281(6):552–557.

Davidhizar, R.E., Brownson, K. 1999. Literacy, cultural diversity, and client education. *Health Care Manager* 18:11.

Davis, T.C., Long, S.W., Jackson, R.H., Mayeaux, E.J., George, R.B., Murphy, P.W. 1993. Rapid estimate of adult literacy in medicine: a shortened screening instrument. *Family Medicine* 25:391.

Doak, C., Doak, L., Root, J. 1996. Teaching patients with low literacy skills, 2nd ed. Philadelphia: Lippincott.

Jastak, S., Wilkinson, G.S. 1993. Wide-range achievement test. Review 3. Wilmington, DE: Jastak Associates.

Lasater, L., Mehler, P.S. 1998. The illiterate patient: screening and management. *Hospital Practice* April 15:163–170.

Mayeaux, E.J., Murphy, P.W., Arnold, C., Jackson, R.H., Sentell, T. 1996. Improving patient education for patients with low literacy skills. *American Family Physician* 53(1):205–211.

National Center for Education Statistics. 1993. Adult literacy in America: a first look at the results of the national adult literacy survey, 2nd ed. Washington, DC: US Department of Education.

National Literacy Act. 1991. 20 USC 1201.

Parikh, N.S., Parker, R.M., Nurss, J.R., Baker, D.W., Williams, M.V. 1996. Shame and health literacy: the unspoken connection. *Patient Education and Counseling* 27:33–39.

Weiss, B.D., Coyne, C. 1997. Communicating with patients who cannot read. *New England Journal of Medicine* 4:272–273.

Williams, M.V., Parker, R.M., Baker, D.W., Parikh, N.S., Pitkin, K., Coates, W.C., Nurss, J.R. 1995. Inadequate functional health literacy among patients at two public hospitals. *Journal of the American Medical Association* 274:1677–1682.

11

Patient Education and Complementary and Alternative Medicine (CAM)

DEFINING COMPLEMENTARY AND ALTERNATIVE MEDICINE

Complementary and alternative medicine (CAM) consists of a number of therapies for maintaining health or treating disease and encompasses a wide range of practices that have roots in vastly different cultures as an integral part of healing. In today's world, the terms *complementary* or *alternative medicine* are usually used to described diverse products or practices that are outside of mainstream Western medical practice for promoting health and preventing or treating disease (Gevitz 1988, O'Conner 1995, Harpham 2001). Despite the differences in origin of various complementary and alternative practices, a common philosophy shared by most is that healing comes from within (Hufford 1997, Josefek 2000). The basic tenet of CAM is the relationship of health and healing to the harmony of the mind, body and spirit. In this context, complementary and alternative methods of treatment stress that the body possesses an intrinsic healing capacity. Rather than using external influences used in conventional medicine, such as drugs or surgery, CAM seeks to enhance the body's ability to fight disease and promote healing from within. Complementary and alternative therapies focus on the patient as a whole, are highly individualized, and are based on the compatibility of the method with the individual patient. The goal of most complementary and alternative therapies is to promote harmony of mind, body, and spirit.

CAM encompasses a wide range of products and practices, and often incorporates a broad spectrum of beliefs (Zollman and Vickers 2000). Complementary medicine and alternative medicine are sometimes described separately. Complementary medicine may be thought of as an approach used together with conventional Western medicine practices. For example, an individual who has chronic headaches may, in additional to using conventional medications for treatment, use biofeedback as a complementary form of therapy to reduce symptoms. Alternative medicine is sometimes thought of as therapies that replace conventional therapy. For example, an individual may elect to use applications of herbal preparations to remove a wart rather than having it surgically removed.

CAM practices range from use of chiropractors, naturopaths, massage therapists, spiritual healers, or folk healers to the self-administered use of herbal remedies, megavitamin therapy, or special diets. Below is a listing of categories of CAM procedures as outlined by the National Institutes of Health's National Center for Complementary and Alternative Medicine (1994).

- alternative medical systems such as homeopathic or naturopathic medicine
- mind/body or behavioral interventions such as yoga or meditation
- biologically-based therapies such as herbs or dietary supplements
- manipulative and body-based methods such as chiropractic manipulation or massage
- energy therapies including biofield therapies such as Reiki and therapeutic touch or bioelectromagnetic-based therapies such as pulsed fields or alternating current or direct current fields

GROWTH OF CAM USE

Complementary or alternative therapies were once viewed by conventional health professionals as countercultural. A common belief was that, although CAM was used by a fringe of the general patient population, CAM practices were not dominant in general. A study by Eisenberg and colleagues (1993) changed this view. Their study indicated that patient use of complementary and alternative therapies was much higher than previously believed. In a follow-up study, Eisenberg and colleagues (1998) found that 42% of adults were found to have used at least one alternative therapy during the previous year, with a significantly higher proportion of patients who saw an alternative medicine practitioner in 1997 than in 1990. There are some indications that the rate of use of CAM is actually greater than most studies indicate (Lazar and O'Conner 1997). As a generally increasing pattern of CAM use has been seen across a range of conditions, recognition of its impact on conventional, mainstream health care has generated significant interest from the conventional health care community.

Use of complementary and alternative therapies remains prevalent. (Owen et al. 2001). Expenditures for alternative forms of treatment have been estimated at more than $21 billion in 1997, an increase of 45% from 1990 to 1997 (Eisenberg et al. 1998). Growth of use of alternative methods by patients stimulated the formation of the National Institutes of Health's (NIH) Office of Alternative Medicine (OAM), which was established in 1993 to evaluate the safety and efficacy of alternative and complementary methods. The OAM was replaced by the National Center for Complementary and Alternative Medicine (NCCAM) under the 1999 Omnibus appropriations bill, enacted by Congress (Josefek 2000). The NCCAM has now grown to be an autonomous center within NIH with ability to fund projects directly (Dokken and Sydnor-Greenberg 2000).

WHO USES CAM: MYTHS AND MISCONCEPTIONS

Preconceived ideas often existed about types of patients most likely to use complementary or alternative methods of health care. It was assumed that patients using these methods were often poorly educated, naive, gullible, or from a lower socioeconomic status (Thompson 1990, Herbert 1997). A number of studies have shown these beliefs to be faulty. Patients more likely to use complementary or alternative therapies tend to be educated, be from a higher socioeconomic group, and are not confined to any one segment of society (Cassileth et al. 1984, Feldman 1990, Eisenberg et al. 1993, Astin 1998).

The assumption that use of CAM was more common in immigrants has also been dispelled. The assumption was that CAM usage was especially common in those groups who were recent immigrants and who might cling to traditional folk health practices of their culture, especially if they had limited financial resources or limited access to mainstream health care (Pachter 1993). Although CAM use is prevalent in this group, use appears to be more prevalent in immigrants who are better educated and in a higher socioeconomic status, not just in groups with limited financial means or limited health care access (Miller 1990).

A common belief held by many health professionals was that patients using conventional care would not use CAM. The converse thought was that patients who used CAM would use those methods solely for health maintenance or treatment of disease. Research has found both of these beliefs to be untrue. Patients have been found to use complementary and alternative therapies even though they also avail themselves to conventional health care resources (Spigelblatt et al. 1994, Elder et al. 1997, Eisenberg et al. 1998) and often seek health advice from conventional health providers as well as advice from alternative health providers at the same time (Spigelblatt et al. 1994, Applewhite 1995, Eisenberg 1998). In addition, patients have been found to often use both conventional or alternative therapies simultaneously for the same condition (Eisenberg et al. 1993).

The once-held view that patients with serious or terminal conditions were more likely to use CAM out of desperation to reverse the disease process has also been found to be inaccurate. Although use of complementary and alternative therapies is common among patients with chronic or end-stage conditions, many of these patients appear to use complementary or alternative methods for general health maintenance rather than as a desperate attempt to cure the disease (Cassileth et al. 1984, Anderson et al. 1993)

Health professionals have often been unaware of the number of patients using CAM and the number of complementary and alternative therapies available to patients. Even if health professionals are aware of CAM use for some medical conditions, there may be lack of awareness that patients may also use CAM for purposes unrelated to their medical condition, such as for general health maintenance. There may be the assumption that complementary or alternative methods used by patients is limited to one type. Types and numbers of complementary or alternative methods used by patients appear to vary widely. According to one study, 73 different types of alternative methods were found to be used by patients in a middle- to upper-middle-class community in the United States. (McQuire 1988). When the extent of CAM use by patients in mainstream health care is considered, the importance of exploration of use of complementary and alternative methods by patients as well as an understanding of how these practices impact patient care is obvious.

PATIENT DISCLOSURE ABOUT CAM USE

Despite widespread use of complementary or alternative methods, studies have shown that most patients do not consult nor inform health professionals about their complementary or alternative practices (Eisenberg et al. 1998, Planta et al. 2000). Although patients frequently express interest in discussing complementary or alternative methods with health professionals and prefer that health professionals take a more active role in using complementary or alternative strategies, they frequently are reluctant to ask questions or bring up the subject (Visser et al. 1992).

Lack of disclosure of CAM practices can be attributed to a variety of reasons. Patients may not approach the subject with health professionals for fear of having their question dismissed or the use of complementary or alternative methods ridiculed or censured. They may be concerned that by admitting to use of or interest in alternative methods they will be categorized as "crocks" or considered to be outside the normal realms of society. Patients may fear that by disclosing their use of unconventional therapies that the health professional will view them as ungrateful or disloyal. In some instances, they may not disclose use because they believe health professionals lack adequate knowledge about CAM and consequently would be unable to answer questions or provide guidance even if the subject were approached (Crigger 2000). In other cases, patients may not believe that CAM therapies are relevant to conventional medical care. Patients may not consider alternative methods as an integrated part of their health care or may be unaware of potential interactions between some alternative and conventional therapies. They may believe that CAM therapies are harmless and consequently insignificant to address with their conventional health professional. They may view conventional health professionals and complementary or alternative practitioners as separate entities, therefore reserving discussion of CAM practices for CAM practitioners.

Of course, another major reason patients do not discuss alternative therapies with health professionals may be because they are not asked. Despite increasing evidence that many more patients use complementary and alternative methods than once thought, many health professionals do not routinely ask patients whether they use CAM or include questions about use of complementary or alternative methods as part of routine health history. Studies have indicated that patients do not necessarily try to hide their use of complementary or alternative methods from health professionals. They have indicated willingness to disclose their use of CAM if the health professional asks (Planta et al. 2000). Including discussion about CAM in routine patient encounters would seem to be a means of facilitating communication and rapport between patient and health professional as well as contributing to general patient care.

ATTITUDES OF HEALTH PROFESSIONALS TOWARD CAM

Attitudes about complementary and alternative approaches to health care vary among health professionals (Berman et al. 1995, Ernst et al. 1995) Whereas some health professionals believe that some forms of complementary or alternative therapy may be effective (Astin 1998, Zollman and Vicker 1999), a number of other health professionals are skeptical or at times hostile to their use (Crigger 2000). Some health professionals may still view CAM as "outside the mainstream" of conventional health care and therefore consider it to be inappropriate. Others may object to complementary or alternative practices because many of these methods are unproven and without scientific evidence of effectiveness. Although concern about proven effectiveness may be valid, it should be noted that some widely used conventional therapies have not been proven, have later been shown to be ineffective in treatment of disease, or in some instances have been found to be harmful (Panush 2000). Likewise, some complimentary and alternative therapies have been shown to be effective in treatment of some conditions and symptoms (Williams et al. 2000).

Some health professionals may avoid discussion of CAM with patients because they lack adequate knowledge of these practices. Most health professionals have had little or no training about complementary or alternative practices. (Eisenberg et al. 1993, Morgan et al.1998). Only recently has training about CAM been included into the curriculum of some professional schools (Rampes et al. 1997). Consequently, health professionals may have limited knowledge about CAM, use of specific therapies, and potential benefits as well as risks of each. Because of inadequate information, health professionals may have negative views of CAM and use of recognized CAM practices.

Whether health professionals advocate or criticize use of complementary or alternative methods to treat disease or to promote health, the data indicate that patients are using them. To work more effectively with patients, it is important for health professionals to put misconceptions aside and learn how to talk with patients about alternative practices. Being aware of the extent of use of complementary and alternative methods by patients who are also using conventional health care resources is a first step. Learning how to approach patients about alternative method use requires an open and nonjudgmental attitude on the part of health professionals. Holding negative and dismissive attitudes toward alternative methods or attempting to coerce patients to abandon their use will not prevent use of these methods but rather tend to discourage patients from being forthcoming about complementary or alternative method use. Open and nonjudgemental questioning of patients may help increase health professionals knowledge of patient use of CAM and help health professionals and patients work together toward better health (Elder et al. 1997). Coming to understand patient motivations for use of alternative methods is of utmost importance in beginning to establish a dialogue with patients about alternative methods.

PATIENT MOTIVATION FOR USING CAM

Each patient brings individual beliefs, expectations, and fears to their experience with health and illness. Patients' decisions to use complementary or alternative practices for treatment of disease or health promotion, either exclusively or in conjunction with conventional health care, are complex. No one theory accounts for the increasing trend toward patient use of CAM for prevention, treatment, or cure of disease. Each patient has a unique notion of perceived vulnerability to disease, a personal family history which may contribute to health or disease, an acquired knowledge base from family, friends, or the media from which beliefs about health and disease are patterned, as well as their own subjective experience with symptoms or disease.

Although patients may at times make decisions to use CAM out of emotion rather than logic, health professionals should recognize that patients' decisions to use complementary or alternative methods are often based on the patient's own unique method of problem solving and rational decision making. If patients had success with an alternative method once, they reason that it will work again. They may not have taken into account the fact that their condition may have had self-limiting symptoms or that success with the alternative method the first time was coincidence. Take, for example, the following case:

Mrs. Schneider's 10-year-old daughter, Pamela, had been diagnosed with leukemia. Pamela underwent chemotherapy, but she experienced severe side effects from the treatment. Mrs. Schneider, distraught by her daughter's diagnosis as well as the side effects of the chemotherapy, was persuaded by her neighbor to try "metabolic therapy" for Pamela instead. Mrs. Schneider, anxious to have her daughter avoid the severe side effects that had been experienced with previous chemotherapy but also anxious to prevent further progression of the disease, took her neighbor's advice and began giving Pamela large doses of vitamins as well as other dietary supplements, rather than having her undergo additional chemotherapy. After a year, there was no evidence of progression of Pamela's disease even though she had not undergone additional chemotherapy. Mrs. Schneider was convinced that the vitamins and dietary supplements were responsible. She did not, however, consider that the initial chemotherapy may have been responsible and that Pamela would have gone into remission regardless of the vitamins and dietary supplements.

Patients may base their decision to use CAM from observations of the perceived success that others have experienced with the treatment. For example, Mr. Lindquist had become increasingly unable to engage in many activities he enjoyed, including hiking, because of osteoarthritis of his right knee. He consulted his physician, who recommended knee replacement. As much as Mr. Lindquist enjoyed hiking, he feared surgery more. He discussed his concerns about surgery and his frustration at the thought of having to give up hiking with a close friend. His friend told Mr. Lindquist that several years earlier he had been faced with the same type of situation, and rather than having surgery, he had opted to try an herbal remedy. The friend assured Mr. Lindquist that within a month of taking Pau d'arco, a South American Indian folk medicine, his knee problems vanished and he was able to continue all the activities he had enjoyed previously. Mr. Lindquist, delighted to receive from a trusted friend such a positive endorsement of a remedy that would help him avoid surgery but still enable him to continue his activities, chose to abandon the idea of surgery in favor of herbal remedy. He was unaware that his friend had actually only had a knee sprain rather than osteoarthritis.

In some instances, patients choose complementary or alternative methods because they have found traditional treatments to be ineffective in producing the desired outcome (Jensen 1990, Lazar and O'Conner 1997). When all conventional methods of treatment have been exhausted with no desired effect, patients may turn to complementary or alternative means. Take, for example, Mr. Gunther. He had experienced recurring shoulder pain, possibly the result of repetitive motion injury related to his job. Dr. Phelps prescribed medication to reduce inflammation and gave Mr. Gunther a referral to physical therapy for consultation. Mr. Gunther took the medication as prescribed, attended the physical therapy consultation, and performed exercises as recommended daily. During Mr. Gunther's routine physical exam several months later, Dr. Phelps asked him about his shoulder. Mr. Gunther disclosed that he had abandoned the prescribed medication as well as the prescribed exercise. He stated that he was now regularly going to see a chiropractor. When Dr. Phelps questioned Mr. Gunther about his reasons for abandoning the prescribed medical treatment he replied: "Well, I did everything that medical personnel told me to do and I still didn't get better, so I went to the chiropractor. I'm continuing to go to him because he's the only one who has been able to help me feel better."

Patients' choice to use alternative therapies may at times be the result of unrealistic expectations for control of symptoms or cure of disease. Health professionals may have neglected to give patients adequate information regarding the length of time after treatment in which patients could expect symptoms to subside, or they may have failed to specify that the purpose of treatment was to control symptoms rather than cure the disease. For example, Ms. Minjeta was seen by her physician because of symptoms of frequency and burning on urination. She consulted her physician, who, after confirming with urine culture that she had a urinary tract infection, prescribed an antibiotic. After 2 days of treatment, however, Ms. Minjeta stopped taking the antibiotic and began self-treatment with St. John's wort. When she confided in her neighbor, Mrs. Jones, who was a nurse, that she had abandoned the physician-prescribed treatment in favor of an herbal remedy, Mrs. Jones questioned her as to why. Ms. Minjeta responded, "I took the medicine for 2 days and I didn't get better so I stopped taking it. Why bother taking medicine when it doesn't work."

In many instances, conventional treatments still have little to offer with regard to curing disease and often are ineffective in controlling symptoms, particularly when chronic pain is associated (Lazar and O'Conner 1997). In choosing complementary or alternative treatments, patients may still be seeking the same effect (e.g., relief of symptoms) or cure they sought but did not receive with standard approaches. For example, Ms. Philbeck had been diagnosed with multiple sclerosis. Ms. Ellis, the nurse practitioner who had been following Ms. Philbeck's case, became concerned after several follow-up appointments were missed. She called Ms. Philbeck who told her plainly that she would no longer be seeking health care at the clinic. Instead she was seeing a spiritual healer and using crystals, as well as a number of other mineral substances because, in her words, "I want my condition to be cured. So-called modern medicine is still in the stone age regarding treatment of multiple sclerosis. When I keep coming to you I keep having exacerbations of my disease. Since I've been seeing the spiritual healer, I've been in remission and I have every reason to believe that I'll be cured."

In other instances, patients may choose alternative methods because they have experienced adverse effects from traditional methods (Cassileth et al. 1984). Mr. Adams was placed on an antihypertensive medication by his physician. After a month, however, he stopped taking the medication and switched to herbal preparations. He confided in a friend that he had stopped taking the prescribed medication because of the side effects he experienced. He stated that he chose the herbal preparation so he would have a smaller chance of side effects.

Patients may find traditional methods to be too complicated or technological (Furnham and Forey 1994) and turn to complementary or alternative methods, which they perceive to be more simple or more easily understandable. Likewise, in a time in which there is growing distrust of the health care industry, and in which patients desire more autonomy or control over their health matters, they may feel that conventional approaches to health care are too authoritarian (Riesmann 1994). Patients may feel they have more control over their health care, feeling a greater sense of autonomy and empowerment when they use CAM. (Kaptchuk and Eisenberg 1998). Health care under conventional practice may be viewed as too fragmented, so that patients seek complementary or alternative methods that they believe to hold a more holistic philosophy of health. Patients may believe that conventional health care treats the symptoms but not the underlying cause of the disease. They may feel that conventional methods do not address spiritual factors in health and may believe that complementary or alternative methods are more congruent with their own health beliefs.

Concerns about toxicity or complications from use of conventional methods may also be a reason patients choose complementary or alternative methods, which they perceive to be more natural. They may feel that complementary or alternative therapies put them at less risk than methods used in conventional care, which they may consider to be mechanistic or synthetic.

The meaning individual patients attribute to pain and disease can affect their ability or inability to cope with their symptoms or disease. CAM may be more consistent with the beliefs some patients have about health or illness (Vincent and Furnham 1996) or may be more consistent with the patient's religious perspectives (Fuller 1989). For example, some religious teachings propose that illness is caused by false beliefs. In this instance, followers of those teachings may believe that healing is possible only through prayer and by replacing bad thoughts with good ones.

Complementary or alternative methods are not always used as a replacement for conventional therapies. At times they are used in conjunction with conventional therapies prescribed to achieve therapeutic goals. For instance, patients may use prescribed anti-inflammatory agents for arthritis while also using meditation. They may take antihypertensive drugs for control of hypertension as well as engage in relaxation techniques to help lower blood pressure.

Some patients may believe that conventional therapies are too expensive and consequently seek complementary or alternative therapies because they believe them to be less expensive (Murray and Rubel 1992). Complementary and alternative methods are not, however, always cheaper. Because many third-party payers do not include CAM as appropriate for reimbursement, many patients are forced to pay out of pocket for complementary or alternative therapies.

Some patients may feel especially vulnerable to disease. They may interpret various body sensations as abnormal and, related to their perceived vulnerability, develop excess concerns about their symptoms. For example, Mrs. Jorgenson had been experiencing pain in her abdomen. After having a medical workup that was negative she began taking Ginseng stating, "The doctor says nothing is wrong but both my mother and grandmother died of stomach cancer. I'm taking Ginseng just in case."

Cultural variations may determine the extent to which alternative methods are used as well as the methods chosen (Hufford 1988, O'Connor 1995). Traditional beliefs of various cultures regarding wellness, sickness, and treatment may be very different from conventional health care treatments. The beliefs, traditions, and customs handed down through many generations may play a principal role in the establishment of individual health practices. Consequently, choosing complementary and alternative methods in health and disease may be because they are more in keeping with the patient's values and beliefs.

To many patients, even those not influenced by a particular cultural group, their own beliefs and values may be viewed as in conflict with the approaches of conventional health care. As a result, a dual health care system may exist, leading to confusion and unsatisfactory results. By exploring and understanding patients' values, beliefs, goals, and differing philosophies of health care, both conventional and CAM practices may be successfully integrated in a way that complement each other and achieve satisfactory results for both. To achieve this result, however, communication about patients' beliefs, values, goals, and use of complementary or alternative health practices must first be addressed.

IMPORTANCE OF DISCUSSING CAM

Given the prevalence of use of complementary and alternative methods, patients should be asked routinely about their use of such therapies. However, many health professionals fail to approach the subject with patients. Omission of the subject may be in part because health professionals are unfamiliar with CAM and consequently they are reluctant to bring up the issue for fear of appearing to be uninformed. To best assist patients make informed choices and use complementary or alternative therapies appropriately, health professionals need to be knowledgeable about them. Health professionals should attempt to familiarize themselves with the philosophy, historical development, underlying concepts, and basic principles of various complementary and alternative practices, as well as attempt to understand more common CAM therapies in depth. In addition to gaining information about CAM practices in general, health professionals should also attempt to understand patients' assumptions and expectations of the CAM methods they may be utilizing. To do this, of course, the subject must first be approached with patients.

There are many reasons why health professionals should be informed of the extent and type of complementary or alternative practices patients use. For instance, some alternative methods have demonstrated beneficial effects, such as pain control by acupuncture (Richardson and Vincent 1986). Research has also shown that using the patient's own physical and mental resources for health and healing can have direct effects on the immune, endocrine, and nervous systems (Cohen et al. 1991, Goleman and Gurin 1993). Once knowledgeable about CAM methods, health professionals can help patients identify therapies that may be most beneficial for their particular condition. In some instances, CAM methods may be used first before more conventional treatments, which may carry greater risks. Not all complementary or alternative methods are devoid of risk, however. In addition to potential adverse effects of some complementary and alternative therapies themselves, when used in combination with conventional therapies, adverse interactions can occur. By being aware of patient use of complementary or alternative methods, health professionals can coordinate efforts so that adverse interactions of methods can be prevented, as well as identify precautions that may need to be taken if alternative and conventional methods are being used simultaneously.

Awareness of patient use of CAM therapies can also help health professionals assist patients in assessing whether the positives of CAM use outweigh the negatives. For instance, although a number of insurers and managed care organizations in the United States now offer alternative method programs and benefits (Pelletier et al. 1997), for many patients, use of complementary and alternative methods constitute a large out-of-pocket expense (Eisenberg et al. 1993). Not all CAM therapies bring about the desired outcomes and may need to be replaced with other options. By identifying patients' CAM practices, health professionals can help patients minimize potential risks by providing the education and guidance so that both CAM and conventional approaches can be utilized in a way that will benefit the patient most.

PATIENT EDUCATION ABOUT CAM

Patient teaching about complementary or alternative methods should focus on safety, informed choice, and shared decision making. Health professionals should be not only solidly grounded in conventional health practices but also possess unbiased knowledge about the value and limitations of complementary or alternative methods.

In initiating the dialogue about patient use of CAM, health professionals should give permission for patients to discuss the topic of complementary or alternative methods by conveying a nonjudgemental, supportive attitude. They should indicate willingness to work with patients, utilizing complementary or alternative methods chosen by the patient in conjunction with conventional therapies when appropriate. Opening discussion of CAM practices might begin with a statement from the health professional such as, "What other things are you doing to stay healthy?" or "Sometimes people have home remedies or other practices they've heard about to treat disease besides those used by their doctor. Have you tried other things to treat your condition?"

Being open and nonjudgmental does not mean that health professionals should condone or refrain from discussion of complementary or alternative methods for which there are safety concerns. Alerting patients to potential hazards, however, should be done in a sensitive manner using sound reasoning and evidence rather than from an emotional basis, which could be construed by the patient as a struggle for authority and control. The goal should be to help patients make an informed choice, not necessarily to have them choose what the health professional thinks is best. As with all instances of patient education, informed choice should be based on unbiased, factual information, not coercion. If the health professional disapproves of the patient's choice of a particularly complementary or alternative method, they should not criticize the patient's use but rather give a rational basis for their concern. The following statement might be used to alert the patient of the health professional's concerns while also informing the patient of safer alternatives:

> I have heard of the herbal preparation you are taking, but I have concerns about its safety. You may have read in the paper about of some of the adverse

effects several people have experienced. There are some other herbal products, however, that you may consider instead.

In instances where there is no major concern about safety of a method but the health professional feels it is inappropriate, the health professional may explain reasons for objection, without deriding the method or discounting the patient's interest in it. In so doing, the health professional communicates respect for the patient's position while at the same time voicing logical concerns. For example:

> Mrs. Clark, although there is no evidence the supplement is harmful, it is very expensive, and I don't think there is clear evidence that its benefits are in keeping with the cost. The final decision, of course, is up to you, but I did want you know my thoughts.

Patients should always be aware that the health professional will continue to care for them despite complementary or alternative use practices. Patients who fear they will be abandoned by the health professional are not as likely to openly share information, which can be important to effective care. By building an open, trusting relationship, the health professional has the continuing opportunity to monitor patient progress.

Helping patients distinguish between legitimate alternative methods and fraud is another important part of patient education about complementary or alternative practices. Health professionals should also be advocates for patients by helping to diminish the potential that they will be casualties of fraud. When patients are seeking care from an alternative care provider, the health professional can help them determine if the individual has some type of certification or peer oversight, the amount of experience the individual has in working with specific conditions, the cost of each visit or treatment, the length of treatment, and the associated risks and benefits. Health professionals should help patients to be aware of warning signs of inappropriate complementary or alternative products or practices, such as therapies that make claims to exclusivity or products that purport secret formulas or ingredients that cannot be revealed. Products or procedures that claim extravagant effectiveness or only personal testimonials as a way of verification of effectiveness should also be called into question.

If health professionals are unfamiliar with a complementary or alternative method, they should be open about their lack of knowledge. They may say, "I'm unfamiliar with that (method; product). Could you bring some information in so I can learn more about it, or tell me where information is available?"

TEACHING PATIENTS ABOUT SAFETY ISSUES REGARDING CAM

When patients consider using complementary or alternative methods, they may look to the health professional for guidance in choosing safe and appropriate approaches. By giving patients factual, unbiased information, the health professional can help patients make logical and informed choices for safer use of CAM. Although many complementary or alternative methods can be helpful, in some instances safety concerns may be present. When patients look for information and guidance, there are several issues of which they should be made aware.

Medicinal plants have, of course, been used for centuries to treat a variety of conditions and symptoms, often with success. They are the original source of many contemporary synthetic medications, and many offer promise of being a source of new drugs in the future. Although some botanical preparations can help or some may be innocuous, not all methods may be safe and, in fact, can be responsible for adverse health effects (D'Arcy 1991, Gordon et al. 1996). Some methods may expose patients to potential harm either directly or indirectly. Direct harm, for example, may result from indiscriminate use of herbal medicines. Patients may believe that because many herbal preparations are labeled as "natural" that they are safe. Some herbs have toxic effects and others can interact with other drugs. Herbs or supplements that have a pharmacologic effect used in conjunction with conventional medications can either potentiate or negate effects of the prescribed drug or cause adverse drug interactions (Lazar 1996). Potential adulterants have also been reported in some herbal medications (Slifman et al. 1998). Patients may also be harmed indirectly if use of a complementary or alternative method draws them away from prescribed medical treatment or if they discontinue using prescribed medications without informing the health professional.

Patients should be helped to realize that there may be considerable variation in the same herbs from different manufacturers. As a result, herbal preparations vary greatly in efficacy and results even if they are taken in the same dose. Patients may view herbal products as more natural than pharmaceuticals and therefore believe that taking more than the recommended dosage can increase the effects from the preparation with little or no risk. Patients should be encouraged to take the recommended dose of herbal preparations and assisted to understand that results should not be expected as quickly as with prescription drugs. Because patients may associate herbal medications with less potent or less harmful effects, they should be helped to understand that even though medicines are herbal, they should not be taken in larger-than-recommended quantities because of the potential for side effects or interactions with other drugs. Patients should be cautioned to read labels of herbal preparations carefully, paying attention to any warnings.

Herbal preparations should not be taken longer than necessary. Patients should be helped to understand that herbs do not necessarily cure all conditions and that herbal preparations should not be substituted for medications that have been prescribed by their health professional without discussion.

Lack of standardization is also a potential problem related to patient safety in using complementary or alternative methods. For example, herbal products are not closely regulated in the same way pharmaceuticals are. In most instances, they are not required to undergo premarket testing and are not manufactured in standardized fashion, nor does safety or therapeutic effectiveness need to be demonstrated scientifically before outcomes are advertised. Likewise, whereas training standards and credentialing are mandated for practicing health professionals in conventional treatment settings, standards and professional standing of alternative practitioners are not well regulated and competence and training received by CAM practitioners may not be consistent.

Patients are often bombarded with information about complementary or alternative methods from personal testimony of family or friends, or from advertisements in the media. They may find it difficult to discern scientifically sound data from that which is based on emotion or on fraudulent claims with no empirical evidence. They may be unaware of possible herb–drug or herb–disease interactions or potential harmful effects of some complementary or alternative methods.

Patients should also be helped to understand that what has been reported to be helpful in the case of one patient may not mean that the same alternative method will be safe or helpful to everyone. Patients should be encouraged to consult several reliable sources for information before making the decision to use complementary or alternative methods. Above all, they should be encouraged to talk with their health professional about any complementary or alternative methods they are using and to promptly report any problems or new symptoms they experience after use.

THE ROLE OF THE HEALTH PROFESSIONAL

Health professionals should become familiar with various complementary or alternative methods, especially those that seem to be more prevalent in their particular geographic area. There should be an awareness that patients' use and interest in complementary or alternative methods may change over time. Consequently, checking only once with patients about whether or not complementary or alternative methods are being used may not be enough. Checks for CAM use should be conducted on a regular basis. The following questions can be helpful in determining whether patients use alternative methods.

- "Have you tried anything else to help your symptoms?"
- "What have you tried on your own to treat your condition?"
- "Is there anything else you have tried besides your prescribed medicine?"

When patients ask about or mention use of specific complementary or alternative methods with which health professionals are unfamiliar, lack of knowledge of the product or method should be admitted. Asking patients for additional information or for resources where additional information can be obtained helps patients feel health professionals are interested in learning more and opens up opportunities for more communication between patients and health professionals. Attempting to gain understanding of patients' rationale for using the alternative therapy also communicates interest and helps build a collaborative relationship.

Patients may use complementary or alternative methods not only for treatment of disease but also for health maintenance. Health professionals can approach the subject with direct statements such as:

Patients use a variety of products and techniques to maintain or improve their general health status. Are you using vitamins, supplements, or techniques such as yoga or meditation to improve your health?

Health professionals should be aware of patients' unmet expectations for care. Patients' underlying vulnerabilities and past experiences should be considered. Understanding patients' expectations helps health professionals better meet patients' needs by providing information to help them make rational decisions and, when necessary, to enter into negotiation regarding patient choices.

Despite open mindedness and willingness to work with patients' expectations, there may be some instances when patients and health professionals disagree on safety or effectiveness of complementary or alternative treatments. When this situation occurs, decisions should be negotiated. Health professionals should express concern, provide sound rational and evidence, rather than fabrications or coercion, and should not use emotional or psychological force. Patients have the right to make informed choices. Health professionals have the responsibility to provide factual information to assure that choices are informed. Health professionals should recognize and accept patients' desire for empowerment. Patients' choices should be accepted and their need for empowerment acknowledged. Health professionals should communicate their availability to patients should questions or problems arise and emphasize the importance of continuing contact and follow up. Disagreeing without humiliating patients or demonstrating hostility offers further opportunity to explore factors involved in patient choices. Health professionals should avoid deriding the CAM modality chosen by the patient, showing respect for patient choices. Patients should not be threatened or forced to choose between continuing care with the health professional and using CAM.

Whereas health professionals may have some difficulty accepting patient use of questionable CAM methods, they may also find patient use of CAM practitioners or therapies threatening. However, if the CAM practitioner's training and credentials can be verified, they can be a good referral source. Health professionals may find it helpful and informative to meet with CAM practitioners to discuss philosophy, training, experience, and cost, and to ascertain ways in which complementary or alternative care may be integrated into conventional care with individual patients.

INTEGRATIVE APPROACHES

Conventional health care has achieved excellence in many realms of preventing, treating, and curing disease. CAM models, however, have also been shown to offer exemplary frameworks for interdisciplinary and holistic health care.

Although most health professionals do not want to abandon conventional approaches to health care, complementary or alternative methods can, in many instances, be integrated into conventional health practices, complementing conventional approaches. Complementary or alternative methods used in conjunction with conventional treatments can help patients gain a sense of control over the effects of their condition and maximize the benefit of self-care strategies. When conditions are seen in the context of individual patients and the impact on their lives, complementary or alternative approaches can supplement conventional therapies, helping patients live with their condition.

Regardless of whether health professionals are enthusiastic or critical of complementary or alternative methods, there is a responsibility to be informed of such approaches and to respond to patients' interest. Although teaching patients about complementary or alternative methods requires additional skills and time, exploring patient use of alternative methods provides health professionals with important information that can ultimately increase quality of care. By not approaching the subject with patients, many opportunities for patient education are lost. Effective patient education about CAM can enrich the relationship between patient and health professional, as well as provide important insights that can help health professionals improve patient care. To effectively teach patients about complementary or alternative methods and to provide guidance that enables patients to make safe and sound decisions about their use, health professionals must also be informed. Utilizing resources for continuing professional development that address different types of complementary or alternative methods and that provide factual information about their use and benefits helps health professionals be better prepared to discuss safety, risks and benefits, and cost effectiveness of various approaches with patients, as well as to discuss how some complementary or alternative methods may be optimally combined with conventional approaches. A first step, however, may be addressing basic attitudes toward complementary or alternative approaches. By re-examining personal values and theories about health care as well as rethinking how to relate to patients regarding alternative methods, health professionals may find that they are able to more fully adapt to patients' expectations and, consequently, are better able to meet their needs.

REFERENCES

Anderson, W.H., O'Connor, B.B., MacGregor, R.R., Schwartz, J.S. 1993. Patient use and assessment of conventional and alternative therapies for HIV infection and AIDS. *Acquired Immunodeficiency Syndrome* 7:561–566.

Applewhite, S.L. 1995. Curanderismo: demystifying the health beliefs and practices of elderly Mexican Americans. *Health and Social Work* 20:247–253.

Astin, J.A. 1998. Why patients use alternative medicine: results of a national study. *Journal of the American Medical Association* 279:1548–1553.

Berman, B.M., Singh, B.K., Lao, L., Singh, B.B., Ferentz, K.S., and Heartnoll, S.M. 1995. Physicians, attitudes toward complementary or alternative medicine. A regional survey. *Journal of the American Board of Family Practice* 8:361–366.

Cassileth, B.R., Lusk, E.J., Strouse, T.B., Bodenheimer, B.J. 1984. Contemporary unorthodox treatments in cancer medicine: a study of patients, treatments and practitioners. *Annals of Internal Medicine* 101:105–112.

Cohen, S., Tyrrel, D.A.J., Smith, A.P. 1991. Psychological stress and susceptibility to the common cold. *New England Journal of Medicine* 325:606–612.

Crigger, B.J. 2000. Alternative and complementary medicine: what's a doctor to do? The Hastings Center Report Jan/Feb. Hastings-on-Hudson, NY: The Hastings Center.

D'Arcy, P.F. 1991. Adverse reactions and interactions with herbal medicines. Part I. Adverse reactions. *Adverse Drug Reaction and Toxicology Review* 19:189–208.

Dokken, D., Sydnor-Greenberg, N. 2000. Exploring complementary and alternative medicine in pediatrics: parents and professionals working together for new understanding. *Pediatric Nursing* 26:383–390.

Eisenberg, D.M., Kessler, R.C., Foster, C., Norlock, F.E., Calkins, D.R., Delbanco, T.L. 1993. Unconventional medicine in the United States: prevalence, costs, and patterns of use. *New England Journal of Medicine* 328:246–352.

Eisenberg, D.M., Davis, R.B., Ettner, S.L., Appel, S., Wilkey, S., Van Rompay, M. 1998. Trends in alternative medicine use in the United States, 1990–1997. *Journal of the American Medical Association* 280:1569–1575.

Elder, N.C., Gillcrist, A., and Minz, R. 1997. Use of alternative health care by family practice patients. *Archives of Family Medicine* 6:181–184.

Ernst, E., Resch, K.L., White, A.R. 1995. Complementary medicine: what physicians think of it. A meta-analysis. *Archives of Internal Medicine* 155:2405–2408.

Feldman, M.K. 1990. Patients who seek unorthodox medical treatment. *Minnesota Medicine* 73:19–25.

Fuller, R.C. 1989. Alternative medicine and American religious life. New York: Oxford University Press.

Furnham, A., Forey, J. 1994. The attitudes, behaviors, and beliefs of patients of conventional vs complementary alternative medicine. *Journal of Clinical Psychiatry* 50:458–469.

Gevitz, N. 1988. Three perspectives on unorthodox medicine. In: Other healers: unorthodox medicine in America. Gevitz, N. (Ed.). Baltimore: Johns Hopkins University Press, 1–28.

Goleman, D., Gurin, J. 1993. Mind-body medicine: how to use your mind for better health. Yonkers, NY: Consumer Reports Books.

Gordon, D.W., Rosenthal, G., Hart, J., Sirotan, R., Baker, A.L. 1996. Chaparral ingestion: broadening the spectrum of liver injury caused by herbal medications. *Journal of the American Medical Association* 273:489–490.

Greenfield, S.M., Innes, M.A., Allan, T.F., Wearn, A.M. 2002. First year medical students' perceptions and use of complementary and alternative medicine. *Complementary and Therapeutic Medicine* 10:27–32.

Harpham, W.S. 2001. Alternative therapies for curing cancer: what do patients want? What do patients need? *A Cancer Journal for Clinicians* 51:131–136.

Herbert, C.P. 1997. Can primary care physicians be a resource to their patients in decisions regarding alternative and complementary therapies for cancer? *Patient Education Counseling* 3:179–180.

Hufford, D.J. 1988. Contemporary folk medicine. In: Other healers: unorthodox medicine in America. Gevitz, N. (Ed.). Baltimore: Johns Hopkins University Press, 228–264.

Hufford, D.J. 1997. Complementary and alternative therapies in primary care: folk medicine and health culture in contemporary society. *Primary Care: Clinics in Office Practice* 24:723–741.

Jensen, P. 1990. Alternative therapy for atopic dermatitis and psoriasis: patient-reported motivation, information source and effect. *Acta Dermato-venereologica* 70:425–428.

Josefek, K.J. 2000. Alternative medicine's roadmap to mainstream. *American Journal of Law and Medicine* 26:295–310.

Kaptchuk, T.J., and Eisenberg, D.M. 1998. The persuasive appeal of alternative medicine. *Annals of Internal Medicine* 129:1061–1065.

Kim, M., Han, H.R., Kim, K.B., Duong D.N. 2000. The use of traditional and Western medicine among Korean American elderly. *Journal of Community Health* 27:109–120.

Lazar, J.S. 1996. Mind-body medicine in primary care: implications and applications. *Primary Care,* 23:169–182.

Lazar, J.S., O'Conner, B.B. 1997. Talking with patients about their use of alternative therapies. *Complementary and Alternative Therapies in Primary Care* 24:699–714.

McGuire, M.B. 1988. Ritual healing in suburban America. New Brunswick, NY: Rutgers University Press.

Miller, J.K. 1990. Use of traditional Korean health care by Korean immigrants to the United States. *Sociology and Social Research* 75:38–48.

Morgan, D.R., Glanville, H., Mars, S., Very, V., The British Medical Association. 1998. Education and training in complementary and alternative medicine: a postal survey of UK universities, medical schools and faculties of nurse education. *Complementary and Therapeutic Medicine* 6:64–70.

Murray, R.H., Rubel, A.J. 1992. Physicians and healers: unwitting partners in health care. *New England Journal of Medicine* 326:61–64.

National Institutes of Health 1994. Alternative medicine: expanding medical horizons. NIH Report No. 94-06. Chantilly, VA: NIH.

O'Connor, B.B. 1995. Healing traditions: alternative medicine and the health professions. Philadelphia: University of Pennsylvania Press.

O,Connor, B., Calabrese, C., Cardena, E. 1995. Panel on Definition and Description, CAM Research Conference, April 1995: defining and describing complementary and alternative medicine. *Alternative Therapy* 3:49–57.

Owen, D.K., Lewith, G., Stephens, C.R., Bryden, H. 2001. Can doctors respond to patients' increasing interest in complementary and alternative medicine? Commentary. *British Medical Journal* 322:154–158.

Pachter, L. 1993. Culture and clinical care. *Journal of the American Medical Association* 27:127–131.

Panush, R. 2000. American College of Rheumatology position statement: complementary and alternative therapies for rheumatic disease. *Rheumatic Diseases Clinics of North American*, Vol. 26, No. 1. Philadelphia: W.B. Saunders.

Pelletier, K.R., Astin, J. A., Haskell, W.L. 1999. Current trends in the integration and reimbursement of complementary and alternative medicine by managed care organizations (MCOs) and insurance providers: 1998 update and cohort analysis. *American Journal of Health Promotion* 14:25–33.

Pelletier, K.R., Marie, A., Krasner, M., Haskell, W.L. 1997. Current trends in the integration and reimbursement of complementary and alternative medicine by managed care, insurance carriers, and hospital providers. *American Journal of Health Promotion* 12:112–122.

Planta, M., Gundersen, B., Petitt, J.C. 2000. Prevalence of the use of herbal products in a low-income population. *Family Medicine* 32:252–257.

Rampes, H., Sharples, F., Mai-agh, S., Fisher, P. 1997. Introducing complementary medicine into the medical curriculum. *Journal of the Royal Society of Medicine* 90:19–22.

Richardson, P.H., Vincent, C.A. 1986. Acupuncture for the treatment of pain: a review of evaluative research. *Pain* 24:15–40.

Riesmann, F. 1994. Alternative health movements. *Social Policy* Spring:53–57.

Slifman, N.R., Obermeyer, W.R., Aloi, B.K., Mussser, S.A., Correll, W.A., Cichowicz, S.M., Betz, J.M., Love, L.A. 1998. Brief report: contamination of botanical dietary supplements by digitalis ianata. *New England Journal of Medicine* 339:806–808.

Spigelblatt, L., Laine-Ammara, G., Pless, I.B. 1994. The use of alternative medicine by children. *Pediatrics* 94:811–814.

Thompson, W.G. 1990. Alternatives to medicine. *Canadian Medical Association Journal* 142:105–106.

Vincent, C., Furnham, A. 1996. Why do patients turn to complementary medicine? An empirical study. *British Journal of Clinical Psychology* 35:37–48.

Visser, G.J., Peters, L., Rasker, J.J. 1992. Rheumatologist and their patients who seek alternative care. *British Journal of Rheumatology* 31:485–490.

Williams, J.W., Mulrow, C.D., Chiquette, E., Noel, P.K., Aguilar, C., Cornell, J. 2000. A systematic review of newer pharmacotherapies for depression in adults: evidence report summary. *Annals of Internal Medicine* 132:743–756.

Zollman, C., Vickers, A. 1999. Complementary medicine and the doctor. *British Medical Journal* 319:1558–1561.

Zollman, C., Vickers, A. 2000. ABC of complementary medicine. London: BMJ Publishing.

Patient Education and Patient Compliance Issues for Older Adults

12

DEMOGRAPHIC CHANGE

The number and proportion of older persons living in the United States increased dramatically during the 20th century. At the beginning of the century, people over the age of 65 accounted for 4% of the population. By the end of the century, this group had grown to 11% of the population with the projection that those 65 and older will reach 17% of the total population by 2020 (U.S. Bureau of Census 1998). This growth, in part, is due to the aging baby boom population; however, much of this growth can also be accounted for by the fact that many other older adults are now living well into their 80s and more and more individuals are living to reach 100 years and beyond (National Institute on Aging 2002). Implications of this growth for health care delivery in general and patient education in particular are enormous. The increased need for patient education both for patients and caregivers is evident, and the need for effective patient education is imperative.

Although many principles of patient education remain the same for all age groups, there are special needs of older adults that must be addressed. Developing more effective approaches to teaching older adults and their families is an increasing challenge for patient education.

DEFINING AGING

Everyone has their own perception of what constitutes the life stage of older age. Older adults, however, are not a homogeneous group and do not share a distinctive and separate culture. A correlation between chronologic and physiologic or functional age cannot be assumed. Aging is a complex multidimensional process beginning at conception with continuing changes throughout life. The initial stages of the continuum consist of growth and development, followed in later stages by gradual deterioration and decline (Schaie and Willis 2002).

Wide individual differences exist in aging and are determined by physical, psychological, social, and economic factors. Even though much diversity exists among older adults and their experience with later life stages, older individuals are often lumped into one group, a tendency that promotes stereotyping. Attempting to place all individuals above a certain age into one "older age" category is problematic for a number of reasons. In addition to discounting individual differences, such a grouping does not take into account the wide age differences at each end of the spectrum. If an arbitrary age of 60 is established at the lower end of the grouping, a 40 year or more time span could exist between those at the beginning and end of the spectrum. The general profile physically, psychologically, and socially of an individual at the age of 60 is much different from an individual who is 100 years of age.

No uniform definition or specification of what constitutes older age exists. There are many definitions. Old age can be defined strictly in chronological terms, based on individual perceptions of the chronological age at which one is considered to be in the older age group. Some people may consider 50 years as the marker for older age, while others may consider the marker for older age to be much later. Legal and economic basis for defining older age also exists. Rules regarding the age at which an individual may retire, the age at which more frequent drivers tests are mandated, and eligibility for withdrawing from pension funds are examples. Older age has also been defined legislatively. Legislation such as the Older American's Act and the Social Security Act have yet other specifications as to what constitutes older age (Atchley 2000). Social groups or organizations can also define old age. The American Association of Retired Persons policies for membership as well as varying ages at which individuals are eligible for "senior discounts" are examples of yet other markers of older age.

In addition to defining older age legally, legislatively, or socially, older age can also be defined biologically, based on physical changes. Outward physical changes that are indicative of older age include postural and gait changes, changes in facial features, hair color, or body fat distribution. Less visible internal signs of aging may include changes in stamina, reaction time, alteration of sleep patterns, or increasing susceptibility to pathologic changes related to disease. The rate and extent to which these changes occur vary considerably from individual to individual and are determined by a number of factors. Whereas some individuals may show significant signs of outward or internal aging by the time they are 50 years old, others may show only minor aging changes well into their 70s.

Old age may also be defined psychologically. An indication of psychological age is the individual's ability to adapt behaviorally to the demands of the environment. Psychological aging includes how old an individual feels and how old they act in response to life events. Psychological aging may be related to individuals' developmental expectations for aging and how they compare themselves to most other people their age. In comparing appearance, interests, or behavior of others of the same age, if the individual feels older they may label themselves as old. If, however, in comparison to others the individual feels more vital and productive, they may denounce the label of old. For example, Mrs. Johnson, at age 75, continues to run her own business and remains active in the community. When she was asked to participate at the local Senior Citizen Center she declined, stating that Senior Citizens Centers were for "old people."

Old age can be defined in terms of social roles or social expectations for behavior for individuals of a certain age with respect to a culture or society. This includes how people dress and how they behave relative to others. Common stereotypes related to psychological aging consist of beliefs that older adults are conservative, stuck in their ways, or resistant to change as opposed to a younger psychological state in which there is receptiveness to new ideas or concepts and the ability to be flexible and to adapt. Other attitudes are specific to behavior in which societal norms or standards dictate types of behavior considered as "age appropriate." Social pressure based on these standards compel older adults to "act their age" even though they may be capable of participating in a number of activities they still enjoy, but which are not considered to be age appropriate. Take, for example, Mr. and Mrs. Atkins. They had always been music lovers. They also loved to dance and throughout their lives had frequented clubs and bars that tended to be popular for jazz, reggae, and rock music. As they reached their 60s however, their son was overheard telling his friends, "I wish mom and dad weren't having so much trouble accepting their age. They still try to act as if they're young by going to clubs that are inappropriate for people their age. They should know when it's time to act their age and just stay home." Although attitudes and expectations of what constitutes age-appropriate behavior for older adults are changing, individuals are not immune to social values, customs, and attitudes that formed stereotypes in the past.

Many terms are commonly used to describe individuals who have reached the later stages of life. Terms such as *elderly, senior citizen,* or *individuals in their golden years* are all terms used to describe adults who have reached their later years. Although these terms are a way of identifying an age group, such terms can also create negative images of individuals who are frail, inactive, or in other ways devalued. Many individuals in later years do not think of themselves as elderly or as senior citizens, and find being lumped into this category offensive. Given the wide range in age that exists in later life stages as well as diversity of the aging experience, such terms used to categorize individuals in later stages of life seem outmoded. What term, then, can best be used to communicate that an individual is in the later stage of life? The term that seems least offensive and that has a more positive connotation is the term *older adult.* This term still communicates that someone has reached the later stage in life but does not create stereotypic mental images that other terms engender.

There is no one correct definition of what constitutes an older adult, nor is there a uniform age marker that indicates when older adulthood is reached. Health professionals should not assume that persons after a certain age fit into a stereotypical category; however, to fully assess individual patient education needs, they must also be aware of specific factors that can be associated with aging and can influence the patient education process and its effectiveness. Treating persons as individuals and appreciating dimensions that are beyond the physical condition and chronological age are important components in effective patient education regardless of the age group. In advancing age, however, social, psychological and physical domains become more interdependent.

RATE OF AGING

Aging is not a disease, but rather a cumulative process resulting from a sum of changes that occur gradually (Christiansen and Grzybowski 1999). Many changes once associated with normal aging are now known to be pathologic conditions rather than part of the normal aging process (Arking 1998). It is therefore important for health professionals as well as patients to distinguish pathologic changes from those changes due to normal aging. When pathologic changes occur, they become superimposed on changes associated with normal aging. As a result, presentation of many conditions, symptoms experience, and response to treatment may be different in older adults than in younger adults with the same condition.

All people do not "age" at the same rate. Some people seem older physically, mentally, or socially at 60 years old than others at 80. Aging is an individual process with different types of aging occurring at different rates. How an individual ages depends on a number of individual factors. Psychological and social stress may accelerate deteriorating changes associated with aging. Environmental factors, such as exposure to extreme temperatures, sun, or toxic substances may also accelerate the aging process. How individuals age is also determined by genetic factors. Although how genetics affects aging is not known, it may determine individuals' susceptibility to certain diseases or may influence functioning of various body organs or systems (Timiras 1994). Socioeconomic status is also a factor because to a great extent it determines access to health care, including preventive treatment and treatment of disease, access to adequate nutrition both in terms of quantity and quality, and levels of stress to which individuals are exposed. Social expectations also play a role in the rate of aging. Individuals who have been devalued or coerced into diminishing roles may exhibit observable changes in behavior, feelings, or attitudes related to older age regardless of other parameters of aging.

Although some changes associated with aging are not reversible, others are, or at least can be retarded. Patient education directed toward prevention can diminish changes brought about by the normal aging process. For example, teaching older adults about the importance of exercise as well as appropriate forms of exercise can help them maintain flexibility and stamina, so that normal changes associated with aging, in the absence of pathologic conditions, have little impact on functional capacity. Teaching older adults about good health practices, including good diet and the importance of obtaining flu shots, can help them to diminish susceptibility to disease. When changes associated with aging do produce permanent functional loss, patient education can help alter deterioration and at times ameliorate the problem. For example, individuals who experience hearing loss due to aging may be taught about ways to maximize their hearing receptivity and, when appropriate, how to use a hearing aid most effectively. If vision is affected, helping patients learn how to maximize their vision and how to minimize accidents due to poor vision may be of use.

ATTITUDES OF HEALTH PROFESSIONALS

Attitudes usually consist of beliefs about or labels of people, behavior, or circumstances that summarize or outline expectations related to people or events. Attitudes are important determining factors in shaping both quality and framework of interpersonal interactions that take place. Attitudes, either negative or positive, effect communication patterns and responses in interpersonal interactions.

Depending on previous experience with older adults, or the type of exposure to attitudes about aging they have experienced, health professionals may have positive or negative attitudes about aging. If attitudes about aging are negative, health professionals will be unable to conduct patient education with older adults effectively. Negative attitudes may be responsible for health professionals' avoidance of patient education interactions with older patients completely.

Positive attitudes about older people facilitate effective patient education. Viewing older people as individuals with values, beliefs and preferences and demonstrating respect for them as individuals builds trust and rapport important to the success of patient education. Health professionals may, however, have attitudes that consist of negative prejudgments about older patients, which in turn thwarts patient education effectiveness. Examples of negative prejudgments may include beliefs about the futility of the potential for changing patient behavior or perceived insurmountable barriers that preclude patient education effectiveness. There may be negative beliefs about the older adult's potential for change, and these beliefs may affect outcome of the patient education interaction. If the health professional expects that the patient education encounter will have limited positive results, then a self-fulfilling prophecy may result. Other examples of negative attitudes may include health professionals' belief that patient education with older adults is not cost effective given the life expectancy of the patient and the extra time that may be needed to conduct patient teaching. Health professionals may believe that, with limited resources, more time and effort should be spent on younger adults who are still in their productive years rather than individuals in later stages of life. Older patients may cause anxiety in health professionals because they remind them of their own aging and mortality. Older patients may remind health professionals about conflicts they experienced with their own parents. There may be feelings of frustration if the patient experiences complex medication problems that are not curable.

Positive attitudes on the part of the heath professional can enhance the patient teaching interaction as well as enhance the possibility of increased compliance. Negative attitudes, however, can also have a negative impact on patient teaching as well as on the degree to which patients follow health advice. Although there has been increased interest in including information about later stages of life in curriculums of health professionals, often information presented focuses on disease processes or on negative aspects of aging, which may result in health professionals developing negative prejudgments about individuals in older age groups.

Attitudes held by health professionals are transmitted to patients they serve. Older patients' perception of the attitude of the health professional is more of a determinant of help-seeking behavior than awareness of illness or perception of the health professional's competence (Nuttbrock and Kosburg 1980). Although communication skills are important in every patient education encounter, even good communication skills cannot camouflage negative attitudes held by the health professional (Engram 1981). Health professionals must acknowledge and confront negative attitudes before patient education can be effective.

AVOIDING STEREOTYPES

Myths and stereotypes about aging are widespread in society despite recent attempts to "normalize" the aging process. Society emphasizes youth, vitality, and productivity and tends to overestimate the number of older adults who are functionally disabled and unable to live on their own and underestimate the number of individuals who are active and independent.

Myths and stereotypes are perpetuated overtly and covertly through humor, literature, media, and advertisements. Humor often projects negative themes in aging, emphasizing decline in physical appearance, sexual dysfunction, or aberrant behavior. Although recently literature as well as films have attempted to portray some older adults as heroes or heroines or as romantic love interests, portrayals of older adults as frail, dependent, disagreeable, and undesirable are far more common. Advertisements directed to older adults also emphasize negative aspects of aging, emphasizing remedies to mask signs of aging through anti-wrinkle cream products or products to cover gray hair, while other products are directed toward problems such as incontinence, aches and pains, or constipation. Even birthday cards directed toward older adults often reflect negative stereotypes about aging and consequently reinforce ageist ideas. Sentiments expressed on greeting cards for older adults often refer to declines in physical ability, appearance, or mental abilities, understating positive traits and abilities while fixating on and generalizing negative characteristics.

Stereotypes diminish the value of older adults. Negative views portrayed by mass media and literature influence the views of younger adults and health professionals, as well as of older adults themselves. As a result, older adults may incorporate stereotypes into their own self-image, accepting negative stereotypes of aging as factual. Because they have incorporated negative views of aging into their self-perception, or because they fear ridicule of younger adults, they may participate in perpetuating negative stereotypes through jokes or negative statements about themselves as aging individuals.

Stereotyping results in compartmentalization of people rather than viewing them as individuals. Stereotypes are harmful to all aspects of social interaction, but they are especially harmful when they impede effective patient education. Take, for example, Mr. Morris, the patient educator for a local senior health project initiative. He had outlined a number of health promotion and prevention topics to be presented at the Senior Citizen Center. When choosing topics, because of his assumption that older adults did not actively engage in sexual activity or would be offended by discussion of sexual topics, he neglected to include information regarding HIV/AIDS prevention through the use of condoms. He was unaware of the inaccuracy of his assumption about sexual interest and activity of older adults and unaware that several participants at the Senior Citizen Center were HIV positive.

The negative effects of stereotyping on individuals' self-perception also has ramifications for patient education. During a routine physical examination, Dr. Jenkins attempted to discuss how to maintain cardiovascular health with Mr. Wylie, an 82-year-old patient. Before Dr. Jenkins could complete the patient teaching, Mr. Wylie interrupted, stating, "Why should I be concerned about this? When you're my age it's too late anyway." In other instances, patients may be influenced by the negative expectations of others. Dr. Ellington was concerned when evaluating Mrs. Boucher, age 85, at a follow-up visit and found that she had not been following the meal plan for her type II diabetes diet. Mrs. Boucher's daughter, who had accompanied her to the office visit, stated to Dr. Ellington that "You just can't teach an old dog new tricks. Older people are naturally forgetful anyway, so how could you expect her to remember what she should have on her diet." A common misperception and stereotype about aging is that older adults are incapable or less able to learn and remember new material than younger adults. In this case, the stereotype was perpetuated by Mrs. Boucher's daughter, and Mrs. Boucher was living up to her daughter's expectation.

Health professionals should remember that there is wide variation in older adults and should not pigeonhole older adults into one group with shared general characteristics. The impact of stereotyping on patient education can be far reaching. Stereotyping can interfere not only with effective patient education but have repercussions on patients' heath and well-being as well.

GENERATIONAL DIFFERENCES

An outstanding feature of the older population is its continual change in character. The older adult of today has had different experiences than older adults of 50 years ago. These differences create different perspectives on social roles, health, health care, and expectations for aging. Likewise, young adults today will have different experiences throughout their lifetime, which will in turn effect their attitudes and perspectives when they reach older age. Each individual has a unique life history, a unique personality, and a unique set of life circumstances, but life experiences are also influenced by the groups within which individuals function and events and circumstances of the times. Specific historic circumstances help shape individuals attitudes and perspectives. For example, a person born in 1920 has had different life experiences from someone born in 1945. Events in history, technologic advances, and social changes will impact on each individual's world view, as well as their view regarding health and illness. Age roles also differ from era to era. Individuals have been socialized regarding appropriate behavior for certain age roles. The expectations the individual born in 1920 has for their role in older age may be much different from the expectations of the individual born in 1945.

Because of the historic period in which people grow up, impressions of aging, as well as impressions of health behavior, may be different in older and younger adults. These factors may distort communication between individuals of different generations. For example, Mr. Byrne, grew up during the depression. Because of the influence of the events he experienced during his early years, he believes in self-sufficiency and that he should be able to overcome problems on his own without asking questions or without seeking service of others. Dr. Karnes, a family practice resident working with Mr. Byrne, found it extremely frustrating when she discovered that Mr. Byrne had delayed on several occasions to seek advice about medical problems he was having, which, if promptly treated, could have been controlled so that complications he is now experiencing could have been avoided. Dr. Karnes neglected to take into consideration that in avoiding medical consultation, Mr. Byrne was not being obstinate but was rather behaving in accordance with the social expectations of his historic past.

In other instances, older individuals may, because of social expectations at the time they were growing up, view the health professional's role as one of paternalism. Consequently, these older adults may have difficulty accepting a more active role in their own health care. In other situations, older adults may be reluctant to talk about emotions, believing that personal and emotional problems are private, not to be shared with those outside the family.

Although generational differences can result in misunderstanding and can interfere with effective communication between patient and health professional, awareness of the possibility of differences can help health professionals adjust their approach to patient teaching, compensating for generational differences to maximize patient education effectiveness.

CULTURAL DIFFERENCES

Cultural differences and their impact on patient education and patient compliance are, of course, important to any age group. Other variables related to culture, which may or may not include ethnicity issues, include social class, nationality, and whether individuals live in a rural or urban environment. Cultural differences can affect patients' views of health and illness, concepts of body function, perceptions of causes of disease, and the use of health care services. These differences may be more pronounced in older adults. Older adults, even though possibly having immigrated many years before, may have clung to cultural customs and beliefs, including use of folk remedies for treatment of disease. Older adults may also have clung to their native language, creating potential communication difficulties when interacting with health professionals.

How age is defined and how age is marked varies among cultures. Age roles differ from culture to culture. Delineating age groups in different cultures may include not only chronologic age but also functions performed by people in different age groups. In some cultures, old age may be defined by altered work responsibilities or retirement. In others, old age may be defined in terms of the status of one's children. For example, in some cultures, becoming a grandparent may be an age marker and bring with it social role expectations for that age.

The role of the family in caring for older adults may also vary in different cultures. Consequently, how social networks, including family, friends, and neighbors, are used to help older patients mobilize resources and how these are applied to health and health care may be of special significance when working with older adults with culturally diverse backgrounds.

Specific cultural differences related to aging are especially important to effective patient education. The chances of developing a chronic disease becomes greater as individuals become older (Ory and Bond 1989) regardless of cultural or ethnic background. Cultural or ethnic variations impact on health and well-being in all age groups. Despite mediating factors, such as socioeconomic status, however, some ethnic groups are more prone to development of certain diseases than others. For example, the rate of diabetes mellitus is higher in Native Americans (Burke et al. 1999), while hypertension and heart disease remain higher in blacks (Harris et al. 1998). Some differences may be associated with poverty and a history of inadequate health care; however, others are rooted in cultural traditions, such as dietary practices. Consequently, awareness of increased risk for such diseases requires special consideration for patient education to older patients from diverse cultural backgrounds.

Cultural issues should be addressed directly. Individual beliefs and values should be respected. Health professionals should be aware that there is significant diversity within cultural groups, with each group containing their own customs and belief systems. These belief systems may extend to how patients view their role in treatment and how they expect to interact with health professionals.

Culture influences the experience of aging, perspectives on health, and relationships. Having an understanding of cultural influences helps health professionals determine potential or actual problems that could interfere with effective patient education. Such an understanding also provides a structure through which various solutions to meet these challenges can be devised.

PATIENT EDUCATION NEEDS OF OLDER ADULTS

Although aging is not synonymous with disease, the incidence of disease and associated disability increase with age (Digiovanna 2000). Over 80% of all older persons report one or more chronic conditions, such as arthritis, heart disease, hypertension, or diabetes (Ory and Bond 1989). With advanced age, several chronic conditions may coexist at one time. As individuals reach later stages of life, chronic and acute illness are superimposed on normal changes of aging, having greater impact on health status. Consequences of chronic and acute illness for older individuals when superimposed on normal changes associated with aging can be more serious and can result in a higher level of functional dependency. The patient's initial disease condition may lead to a cascading effect of a secondary complication or problem, which then contributes to a yet a third problem. Take, for example, Mrs. Barnes, age 89, who had made a concerted effort to walk and exercise on a regular basis after her myocardial infarction, which had resulted in mild congestive heart failure. Because she also had osteoarthritis of both knees, however, she experienced increasing pain when walking and, as a result, was unable to maintain her exercise program. Because of her inactivity she become constipated, feeling bloated and nauseated, so that she no longer had adequate intake of fluid because she felt it increased her bloating. As a result of her decreased fluid intake, in combination with the diuretic she was taking for the mild congestive heart failure, she became dehydrated. Her dehydration resulted in orthostatic hypotension, so that one day when getting up from her afternoon nap, she lost her balance, fell, and broke her hip.

In some instances, one disease may mask or alter the presentation of another. For example, Mr. Roberts, because of his arthritis, was unable to perform major exercise. Because of his decreased level of activity and consequent lack of increased oxygen demand, it was not discovered that he also had angina pectoris until late into the course of the disease. Mild symptoms he had been experiencing due to his coronary artery disease had been attributed to indigestion. He was not aware that his symptoms could be due to another disease process.

In other instances, one disease may exacerbate the symptoms of the second. Mrs. Little was in the early stages of Alzheimer's disease, although still able to function somewhat independently. Mrs. Little's son, who checked on her daily, mentioned to his neighbor, a nurse, that he was surprised at how quickly his mother's Alzheimer's disease was progressing, stating that one week she was able to function on her own and suddenly she was unable to perform most of the tasks she had still be capable of performing. Mrs. Little's son had not been informed that sudden changes in cognitive function could indicate the presence of another disease condition. His neighbor encouraged him to consult his physician. When Mrs. Little was evaluated by the physician she was found to have a urinary tract infection that had not been identified, but which was exacerbating her symptoms of confusion.

Standard treatment for disease conditions may also need to be altered because of coexisting conditions. Mr. Simmons underwent coronary bypass surgery. Although normally the rehabilitation process would encourage exercise, Mr. Simmons had preexisting osteoarthritis of his left hip and knee, which made walking very difficult. Consequently, patient teaching was directed to helping Mr. Simmons find other ways to increase his exercise tolerance.

Conditions such as arthritis, poor eyesight, or memory problems can interfere with older patients' ability to take medications appropriately. Patient education efforts may need to be directed to devising strategies that can make taking medication less difficult. Instructing patients to ask the pharmacist for medication bottles that are easily opened, use of a magnifying glass for medication identification, or development of charts to assist patients in keeping track of when to take medications are examples of patient education interventions that can maximize the older adults ability to follow treatment recommendations accurately.

Coexistent chronic disease frequently involves an increased use of medications. Patients may be unaware of the potential for side effects or for drug interactions. They also may be unaware of the potential for interactions with over-the-counter medications. Patient teaching that helps patients identify potential drug interactions as well as alerts them to interactions with other over-the-counter medications can help them avoid adverse effects, complications, and further disability. Older adults, just as younger adults, should be knowledgeable about the medications they take and about potential side effects. They should be encouraged to check with the appropriate health professional when they have questions or if they experience problems with the medication. Like all patients, older patients should be informed about why they are having the medication prescribed, the anticipated effect of the medication, and possible consequences of taking the medication.

The implications for patient education in helping individuals and caregivers learn to manage disease is obvious. The differentiating factor in teaching older adults with chronic disease is concomitant changes due to normal aging, which may impact on the individual's ability to maintain function and independence. Consequently, the patient education needs of older adults may become expanded in order to assist them in managing chronic disease in the context of changes brought about by normal aging. Patient education may also be directed toward helping older adults maximize function and independence, and toward preventing complications which could cause further disability from occurring.

Older adults often believe themselves to be in good health despite the simultaneous presence of chronic disease (Cockerham 1997). Older adult's assessment of their own health is frequently more related to their ability to maintain activities and independence than to actual diagnosis and treatment of disease. A goal of patient education for older adults is to maximize both the quantity and quality of life. Therefore, another patient education need is to assist individuals to maintain maximum health and function by preventing development or progression of disease as much as possible and by avoidance of acute illness or other events that could result in functional decline or disability. A simple example of patient teaching related to prevention may be assessment of the accident potential in the patient's living environment and accompanying instruction to the patient and/or caregivers about how to prevent falls from occurring. In some instances, patients may be taught alternative techniques for treatment of disease other than medication. For example, patients with arthritis pain may be able to reduce the amount of medication they use if they are instructed about the use of heat and massage as treatment modalities. Teaching patients about the importance of fiber, fluids, and exercise to prevent constipation may help them avoid use of laxatives.

A more subtle form of prevention teaching may involve teaching the patient and/or caregiver how to differentiate the normal aging process from treatable diseases. Older patients and their families may attribute symptoms they experience to normal aging when actually symptoms are associated with disease or medication side effects. Consequently they may delay seeking medical treatment and as a result develop more serious consequences of disease that might have been contained if treated earlier.

BARRIERS TO EFFECTIVE PATIENT EDUCATION WITH OLDER ADULTS

Although many principles of patient education remain the same, regardless of patients' ages, when teaching older adults, a number of factors specific to older age can hinder communication. Attitudes, both on the part of older patients and health professionals, can interfere with effective communication regarding health-related matters. Attitudes of health professionals and the impact on effective patient education have been discussed previously. Attitudes of older patients can also play a role. Although older patients should be treated as individuals, rather than as a part of a stereotypical group, there are some commonalities of which health professionals should be aware.

Not all older patients feel "old." Patients may resent being categorized as "old" or having terms such as "senior" applied to them. Consequently, instructions regarding specific safety measures, screening procedures, or other medical interventions that they believe are being directed toward them because they are "older patients" may be rejected.

The experience of the older adult in the context of the social milleau in which they have lived during the time period of their younger and middle years with resultant social expectations about aging may be different from that of the experience of health professionals working with patients today. Consequently, expectations of the interaction may differ. Some older patients may place health professionals on a pedestal, expecting health professionals to take a paternalistic approach to health care. Older patients may be reluctant to ask questions or be active participants in their care, desiring to take a more passive role. Older patients may believe that health professionals should not be bothered with what the patient considers as "trivial concerns." Older patients may refrain from asking questions for fear of offending the health professionals or fear that their questions will be perceived as a challenge to the health professionals' recommendations or judgement. Some older patients may be reluctant to share information that they consider to be too private or personal to discuss with others. This may be especially true of issues such as incontinence, impotence, or other sexual concerns.

Older adults may have different perceptions of health and illness and may define health differently than health professionals. To older adults, remaining independent and active may be defined as healthy, despite chronic illness and symptoms. They may believe that many of their symptoms are to be expected as a part of aging and may avoid seeking medical attention or following medical advice because they believe symptoms to be a natural consequence of aging. They may fear that by sharing all their symptoms and concerns with health professionals they will be labeled as a hypochondriac or as a complaining old person. In other instances, they may not mention their symptoms to health professionals because they believe tests or treatment will be too expensive, or that treatment could involve giving up independence and perhaps even being moved from their own home.

Auditory and/or visual impairments vary in degree in older adults. Hearing loss and loss of visual acuity can interfere with effective patient education as well as the patient's ability to follow treatment recommendations, especially if appropriate assistive devices are not being utilized. Hearing or visual loss may not have been identified or may be denied by the patient. Assessing the presence of these conditions and the degree to which they impact on function as well as on the patient education process can assist health professionals in altering communication approaches as well as guide them in providing patient education information that helps older patients to maximize function through use of appropriate assistive devices.

BARRIERS TO PATIENT COMPLIANCE IN OLDER ADULTS

Patient education activities with older adults may range from teaching them about how to prevent illness or complications from occurring to assisting older patients and their families acquire skills in self-management of chronic illness. Patient education issues may also involve helping patients make choices about different living environments as well as decisions about end-of-life issues. Regardless of the patient education topic, health professionals should keep in mind special needs of older adults, which influence the degree to which older patients are able to carry out recommendations given.

For example, prevention teaching, which may address topics such as fitness, nutrition, stress management, personal health care management, or accident prevention, cannot be totally effective unless various other factors are considered. Merely giving older patients information about prevention practices may be insufficient to ensure that the practices can be carried out. For instance, teaching patients about the importance of exercise through walking may not be adequate without also assessing potential barriers that could preclude patients from following the recommendation. Does the patient have a place in which to walk safely? Do they live in a high-crime area, which would place them in jeopardy? Are there sidewalks in their neighborhood, and if so, are they in good repair? If there is a mall nearby in which older adults routinely walk, and does the patient have the means to get there? Does the patient have another condition, such as arthritis or foot problems, which may prevent them from walking as recommended?

Likewise, it does little good to teach older adults how to eat nutritiously without also assessing their ability to afford the foods recommended or their ability to obtain and prepare them. Does a coexisting medical condition makes food preparation difficult? Are assistive devices needed? If the patient lives alone, is eating alone or preparing food for themselves an issue? Are there other services in the area, such as transportation services, meals on wheels, or communal food programs for older adults that can be used to help patients follow the food recommendations? In addition, if patients are being taught about stress-management techniques, it may be insufficient to teach techniques without also evaluating the source of the stress and helping older patients identify ways the source of the stress can be reduced or eliminated.

Health professionals must be aware of social and economic needs of the older adult. Physical handicaps or other factors such as fixed incomes, limited insurance reimbursement, or transportation problems may make it more difficult for patients to follow recommendations given by health professionals. Does the patient have support from family members or friends? Do they have transportation to reach health care facilities for appointments? Is the older adult able to afford medication prescribed? Does the patient have physical problems that interfere with following recommendations given in patient teaching? Is there need for modifications to help older individuals compensate for any sensory or physical problems?

To help patients remain at their maximum functional capacity as well as carry out recommendations, patient teaching may be directed toward teaching patients about the availability and use of self-help devices to compensate for physical need. Many simple and inexpensive adaptive devices are available to help promote independence. For example, in the case of arthritis, which can impede manual dexterity, Velcro closures can eliminate the need for buttons or zippers. For kitchens there are specially designed cooking tools, such as cutting boards with finger guards or sticky materials to hold plates in place. Individuals with visual impairment may find large-print stove dials or magnifying devices useful. All of these devices not only serve as aids to independent living but can also help the older adult follow through with patient education recommendations.

Health professionals are not expected to be able to solve all problems related to older patients' ability to follow recommendations, but an understanding of the limitations patients experience and the availability of means to overcome limitations promotes better planning and enhances the opportunity for compliance. Many organizations and devices are available to assist older adults. These services and tools are often the critical factors that enable older patients to maintain maximum independence. Consequently, health professionals' knowledge of the availability of services and devices and ability to pass this information along to patients and their families is an important aspect of providing effective patient education to older patients.

SPECIAL TEACHING NEEDS OF OLDER PATIENTS

When teaching older patients about specific conditions, health professionals should be aware that there are differences in approaches to older adults and younger adults, even though they may have the same diagnosis. Although the diagnoses may be the same, teaching needs of younger and older adults may be different. The overall health status of every individual, young or old, represents to some degree a synthesis of medical, psychological, and social domains. In older adults, however, these domains become more interdependent. Differences both in physiology in advanced age as well as the patient's life circumstances may not only alter the course of disease but the patient's response to treatment as well.

Older adults, just as all other patients, require patient education that considers comprehensive, individually tailored information and takes into account the whole person including the physical and psychological environment in which they live. Although many older adults remain active and in relative good health, function is compromised to some degree with advanced age or with additive effects of disease. Patient teaching with older adults then should be directed not only to prevention or management of any chronic or acute condition they may be experiencing but also toward maximizing functional independence. This means that the approach toward older patients may be more complex. In advanced age, changes due to normal aging, chronic disease, or a combination of both precipitate additional competing risks that raise additional questions of prolongation of life versus quality of life. These factors add to the complexity of patient teaching as well as decision making.

Most older individuals are not institutionalized, and most do remain in their own homes, however the incidence of chronic disability requiring some type of assisted-living arrangement increases with advanced age. When disease results in functional dependency so that patients are unable to carry out one or more major activity such as eating, hygiene, or dressing, or when safety becomes an issue, alternative living arrangements may be necessary. A realistic assessment of affordability, available support systems, and the patient's physical environment are critical components in determining when a change of living arrangements may be necessary. Although physical and/or cognitive disability are not necessarily a normal part of aging, when physical or cognitive limitations make independent living for older adults less feasible, helping patients and families determine when different living arrangements are needed as well as informing them about housing options available are important parts of patient education. Choosing a housing option can be confusing and overwhelming for both the patient and their family. By helping patients and families identify preferences, recognize the level of need for assistance, and determine resources available, health professionals can assist patients and families choose the living arrangement most appropriate for them.

INVOLVING A THIRD PARTY IN PATIENT TEACHING

Patient teaching with older adults sometimes necessitates involvement of a family member or caregiver (Brown et al. 1998). Inclusion of a third person into the medical encounter changes and influences the relationship between patient and health professional (Stewart et al. 2000). Having a third party present can have a positive effect on the relationship as well; through assistance they are able to provide by helping the older adult recall information. The third party may also be useful in helping older adults later recall recommendations they have been given by health professionals if memory is a problem.

When a third party is present in the interaction with the health professional, issues of autonomy are also present. Older patients have a right to patient education information about prevention, disease conditions, and treatment and to make decisions about the degree to which recommendations will be followed. Health professionals should talk to the patient, not to the third party as if the patient were not present.

The patient and third party may disagree about the recommendations being made or the extent to which the older patient can carry them out. Family members or caregivers may request to speak with the health professional alone and then attempt to collude with the health professional to withhold concerns or other information with the patient. It can be difficult to respect the concerns of the family member as well as to respect autonomy of the patient. Older patients should, however, be approached with the same respect and concern that would be given any other patient. Although it is important to be sensitive to family or caregivers' concerns, it is also important to stress patients' rights to be fully informed about their treatment and condition.

The patient's autonomy should be respected as much as is reasonable. The health professional's primary obligation is to the patient. This means that in some instances, patient education may involve helping the family member or caregiver understand the patient's rights to information and to determine treatment. For example, Mr. Jackson, at 82, was shown to have elevated cholesterol. His daughter insisted he follow a strict diet, which he found unpalatable. Ms. Freeburn, the nurse conducting patient education, helped Mr. Jackson's daughter see that following the diet in moderation while still allowing him to have foods he enjoyed may be more important than lowering his cholesterol.

MAXIMIZING COMMUNICATION EFFECTIVENESS
WITH OLDER ADULTS

Patient education information should be provided to patients in a way that they will be able to understand. Health professionals should be alert for clues about the ability of the older adult to comprehend information, whether these clues relate to level of alertness, cognitive ability, or decreased hearing ability or vision.

As much information as possible about the patient should be gathered before the patient education intervention. Health professionals should assess the patient's general level of alertness. For instance, if patients are sedated they will be unable to focus attention on the information being presented. Being aware of patients' thought process and content can help health professionals assess the detail of information that needs to be given and whether a caregiver should also be present. Older patients may be unable to process complex information as swiftly and efficiently as younger patients and may need more time to conceptualize and organize their thoughts. Health professionals should not interrupt or try to put words into the patient's mouth. More time may be needed to allow patients to process the information appropriately.

Health professionals should not show annoyance if patients ask questions or ask to have information repeated. Patients' questions should be responded to appropriately. If patients perceive annoyance on the part of the health professional, they may be more reluctant to ask questions or may pretend to understand even when they don't. Health professionals should look for clues of misunderstanding and restate what they said if needed. If much information is being provided, patients should be given the opportunity to rest, or the patient education intervention should be broken up into several sessions.

When memory problems are present, the health professional should assess the degree of memory impairment and tailor patient activities accordingly. If patients become distracted from the topic being discussed, they may need to be gently reminded of the topic at hand before continuing. Repeating and reinforcing information that has been given is important in helping patients incorporate patient teaching points. Written materials that the patient can review at home may also be of help. Various prompts may also be used for helping patients remember treatment recommendations.

Because of normal aging changes in the eyes, visual acuity and the perception of color, as well as degree of illumination for different tasks, may be altered. Color perceptions may change, making it more difficult for older individuals to distinguish between certain colors. Consequently, patient education materials should be evaluated based on their readability, both in terms of color contrasts and size of print. When conducting patient education, health professionals should also make sure that sufficient lighting is available, especially if patient teaching involves demonstration of tasks. Lighting that minimizes shadows and reduces glare is optimal. When conducting patient teaching, health professionals should position themselves in light, facing the patient, and preferably at eye level.

Varying degrees of hearing impairment may also be experienced by older adults. Patients cannot follow recommendations that they are unable to hear. Patient education is best conducted in a room free of excessive and background noise. If the patient does not see the health professional enter the room, the patient's attention should be obtained by touch or verbal greeting. Health professionals should talk with the patient in a normal tone of voice, speaking slowly and distinctly. Excessive body movements or exaggerated movements should be avoided. Raising the voice causes distortion, making it more difficult for the patient to hear. Health professionals should face the patient when they speak. Not only is this polite, it provides better sound and enables patients to pick up visual cues. Health professionals should avoid covering their mouth when they speak and should look directly at the patient when they speak. They should maintain a comfortable distance from the patient, not being too close, which can distort sound. Speaking directly into the patient's ear should also be avoided.

Because much of the effectiveness of patient education is dependent on the therapeutic alliance built between patient and health professional, conveying respect for the patient early on in the intervention is crucial. Health professionals should avoid calling older patients by their first name unless invited to do so. Likewise, terms such as "sweety" or "honey" should be avoided. Using touch on the hand, arm, or shoulder of the patient can also convey reassurance and help put the patient at ease.

Health professionals should be flexible in following the patients' train of thought and pace the patient education session. Patients should be given ample opportunity to express concerns, and their most pressing concern should be addressed even though it may be different from that of the health professional.

EFFECTIVE PATIENT EDUCATION WITH OLDER ADULTS

Special sensitivities and skills are required for effective patient education with older adults. As discussed previously, definition of "older" varies with the individual. Some individuals are relatively healthy and active in their 80s, whereas others have significant functional limitations and consider themselves old in their late 60s. There are no specific rules or definitions of when a person is considered old. The approach to teaching older adults must, therefore, be individualized and based on individual patient need. Patient education should be geared to specific patient circumstances, rather than chronologic age.

An evaluation of patient education potential should be performed routinely. Patient education must be conducted within the context of a multidisciplinary plan that considers additional medical problems, potential side effects of treatment, and special arrangements that may need to be made so the individual has the best opportunity for carrying out the patient education plan. As with all patient education encounters, the health professional must work to establish a therapeutic alliance with the patient.

Assessing patients' perceptions about their concepts of aging provides health professionals with beginning information that can be helpful in patient teaching. Patients may attribute symptoms to normal aging even though symptoms may be indicative of side effects of treatment or of a specific disease. Likewise, symptoms related to disease may present more subtly in older adults than in younger adults. If symptoms are ignored or unrecognized, a treatable condition may go untreated and complications may result. Older patients may be reluctant to share symptoms because they fear they will be categorized as complaining. Helping patients understand the importance of reporting symptoms and reporting them accurately is an important first step in patient education.

Distinguishing acute symptoms from those that are chronic provides important information that can be used as a guideline for patient teaching. For example, if the patient complains of incontinence, patient teaching takes a different approach depending upon whether the problem has existed for years or whether the symptom is new. If incontinence has been ongoing and has been appropriately evaluated, depending on the cause of incontinence, patient education may involve teaching patients to use easily removable garments that facilitate toilet use or teaching patients behavior techniques that can help them learn to control their bladder and pelvic muscles. If the condition is new, however, patient education may involve teaching patients that incontinence is not a normal part of aging and helping them obtain a referral for evaluation.

Content of patient education may be different as well. The need to assess functional status in terms of everyday activity and their ability to carry out recommendations may need to be more detailed in the older adult. For example, teaching younger patients about medications and potential side effects as well as their ability to obtain the medication is important. In older adults, however, depending on circumstances and other disease processes, patient education about medication may also include strategies for remembering to take the medication. If visual problems exist, the patient may need to be taught how to distinguish one medication from another, or if physical limitations exist, what devices or solutions may be used to help patients carry out recommendations.

Patient education for family members may also be important. Although the goal may be to help the patient maintain independence, family members may be overly protective. Families may need to be helped to accept the patient's feelings and need for maintaining maximum independence while at the same time allaying family members' anxiety by identifying potential services and resources that enhance independence while assuring safety. In other instances, patient education interventions for family members may be directed toward helping them reduce their burden of care. Resources regarding respite care or other services can be helpful.

Patient education should be structured with problem-focused, well-defined goals. The health professional should emphasize patients' strengths, supporting preexisting positive coping patterns. Emphasis should be placed on current concerns of the older adult, and practical solutions should be considered. As with all patient education encounters, the best predictor of compliance is concordance between the health professional and patient regarding goals. This is especially true when working with older adults because much variability exists in cognitive ability, verbal skills, medical problems, and degrees of social support.

The health professional should be flexible in patient teaching, tailoring teaching to the patient's specific needs and orientation. If the patient's major concern is maintaining independence, this need should be addressed first, even though the health professional may believe another aspect of patient teaching to be more important. Establishing plans for maintaining contact with the health professional through return visits or phone calls for short-term follow-up may be even more important with older patients than with younger patients so problems or concerns can be identified early and appropriately addressed.

A goal of patient education is to effectively integrate physical as well as social and psychological aspects of each individual patient. Using an interdisciplinary team approach can increase resources available that support health professionals in working with older patients with a variety of social and interpersonal problems related to their care. The older patient should be an equal member of the team. Continued reevaluation and treatment should be ongoing. Most of all, health professionals should treat older patients as individuals and with respect. The older patient's life as an independent person with unique likes, dislikes, values, and choices should not be discounted.

REFERENCES

Arking, R. 1998. Biology of aging. Sunderland, MA: Sinauer Associates.

Atchley, R.C. 2000. Social forces and aging. 9th ed. Belmont, CA: Wadsworth.

Brown, J.B., Brett, P., Stewart, M., Marshall, J.M. 1998. Roles and influence of people who accompany patients on visits to the doctor. *Canadian Family Physician* 44:1644–1650.

Burke, J.P., Williams, K., Gaskill, S.P., Hazuda, H.P., Haffner, S.M., Stern, M.P. 1999. Rapid rise in the incidence of type II diabetes from 1987–1996: results from the San Antonio Heart Study. *Archives of Internal Medicine* 159:1450–1455.

Christiansen, J.L., Grzybowski, J.M. 1999. Biology of aging: an introduction to the biomedical aspects of aging. New York: McGraw Hill.

Cockerham, W.C. 1997. This aging society. 2nd ed. Upper Saddle River, NJ: Prentice Hall.

Digiovanna, A.G. 2000. Human aging: biological perspectives. Boston: McGraw Hill.

Engram, B.E. 1981. Communication skills training for rehabilitation counselors working with older persons. *Journal of Rehabilitation* 47(4):51–56.

Harris, M.E., Flegal, K.M., Cowie, C.C., Eberhardt, M.S., Goldstein, D.E., Little, R.R., Wiedmeyer, H.M., Byrd-Holt, D.D. 1998. Prevalence of diabetes, impaired fasting glucose, and impaired glucose tolerance in U.S. adults: the Third National Health and Nutrition Examination Survey, 1988–1994. *Diabetes Care* 21:518–525.

National Institute on Aging. 2002. Aging in the United States: past, present and future. 1960–2020. Washington, DC: U.S. Department of Commerce.

Nuttbrock, L., Kosburg, J.I. 1980. Images of the physician and help seeking behavior of the elderly: a multivariate assessment. *Journal of Gerontology* 35(2):241–248.

Ory, M.G., Bond, K. 1989. Aging and health care. London: Routledge.

Schaie, K.W., Willis, S.L. 2002. Adult development and aging. 5th ed. Upper Saddle River, NJ: Prentice Hall.

Stewart, M., Meredith, L., Brown, J.B., Galajda, J. 2000. Communication between older patients and their physician: the influence of older patient physician communication on health and health related outcomes. *Clinics in Geriatric Medicine* 16(1):25–36.

Timiras, P.S. 1994. Physiological basis of aging and geriatrics. 2nd ed. Boca Raton: CRC Press.

U.S. Bureau of Census 1998. Current population reports, Series P20-514. Washington DC: US Government Printing Office.

Patient Education About End-of-Life Issues

13

IMPORTANCE OF TEACHING ABOUT END-OF-LIFE ISSUES

Patient education is usually characterized as a process by which patients are provided with information about causes and treatments of health problems, are counseled about risk factors, or are given information about prevention of disease or complications. The focus on patient teaching is to help patients maintain or improve health by achieving long-range outcomes or life-style changes. Another focus of patient education is to enhance patients' ability to make informed choices about health and health care.

Patient teaching about end-of-life issues is rarely considered a part of the general concept of patient education. Although less recognized, patient education about end-of-life issues is vitally important to assist patients to make informed choices and to enhance quality of life, whether death is imminent or a distant possibility.

As technologic advances and treatment interventions that extend the life of those with life-threatening disease multiply, as the aging population grows, and as awareness of the need for compassionate and respectful care of individuals with terminal conditions increases, the need for effective ways to teach patients and families about end-of-life issues becomes even more important (Schears 1999). Discussion of living wills and advance directives is important even when patients are in the best of health because no one can predict when a devastating accident or serious illness may necessitate decisions about approaches to dying and death. Whether preparing for the future in the absence of disease, living with a life-threatening disease, or coping with terminal illness, patients may have distinct preferences about treatment, about procedures they would or would not want to have performed at end of life, and about how, under those circumstances, they would prefer to spend the remaining days of their lives. Information about end-of-life issues can provide patients with a sense of preparedness and control, whether death is a distant possibility or more imminent.

Although health professionals have become more aware of the need to employ a holistic, family-centered approach to death and dying, in many instances emphasis still often remains on patients' physical needs. Even when issues of death and dying are addressed from a psychological or social perspective, patient education needs of the patient may not be adequately addressed. Addressing patients' medical, psychological, or social needs without also providing them with information and skills needed to make end-of-life decisions or to manage care at end of life thwarts their control and autonomy and inhibits patients' ability to fully participate in their own care and decisions.

Whether engaging patients in proactive planning about end of life before a crisis event or discussing end-of-life issues during terminal stages of disease, health professionals should not make assumptions that their personal beliefs coincide with patients' preferences. Given vast differences in individual values related to end of life, the only way to determine patients' preferences is to participate in active discussion with them.

Increasing the patient's state of well-being through provision of complete and honest information underpins all patient education. Nowhere is this ideology more important than when discussing issues related to end of life. Discussions should be individualized and should be directed toward helping patients gain information that enables them to make informed choices, to maximize quality of life at end of life, and to die with as much comfort, dignity, and freedom from anxiety as possible.

In view of the individual nature of beliefs and feelings about death and dying, health professionals face a special challenge when teaching patients and their families about end-of-life issues. The challenge can be met, however, if there is a basic understanding of pertinent principles and dynamics involved, and if health professionals reflect, understand, and acknowledge their own beliefs and feelings about death and dying.

RELUCTANCE TO TALK ABOUT END-OF-LIFE ISSUES

Discussions with patients about end-of-life issues are not always conducted when the opportunity presents itself. Health professionals may have feelings of discomfort with the topic or may feel they are inadequately trained to communicate with patients about death and dying (Elder 1996). Health professionals are often action oriented, having been trained to focus on saving lives, curing, preventing, or stabilizing conditions. Consequently, accepting and acknowledging the realities and finality of death may be difficult (Dangler et al. 1996). When working with generally healthy patients, health professionals may not view such discussions as being relevant or may not think this type of patient teaching is within the general framework of their role. Consequently, health professionals may neglect to bring up the topic altogether. When confronted with patients with terminal illness, health professionals may also avoid discussion of end-of-life issues because they feel a sense of helplessness or because they believe there is little left that they have to offer professionally.

Death and dying may be perceived as a highly ambiguous issue with no clear reference points. Health professionals who have a low tolerance for uncertainty may experience discomfort in end-of-life circumstances that present complex or contradictory situations (Kvale et al. 1999). In these cases, they may find it difficult to confront their own values, beliefs, and attitudes about death and dying, and neglect to focus on more passive, reflective approaches. When patients have beliefs and values that differ from those of the health professional, the situation may be even more difficult.

Discussing death and dying with patients can be emotionally painful, distressing, and sometimes threatening, especially if the patient's condition is incurable or when death is imminent. Under these circumstances, patient education may elicit anxiety in health professionals, hindering their ability to effectively help patients and families cope. High degrees of death anxiety may cause health professionals to distance themselves from discussions of end-of-life issues and to focus on patients' physical needs rather than on the emotional aspects of care (Garfinkle and Block 1996). In some instances, health professionals may minimize patient contact or avoid interacting with patients with life-threatening or terminal conditions altogether.

Reaching a level of comfort with discussion of end-of-life issues requires health professionals to explore their own feelings and attitudes about death and dying. Just as patients' reactions to death and dying are determined by culture, family attitudes, religion, and past experiences with death, so are reactions of health professionals. Issues of death and dying may engender anxiety in health professionals because these issues arouse thoughts about their own mortality or of the fragility and vulnerability of loved ones who could be lost to death.

Anxiety may be provoked by thoughts of the dying process rather than by death itself. Health professionals may experience feelings of inadequacy or failure when faced with patients with life-threatening or terminal conditions. They may also experience feelings of guilt about whether more could have been done to postpone or reverse the dying process.

Some health professionals may focus on personal experiences with the death of loved ones, projecting feelings and experiences onto patients and their situation. Take, for example, Lana, who had provided nursing care for Mrs. George throughout her postoperative course after surgery for colon cancer as well as during chemotherapy. Despite surgery and chemotherapy metastasis resulted. Mrs. George's physicians informed Mrs. George and her family that her prognosis was grave. They offered her the possibility of additional chemotherapy but also advised her of potential adverse effects she might experience. They informed Mrs. George that despite additional chemotherapy, chances of cure or remission were only slight. After discussion with her family, Mrs. George elected to forego chemotherapy, choosing to return to her home, enlisting the services of Hospice. Lana, although maintaining a professional demeanor with Mrs. George, went to her supervisor and requested a change of assignment because she could not understand Mrs. George's resistance to treatment and did not agree with Mrs. George's "not trying." Although Lana was unaware of the underlying cause of her strong feelings at the time, she later realized that she was associating Mrs. George's situation with that of her own mother who had died of colon cancer several years earlier.

Caring for patients with life-threatening or terminal illness can revive memories of unresolved losses health professionals have sustained in their life. Had Lana understood how her own situation impacted on her feelings about Mrs. George's situation, or had she resolved her feelings about her mother's death, she may have been able to use her own experiences to provide information and support to Mrs. George and her family. Resolving prior conflicts can provide health professionals with valuable insights that can be useful and helpful in the patient education intervention.

In some instances, reluctance to discuss end-of-life issues with patients may be due to fear of the inability to maintain emotional composure or fear of losing control in front of the patient. Although maintaining a professional demeanor with patients is important, displaying a cold, unfeeling exterior in the face of news that is devastating to the patient can do more harm than good. Patients are often touched and feel solace when health professionals demonstrate sincere emotion and concern when discussing serious issues with patients and their families (Buckman et al. 2000).

Health professionals may also fear that discussion of end-of-life issues will be upsetting to patients and their families and consequently avoid such discussions altogether. Avoiding discussions, especially in the case of life-threatening or terminal conditions, can cause even more anxiety in patients who may not know what to expect or feel they have lost control of their own destiny. Frank and compassionate discussions with patients during this time can be a source of empowerment and help patients to more fully participate in their own care and decisions.

For health professionals to reach a comfort level that would enable them to initiate and conduct effective dialogue with patients about end-of-life issues, feelings and attitudes about death and dying must first be explored. Examining these feelings and attitudes assists health professionals to recognize their limitations as well as areas of strength in conducting patient education about end-of-life issues. Through awareness of their own feelings related to death and dying, health professionals will be better able to approach patients' feelings and preferences about care at the end of life with sensitivity and compassion.

Awareness of personal beliefs, feelings, and attitudes about death and dying is an important first step to effectively conducting patient education about end-of-life issues. Despite self-exploration and awareness, however, resolution of all personal issues may not be reached. Not everyone can work adequately with all types of patients with life-threatening conditions. Jane, a 4th year medical student, lost her own child to leukemia before entering medical school. The event was devastating for Jane, who went into medicine with the hope that she could help others who had been touched by life-threatening conditions. When choosing the medical field in which she wanted to specialize, she determined that pediatrics would not be a choice. Despite her desire to help others, she was aware of potential difficulties her own experiences might cause if she were providing care for children with life-threatening conditions. She realized, however, that by choosing a specialty such as internal medicine, she could use her own experiences and insights to offer support and understanding to adult patients should they be confronted with a situation similar to that which she had experienced in the past. Jane was able to recognize not only her limitations but her strengths in dealing with end-of-life issues and was able to use this knowledge productively.

When health professionals feel unable to provide appropriate information or support to patients regarding end-of-life issues, referrals should be made. Health professionals can still convey concern to patients without compromising their own feelings and without causing patients to feel abandoned. Statements such as the following can help patients feel that the health professional is still providing the support they need but not deserting them when making a referral:

> In this situation, I want to make sure that you have the very best support possible. Although I will continue to be a resource for you, I would like to refer you to Mr. Walker, the social worker, who has special training in helping with these issues and, consequently, may be better able to meet your specific needs right now.

CULTURAL VARIATIONS IN DEATH AND DYING

Culture is more than race or ethnicity. It can be broadly defined as a common social experience containing a shared belief system, shared expectations, and shared behaviors and rituals (Hallenbeck 2001). Cultural differences have an impact on all aspects of health care. Because culture permeates life, all aspects of end-of-life issues have a cultural component. Cultural beliefs, rituals, and attitudes impact upon concepts and reactions to death, and upon end-of-life care and decision making regarding preferences to care. Whereas Eastern philosophies tend to accept death as part of the natural rhythm of life, Western cultures tend to view death as an event to be postponed as long as possible (Klessig 1998). Concepts of death in our society often focus on Euro-American and Judeo-Christian values rather than incorporating beliefs of other ethnic and religious groups. Some cultures encourage truth telling, whereas other cultures expect the truth to be hidden from the patient. Some cultures value individual autonomy in decision making, whereas other cultures traditionally view families as the decision makers.

Racial, religious, and cultural differences influence views of end of life held by health professionals, as well as those held by patients and their families (Vincent 2001). Therefore, basic understanding of cultural issues involved in death and dying and sensitivity to interpersonal relations in the context of culture are key to effective patient education about end-of-life issues.

When patients' skin color, mode of dress, facial features, or language are different from those of health professionals, the possibility of cultural differences is easy to recognize. Cultural differences may be discounted, however, when patients share many of the same cultural attributes with health professionals even though their culture may still differ in significant ways. Not only are there variations within the same culture, but every individual within a culture is unique unto themselves (Safonte-Strumolo and Dunn 2000). Sensitivity to individual differences related to culture, even in situations where culture differences are not immediately recognized, helps health professionals avoid misunderstandings and cultural conflicts and facilitates communication about end-of-life issues.

Before initiating patient teaching about end-of-life issues with patients from a different culture, health professionals may find it useful to inquire about concepts and practices about death and dying within the patient's culture. Some cultures have taboos against direct, verbal communication about death related to a specific individual. There may be fear that discussion of death and dying increases the chance of death for the patient or that talking about death will have unfortunate consequences for family members (Hallenbeck 2001). If this is the case, patient education interventions that include end-of-life discussions may be resisted by patients. Health professionals can still introduce the discussion while respecting patients' beliefs with a phrase such as:

> I am unfamiliar with your culture, but would like to learn more. Talking in general terms, what is your culture's belief or practice surrounding end of life?

Such an inquiry helps health professionals approach the subject and learn more about cultural beliefs of the patient while avoiding direct discussion of death related to a specific patient.

If patient teaching involves a situation in which death is imminent, but discussion of death and dying remains a sensitive issue, health professionals may ask the patient or family members if there are specific concerns about activities or procedures health professionals may carry out at this time that could violate cultural taboos. By asking for specific ways in which the patient's cultural integrity can be maintained, health professionals communicate concern and respect for the patient and family's cultural priorities.

Cultural differences about the role of family in end-of-life decision making varies greatly. Some cultures focus mainly on the family, protecting it from outsiders (Vincent 2001). In these instances, participation by health professionals in end-of-life discussion or decision making may be viewed as an intrusion or violation of family privacy. Family members may be reluctant to discuss end-of-life issues for fear of appearing to be disloyal to the family unit. Approaching the family in a nonjudgmental and nondefensive way builds trust and shows regard for the patient's cultural concerns.

Some cultures value individual participation and involvement in end-of-life issues, whereas other cultures prescribe that close relatives, rather than patients themselves, are involved in decision making and given details about the patient's condition. When health professionals are from a culture that values patient autonomy as an important part of medical care, withholding information from the patient may seem like a violation of patient rights. Under these circumstances, health professionals may approach the family request for withholding information by clarifying reasons for the request with statements such as:

> I know different people have different beliefs about how situations such as this should be approached. In my country, we generally believe that it is the patient's right to know about their condition and to participate in decision making about their care. Could you tell me more about your culture's beliefs?

If family members confirm that in their culture it is appropriate to allow family members to be given medical information about the patient and to make decisions without patient input, health professionals need to confirm this belief with the patient. The patient may be approached with a statement such as:

> I've been trying to understand more about your culture so I can provide care that does not violate your beliefs or values. I understand in your culture details about a patient's medical condition as well as decisions about how care should be managed is discussed with the family and that the family, rather than the patient, usually makes decisions. Is this the way you would like for me to handle this in your case?

If the patient agrees, their wishes should be respected. If the patient confirms that this is the practice in the culture, but also acknowledges that they would prefer to understand their own condition and be involved in making their own decisions, the health professional should honor the patient's wishes. In this instance, further discussion with the patient about how they would like this situation to be approached with the family, as well as further discussion with the family, should be undertaken.

Patients can be from a different culture but still share a common language with health professionals. In instances where there are language differences, however, a significant barrier to communication exists. Unless information can be translated competently and completely, patient education interventions will be ineffective. If possible, services of a professional medical translator should be requested. Health professionals should be aware that translations can be skewed, misinterpreted, or filtered when family members or others who only have a working knowledge of the language are utilized as translators.

Cultural history can also influence patient education about end-of-life issues, especially where there has been a history of inequities and conflict between cultural groups or where mistrust, prejudice, and discrimination have existed. For example, in discussions about advanced care planning and end-of-life decision making, patients in some cultures may be more likely to desire full and prolonged life support, for fear of premature termination of life based on prejudice, whereas individuals in other cultures who have not experienced the same degree of prejudice or discrimination may prefer limited intervention or withholding treatment when death is imminent.

Health professionals must always be aware of cultural influences and how these have shaped their lives and practices. They should also be aware of possible differences between their own beliefs and those of patients from cultures different from their own. In addition to awareness of cultural differences, health professionals should be aware of intergenerational differences in beliefs, reactions, and adherence to traditions about end-of-life issues, even within the same culture. Culture is not stagnant but rather is continually evolving. Consequently, health professionals should not assume that values, beliefs, and traditions that a culture held relevant many years ago are necessarily still prevalent today. Patient education about end-of-life issues with individuals from different cultures should focus on respect for individual differences, promoting mutual understanding.

Even when individuals from other cultures may have become acculturated into a new society, it is important to note that in death, people often revert to their own cultural roots. Health professionals should not assume that individuals who have apparently incorporated beliefs and values of a new culture into their own life have necessarily abandoned their own cultural beliefs, especially in discussions of death and dying. Clarification of values without making assumptions helps health professionals avoid misunderstanding in these instances.

Although maintaining cultural sensitivity is important, individual variations exist within each culture. Factors such as educational and socioeconomic status as well as other individual factors can impact a patient's cultural beliefs and values. The same approach may not be appropriate to all patients, even when they are from the same culture. Consequently, approaches to patient teaching about end-of-life issues should be adapted to fit the patient's cultural norms and individual needs.

UNDERSTANDING DEATH AND DYING IN THE CONTEXT OF THE PATIENT

Health professionals' awareness of their own personal feelings about death and dying is an important component of effective patient education about end-of-life issues; however, another important consideration is understanding the meaning death and dying has to individual patients (Bone 1997). Not everyone shares the same concept of the meaning of death. Likewise, not everyone's outward report of their concept coincides with their unconscious or internal beliefs.

There is no standard meaning of death. Each patient brings a unique perspective to death and dying. This individual perspective is dependent on culture, religion, past experiences, and general philosophy of life. When conducting patient education about end-of-life issues, health professionals must be ever mindful of individual differences, considering the patient's perspective. To be maximally effective, patient education information about end-of-life issues should be presented within that context.

REACTIONS TO BAD NEWS

Receiving news of a life-threatening or terminal condition is not only an individual experience. It has multiple dimensions involving patients, their family and friends, as well as health professionals. Not all patients react to the diagnosis of life-threatening or terminal illness in the same way, nor do they progress in their reactions to the diagnosis in predictable stages (Peteet et al. 1991). Although the way patients react to bad news is individual, most patients experience cognitive, emotional, behavioral, and physical reactions to the information. Health professionals should remember, however, that "bad news" is contextual—it is not interpreted in the same way by everyone. How news is interpreted may depend on the nature of the news and the meaning the individual attaches to the news. Take the following case as an example:

Marla had been having vague symptoms for the past 8 months. Sometimes she felt dizzy; sometimes she felt too weak to go up a flight of stairs; other times she had difficulty with fine motor movements. She made an appointment with her physician, but there were no physical findings that accounted for her symptoms. Her symptoms would subside for a while but then reappear. She sought opinions from a number of physicians, all of whom could find no reason for her symptoms. One physician suggested that her symptoms were due to work-related stress, although she insisted she loved her job as a teacher. Her family also began to doubt the physical nature of her symptoms, suggesting that it appeared her symptoms seemed to flare up only when there was something she didn't want to do. Marla became very discouraged and withdrawn. Finally, she decided to attempt one more time to solve the mystery of her symptoms, seeking an opinion from yet another physician. After listening to her symptoms and history, and conducting an examination, the physician finally concluded that Marla had multiple sclerosis. In preparing to tell Marla of the diagnosis, the doctor told a colleague, "I really dread giving this type of diagnosis. I never like giving bad news." The physician was surprised, however, when Marla responded to the news with relief. "I am so relieved that there is a physical cause for what I've been experiencing. Not knowing why I felt like I did, and having everyone think I was crazy or that I was making the symptoms up was really getting to me. Now I know the cause, even though it is a progressive condition, I can at least plan accordingly."

Marla's condition wasn't immediately life threatening or terminal, however the news still implied potential loss. Despite the chronicity of her condition and losses she could be expected to experience, she felt relief now that she knew the diagnosis and could plan accordingly. Although different reactions and issues may be associated with life-threatening or terminal conditions, patients may also react in a way similar to Marla, putting energy into planning for the future.

Fear

A natural first reaction to a diagnosis that threatens existence of self is fear. Patients may fear death, but also, more than death itself, they may fear the dying process. Fear may lie in the uncertainty of what the dying process holds. Many patients fear potential pain and discomfort associated with dying. Assuring patients that all measures will be taken to keep them as comfortable as possible and providing them with practical information about how symptoms they may be experiencing can be controlled can help decrease fear.

Patients may also fear being deserted by family, friends, or perhaps even by health professionals. Although there is no way of predicting reactions of family and friends, promoting active inclusion and participation of those individuals to whom the patient feels close helps strengthen relationships and bonding between individuals. Active collaboration and building a partnership between patient and health professional also helps to decrease fears and reassures the patient that help will be provided when they need it most.

Fears of loss of dignity and/or loss of control can be lessened by encouraging and respecting patient autonomy and authority in their own care and by exploring and maintaining as many areas of control for the patient as possible. If the patient had previously addressed end-of-life issues through a living will or advance directives, reassuring patients that their wishes will be adhered to can also reduce fear.

Patients may fear that medical costs could jeopardize continued medical care or treatment, or could cause significant financial burden to family. Referrals to appropriate personnel and social agencies can help patients sort out their concerns and help them determine how financial concerns can be addressed.

Denial

Some patients react to the life-threatening or terminal nature of a condition through denial of implications of the diagnosis. Denial, especially in the initial stages can be one of the most pervasive and persistent responses to dying. Denial, however, expresses itself in different ways. Individuals may totally avoid admitting anything is wrong, or they may acknowledge the seriousness of their diagnosis, but deny the terminal nature of the condition. This reaction is not uncommon, especially initially. Patients may be unable to accept or assimilate the seriousness of their condition, such as was the case of Mr. Kottke. After undergoing a liver biopsy, Mr. Kottke was found to have end-stage nonalcoholic fatty liver disease.

Liver transplantation was recommended. He declined the procedure stating, "Oh, I'm sure that can't be a correct diagnosis; I just had a physical exam last year and everything was fine."

Patients may also react by distorting the facts and placing a more favorable prognosis on the diagnosis than is warranted. Mrs. Jameson's physician informed her that she had an inoperable malignant tumor of the brain. When she told family and friends about her diagnosis, however, she was heard to say, "The doctor said I have a tumor on the brain, but luckily didn't say I had cancer, so although it's serious, I think I'll be alright."

Denial can be a protective mechanism when the diagnosis causes more stress than the patient can cope with at the time. Unfortunately denial can also result in avoidance of medical care and treatment that could prolong life or make life more comfortable for a longer period of time. In some instances, although the seriousness of the condition isn't denied, the terminal nature of the condition may be, causing patients to frantically seek other medical or nonmedical options, which can be costly and at times harmful, causing additional suffering or even earlier death.

Patients who deny the terminal nature of their condition may be unable to cope with the pain and anxiety associated with the reality that accompanies the threat of loss of self. Acceptance of patients' feelings builds trust and provides time for patients to begin to assimilate the diagnosis and work toward acceptance. Forcing patients to face the reality of the diagnosis before they are able to accept it only increases anxiety and alienation, fracturing trust and potentially delaying the possibility of helping patients accept their diagnosis. By expressing care and concern as well as offering patient support, health professionals provide patients the opportunity to gradually accept the threat of the diagnosis so they may adjust to the terminal nature of their illness.

Anxiety

Anxiety is a universal reaction to threat and is a common reaction to a diagnosis that implies potential or imminent threat to life. One source of anxiety is related to loss. Health professionals can help patients deal with their sense of loss by being available to them and understanding what loss means to them and how it effects them.

No one knows exactly what it is like to die. Death is an unknowable and irreversible experience. A major source of anxiety about death in some patients may stem from loss of the known. Questions of what lies ahead, the thought of nothingness, or the concept of ceasing to exist can all be sources of anxiety for the patient. Health professionals can reduce patient anxiety by demonstrating willingness to listen to patients' fears and concerns. Approaching patient concerns in a nonjudgmental manner creates an atmosphere of trust and confidence, thereby decreasing anxiety.

In other instances, patients' anxiety may be related to fear of separation from loved ones or loss of the comfort and self-esteem such relationships provide.

Exploring the significance of patients' relationships and acknowledging their importance helps establish a sense of continuity and meaning. Fostering interactions between patients and those they hold dear, as well as encouraging involvement in life and with other people, can be a source of strength for all concerned. If conflicts between the patient and family members exist, helping patients identify resources that enable them to explore opportunities for resolution can also allay anxiety.

Patients' anxiety may, in some instances not be due to loss of contact with loved ones but because of fear about the consequences the patients' death will have on those they care about. Patients may perceive their death as loss of ability to provide assistance or support to family members. Take, for example, Mr. Pearson. At the age of 90, he stated he felt he had lived a successful, productive life, and did not fear his own death per se. He did, however, relate that he felt considerable anxiety because after his own death he feared what would happen to his wife who had dementia. Another example is that of Mr. Appleton. Mr. Appleton's wife and three children appeared to have accepted the terminal nature of his condition and offered him considerable support and consolation. Despite his close-knit family, Mr. Appleton continued to experience considerable anxiety. He stated that he worried constantly about the impact he feared his death would have on his family's financial stability. In the case of both Mr. Pearson and Mr. Appleton, identifying and acknowledging their fears and then assisting them to identify resources that could be used to help them plan for the future provides a mechanism through which potential solutions can be reached, thus decreasing anxiety levels.

Other patients experience anxiety when confronted with end-of-life issues because of fear of loss of dignity and integrity. They may fear loss of control of their life, of their self, of their body, or of the ability to master their own fate. Patients can be helped to explore remaining areas in which they do have control or in which they can take more control. Providing patients with information about how to control symptoms, as well as collaborating with patients in the management of their care can help them gain a sense of control and consequently reduce anxiety. By respecting and encouraging patient autonomy and authority in those matters in which they can make choices, a sense of control and freedom can be fostered.

If patients have not planned advance directives, helping them outline specific wishes and assuring them of cooperation and support of health professionals in carrying out their wishes can also be a means of reducing anxiety. If the patient has already prepared advance directives, reviewing the directives with the patient and providing reassurance can also bring a measure of peace.

Grief

Grief is a normal reaction to loss. It is to be expected that patients who experience a life-threatening or terminal illness will also experience grief to some degree. Grief can be manifested in a number of ways, from physical symptoms to psychological symptoms including depression. Health professionals can help patients through the grieving process by acknowledging grief and teaching patients ways to deal with it. A first step is to listen and acknowledge patients' expressions of feelings. Teaching patients that grief is an expected reaction to loss helps them to recognize symptoms that may be related to grief as well as helps them normalize reactions they may be experiencing. The following types of statements may be helpful:

> Grief is a natural and normal reaction to loss. We've just talked about some of the losses you feel you will be experiencing because of your diagnosis. Grief is a reaction to those experiences and feelings that you have in response to the losses. As painful as grief is, however, it can be used to learn new approaches to living and to relating. There is no one right way to grieve and there is no timetable associated with it. It is an individual process that each person experiences differently.

Health professionals can help patients identify sources of support, such as family, friends, church, or other social groups. Patient support groups can also help patients be in touch with others with similar experiences. Sharing feelings in an atmosphere of understanding can help patients work through their grief and reach acceptance.

Helping patients review and identify their strengths and abilities can also promote confidence in their ability to cope. Other interventions that can help patients cope are providing written information, acknowledging reactions and feelings, and providing opportunities for patients to express feelings. Some patients may find it helpful to record their thoughts and experiences in a journal. Writing out thoughts can help patients express feelings as well as clarify issues that they may otherwise find difficult to bring into focus or to express verbally.

Anger

When threatened with the potential or imminent loss of life, patients may react with anger. Angry outbursts may be directed toward those individuals closest to the patient or toward health professionals most involved in an attempt to help.

Take, for example, the case of Mr. Lovelace. Mr. Lovelace was unaware he was HIV positive, although he had had significant weight loss and had begun to experience other symptoms that he couldn't explain. When he was admitted to the hospital for elective surgery, results of routine preoperative surgical lab tests showed him to be HIV positive. In conducting the preoperative interview, it was noted that he already had begun to experience symptoms consistent with the diagnosis of AIDS. When the physician discussed the diagnosis with him, Mr. Lovelace became extremely angry. His anger was directed not only toward his physician but also toward the nurses responsible for his care. He insinuated that they were incompetent and threatened to sue the physician for defamation of character. Mr. Lovelace's expressions of anger, although directed at health professionals, were actually a reflection of anxiety related to his diagnosis. Although his physician and nurses were not responsible, nor could they cure his condition, Mr. Lovelace's anxiety about the condition caused him to lash out at those most readily available to help.

Reactions of hostility, anger, or defensiveness may be difficult for health professionals to accept. Hostility or anger, however, should be viewed as a symptom with meaning that should be explored, not ignored or avoided. Communicating understanding of the distress brought about by the situation helps patients gradually come to grips with their anger and reach acceptance of the situation at hand. Although communicating understanding may not help patients immediately resolve their anger, it affords patients the opportunity to work through their anger in a supportive atmosphere, increasing the likelihood that a helping relationship can be established.

Retreat

Patients may also react to bad news through retreat. Ms. Castilano, who had surgery for breast cancer, underwent radiation and chemotherapy after surgery. After treatment, she was relieved to hear from the physician that she was 95% sure that all cancer cells had been eradicated. When Ms. Castilano began experiencing symptoms several years later, she was again evaluated by her physician. The cancer was found to have metastasized to the extent that only palliative treatment could be of benefit. Ms. Castilano accepted the diagnosis calmly and returned to her apartment where she stayed for weeks, refusing to go out, refusing to answer the phone, and refusing to answer the door.

Reflection

Other patients may use the diagnosis of life-threatening or terminal conditions to reexamine goals and values, altering both to reach a higher level of growth. Such individuals may become more acutely aware of their environment and those in it. They may become more compassionate and caring, directing their life toward the needs of others. For example, Mr. Fang experienced severe heart disease. He received a heart transplant but was told that in all likelihood the transplant would help him survive no longer than 5 years. "I feel like I have a new lease on life," he told friends. "All the things I once through were important, such as my social status and advancing in my profession no longer seem so important. I may have limited time, but I'm going to make the best of it. I want to spend more time with my children. I want to volunteer at the Senior Citizen Center, helping others; things I never took time to do before."

Humor

Individuals who have used humor as a coping mechanism in their healthier life, or those who see humor as a way of maintaining a sense of self, may react with humor in face of adversity, a reaction some health professionals may interpret as inappropriate. Patients using humor in this way should not have their efforts thwarted but rather should be encouraged to continue to use humor as a coping mechanism, if it is appropriate for them. As an example, Mr. Andreasi, upon learning from his physician, Dr. Lawrence, that he had ALS responded by saying, "That sure won't do much for my golf game." Dr. Lawrence was shocked by the response and later said to the nurse, "Mr. Andreasi obviously is denying the seriousness of his condition," when in fact, Mr. Andreasi was well aware of the seriousness and implications of his condition and was merely using humor as a way to cope with news, which he found devastating. Humor should not, of course, be imposed on the individual by health professionals. Health professionals should be sensitive to patients' needs, taking cues from the patient and participating in humor to the extent the patient continues to do so. Health professionals should be cautious, however, that patients are not made to feel they have to continue to approach their condition in a humorous way to keep up appearances or for the sake of others. Being available, open, and sensitive to patients communicates willingness of health professionals to accept them as they are, whether or not humor is used.

UNDERSTANDING END-OF-LIFE ISSUES IN THE CONTEXT OF THE FAMILY

In an attempt to approach patient teaching about end-of-life issues from a holistic approach, health professionals may tend to think of families as a single entity, as if all members of the family share the same views and values. Health professionals should be continually mindful, however, of individual differences regarding adaptation and coping with crisis in general and in issues related to death and dying in particular. Consequently, assumptions about shared values within a family should not be made. It may not be possible to approach all family members in the same way. By considering individual differences, health professionals can better help family members understand and appreciate each other's perspectives as well as the perspective of the patient. Sensitive intervention can increase families' tolerance for variation of perspectives among family members.

Each family member is involved, to some degree, in the overall functioning of the family, whether financially, emotionally, or by merely being a physical presence. The roles and contributions each family member makes to the overall functioning of the family is determined to a large part by the age of the individual as well as other factors. When a family member becomes ill, and especially if illness is life threatening or terminal, family roles are disrupted. The family member who has the life-threatening or terminal condition may have decreased ability to contribute to the family emotionally and may be unable to participate in daily tasks once associated with their role. They may also be unable to contribute financially to the family. Consequently, other family members may need to assume additional responsibilities, thus potentially increasing stress on individuals within the family unit.

Families may react to a diagnosis of life-threatening or terminal illness in a myriad of ways. Some reactions are determined by personality or temperament of individual family members. Reactions may also be determined by the role the patient played within the family unit. For example, if the patient was the authority figure and decision maker of the family, family members may feel insecurity and instability if the patient is no longer able to function in the leadership role.

Intergenerational differences, integrated with gender and cultural factors can also alter views of end-of-life issues. It is important for health professionals to affirm values of protection, respect, and loyalty, and identify with the family to enhance the ability of the family to accept and understand individual differences, thus facilitating positive communication about issues of death and dying.

How family members react to the diagnosis can impact on their response to the patient and in turn to the patient's response to their diagnosis. While some families may be supportive and open in communication with the patient by helping them process and accept the information, other families may attempt to shield patients from what they consider trauma of the news. They may play down the serious nature of the condition or attempt to withhold additional information from the patient. In some instances, families become angry, blaming the patient for the diagnosis. At times, due to their own fear and anxiety, family members may withdraw from the patient completely. In other instances, withdrawal is due to family members' perceived inadequacy of no longer knowing what to do or what to say.

Health professionals, sensitive to the family members' needs, can help families cope by providing information related to reactions to life-threatening and terminal conditions of family members, helping them learn how to assist in the care of the patient, and by increasing their awareness that often it is not merely what they say or do but their very presence that is the most important to the patient.

Although the presence of family members can offer solace to patients, health professionals should not make the assumption that family members are a source of strength and support for the patient. At times, depending on the relationship and the patient's and family's reactions to the diagnosis, family members can cause the patient additional stress. Relationships that were strained before the illness can become more strained because of the diagnosis of a life-threatening or terminal condition. Family members with strong, opposite preferences can cause increased conflict. Patient preferences regarding involvement of family members should be assessed and their wishes should be respected.

Just as patients have rights and responsibilities that should be respected, so do family members. Health professionals can help family members recognize that they have the right not to be blamed for the patient's diagnosis and that they have a right to maintain as normal a family life as possible. By helping families gain information about illness and treatment, as well as helping them understand what might be expected, health professionals enable families to cope with the situation at hand. Health professionals should remain nonjudgmental when working with families of patients with a life-threatening or terminal condition. The goal should be not only to help families accept the patient and their diagnosis but also to help them accept patients' rights to their own preferences and decision making, especially should those preferences and decisions differ from those of the family.

COMMUNICATION SKILLS IN TEACHING ABOUT END-OF-LIFE ISSUES

Good communication skills are essential to forming an open and trusting relationship with the patient. Also important is demonstrating sensitivity to individual patient needs. These skills are the foundation of all effective patient education. Never are these skills more critical, however, than when discussing end-of-life issues with patients and their families. Patients who feel accepted as individuals are more likely to divulge feelings and thoughts about issues and preferences surrounding death and dying. They will also be more receptive to information they are given (Detmar et al. 2001).

When teaching about end-of-life issues, it is important to use responses that communicate that the health professional both hears and understands what the patient is saying and experiencing. Patients should not be interrupted while they are attempting to express feelings or explain their views; however, health professionals should convey a sincere desire to grasp what patients are saying. This can be accomplished by clarifying the meaning of what the patient is expressing. For example, if the patient makes a statement such as, "I'm just not sure I can tell my mother about the serious nature of my diagnosis," the health professional may respond with a statement such as, "Do you mean you're afraid of how you might respond when telling her, or that you are afraid of how she will react?" By making such a response, the health professional communicates the desire to understand the patient's concerns by asking for additional clarification. If, however, in the same scenario, the health professional knows from previous interactions that the patient's main concern is the emotional fragility of the mother, the health professional may respond with a statement such as, "You're really concerned that this may be very hard for your mother." This statement conveys not only the health professional's desire to understand but that they actually do understand the meaning of what the patient said.

Responses that restate and reflect feelings the patient has expressed communicate both understanding and caring. For example, if a patient were to make a statement such as, "I feel so self-centered because it seems all I do is think about my future right now," an appropriate response may be, "It sounds like you're feeling selfish, when in fact it is perfectly natural to have feelings of concern. That's really important for you to do right now." Such a response communicates acceptance, gives reassurance, and encourages the patient to further discuss feelings and concerns. Health professionals who actively listen to patients, observing both verbal and nonverbal cues, increase effectiveness of patient education about end-of-life issues.

TEACHING ABOUT ADVANCE DIRECTIVES

An advance directive is a legal document in which patients exert their right to accept or refuse medical care even if they should be incapacitated and unable to make their own decisions (Levenson and Feinsod 1998). The document came out of a Supreme Court ruling, which was followed by the Patient Self Determination Act. Under the Patient Self Determination Act, health care facilities are obligated, among other things, to educate patients about advance directives and about their right to accept or refuse treatment (Lynn et al. 1998).

There are several types of advance directives but the most common are the living will and durable power of attorney for health care (Parkman and Calfee 1997, Emanuel et al. 2000). Living wills enable patients to describe the type of health care they would or would not wish to receive in certain medical situations. Durable power of attorney for health care enables patients to specify what type of care they would or would not want to receive in certain medical situations, as well as to appoint an individual or proxy to make decisions for them if they are unable to do so.

The ultimate goal of advance directives is to provide patients with autonomy to make their own decisions about end-of-life care and to communicate these choices clearly to family, friends, and health care providers (Arenson et al. 1996). Having advance directives can help to ward off potential disagreements between family members who may have different perceptions about what they think the patient wants. Advance directives can also ease the burden of decision making for the family.

Patients may not be aware of the importance of engaging in end-of-life discussions, especially if they are not currently faced with a life-threatening or terminal condition. They may be unaware that they have the right to be involved in end-of-life decision making. Patients may also be reluctant to initiate discussion of end-of-life issues because they believe health professionals do not have the time or are unreceptive to taking time for this type of discussion. Raising patients' awareness of their right to be active participants in end-of-life decisions, and creating an atmosphere that conveys receptivity on the part of health professionals to this type of discussion, can be done easily. Patient education information about advance directives can be obtained from local, state, and national organizations. Flyers, brochures, or posters that encourage patients to ask their health care provider about advance directives or other end-of-life issues can be displayed in waiting rooms of physician offices, health clinics, or hospitals. Information can also be disseminated when patients are discharged from the hospital, at health clinic checkouts, or with regular mailings patients receive. Actively attempting to provide patients with information conveys the importance of this type of planning and communicates openness and willingness on the part of the health professionals to engage in discussion about end-of-life issues.

Ideally, patients initiate end-of-life discussions on their own from interest in and willingness to attend to practical issues in the event they are faced with a life-threatening or terminal situation. In many instances, however, despite efforts to communicate with patients about end-of-life issues, patients may be unaware of the importance of advance planning. In these cases, the health professional may choose to instigate the discussion. Health professionals can take the initiative and approach the subject with the patient with a statement such as:

> We all have the right to participate in making decisions about medical care and treatment at the end of life. The best time to make those decisions is before the situation occurs, when we can discuss possibilities rationally. Even though you aren't currently faced with a life-threatening situation, none of us know when we could be faced with a disease or an accident in which end-of-life decisions need to be made. If that situation would occur, have you thought of how you might like things handled, or what you would or would not want to have done medically?

Discussion about advance directives can be directive or nondirective. Nondirective approaches facilitate communication with the patient. Patients should be encouraged to express concerns and questions freely so that a clear understanding of what advance directives mean can be reached. Direct approaches to discussions focus on problem solving, helping patients identify or clarify specific problems and issues, and on identifying how those problems and issues might be resolved. Patients may not have given thought to their values, beliefs, and priorities should they be faced with a life-threatening situation. In these instances, it may be helpful to help patients explore their attitudes about life and death, identifying what is important to them. Although patients can be helped to clarify their values through discussion, several "values history forms" are also available to help patients clarify values (Doukas and McCullough 1991). Values history forms contain a list of values from which patients can identify values that are most consistent with their own definition of quality of life. Whether engaging in discussion with patients about their values or using a values history form, in all instances, patients should be allowed to set the pace and agenda.

The focus of communication about end-of-life issues should be on developing a mutual understanding between the patient and health professional so that patients' preferences about end-of-life care are identified and correctly interpreted (Kassirer 1994). Reaching this type of understanding helps to prevent potential conflict between patients, family, and health professionals when a life-threatening or terminal condition does occur. Patients should be encouraged to discuss their values and preferences with their family. If there is a religious affiliation, patients may also want to discuss end-of-life issues with members of their religious community.

At times, advance directives can be so general that their content is open to wide interpretation (Siegler and Levin 2000). For instance, an advance directive that states that "no extraordinary means should be taken" can be interpreted in a number of ways, depending on individual perceptions of the meaning of "extraordinary." To be useful, advance directives address patient preferences specifically, in language that is clear, concise, and free of multiple interpretations. Patients should be taught about life-sustaining measures such as cardiopulmonary resuscitation, artificial ventilation, hydration, and nutrition. They should be helped to understand that they have the right to refuse all of the treatment, or only some of it.

Health professionals should ensure that patients have a clear understanding of the meaning of what the advance directive means. The health professional should also make sure they themselves understand exactly what the patient means when they state their wishes. For example, Dr. Adams had engaged in a long discussion with Mr. Hadley about advance directives. Mr. Hadley was adamant about wanting everything done for him during end-of-life care. Dr. Adams interpreted this to mean that Mr. Hadley wanted life-support measures instituted. At a later visit, the nurse discovered, in reviewing the advance directives with Mr. Hadley, that by "everything" Mr. Hadley meant he wanted to be kept as comfortable and pain free as possible, not to be kept alive by artificial means. In another instance, Mrs. Coleman told Ms. Donnley, the nurse, that she wanted no artificial life support. As Ms. Donnley further questioned Mrs. Coleman, however, it became evident that Mrs. Coleman only meant mechanical ventilation when referring to life support, not nutrition and hydration.

Teaching patients about end-of-life issues may take place over several visits. When patients are unfamiliar with advance directives or living wills, they may be sent home with sample copies as well as with information explaining advance directives, living wills, and their purpose. Patients may need time to reflect on preferences for end-of-life care, on who they would name as a durable power of attorney, and whether different disease scenarios may warrant different procedures. More detailed discussion can then take place during subsequent teaching sessions after patients have had the opportunity to read the material, think about their values, and clarify their preferences for end-of-life care.

Patients' treatment preferences and priorities regarding end-of-life issues may change over time. Periodic review of advance directives, preferences and priorities, and specifications for durable power of attorney for health care helps assure that the type of care the patient has specified is up to date and current with their current wishes.

Teaching patients about advance directives and helping them clarify their values so they can make decisions about life-sustaining treatments before a crisis is an essential skill for health professionals. Health professionals should have an understanding of legal and ethical issues as well as practical issues involved in individual situations. They should also be aware of specific laws in their state regarding withholding or withdrawing life-sustaining treatments. In all instances, plans should be customized to the patients' individual needs and desires.

BREAKING BAD NEWS

Giving patients bad news is a difficult task for most health professionals. From patients' perspectives, receiving news about progression of a chronic condition, receiving a diagnosis of a life-threatening condition, or receiving news that they have a terminal condition is a traumatic event. The extent of negative impact of bad news is often related not to the information itself but to how the information is delivered. How the news is presented can impact on the way patients respond to recommendations for future care and treatment and can set the tone for how the entire illness experience is handled by patients and their families (Ptacek and Eberhardt 1996).

What constitutes bad news is subjective (Ambuel and Mazzone 2001). Bad news can be defined as news the patient doesn't want to hear. Patients and health professionals may have differing views as to the meaning of the news. News considered as benign by health professionals may be considered catastrophic by the patient and visa versa. Take, for example, Mrs. Lopez, who had come to the health clinic for a pregnancy test. The nurse, assuming that a positive test would be joyous news for Mrs. Lopez excitedly announced to her that the test was positive and indeed she was pregnant. Mrs. Lopez burst into tears, obviously upset with confirmation of the diagnosis. Because of different meanings news may have on patients and health professionals, health professionals need to be sensitive to patients' perspectives and reactions before making assumptions about the impact. Health professionals should be ready and available to tend to patients' emotional needs and reactions, no matter what they are.

The amount of information patients want about their condition, especially if the diagnosis is unfavorable, is frequently underestimated by health professionals (Covinsky 2000). Most patients want to be given information about their condition even if the news is bad (Peteet et al. 1991). Evidence suggests that although patients may initially experience a negative emotional impact from bad news, they generally adjust well in the long term.

Because breaking bad news can be a difficult task, providing patients with bad news may be delayed, or the responsibility for giving bad news may be passed from health professional to health professional. As a result, patients receive scattered, and at times inconsistent, information. Generally, the health professional who delivers the bad news should be an individual who has had or who will continue to care for the patient. In some instances, more than one health professional may participate in relaying the information, especially if there have been several health professionals closely involved with the patient. Information should be presented in a manner appropriate to the individual patient and should be presented in a compassionate, direct manner.

In most instances, patients should be given the news directly, and in person. In most cases, giving patients or family members bad news over the phone should be avoided. There may be circumstances, however, in which giving bad news over the phone is the only option. Under these circumstances, information should be provided in the same sensitive way as if it were being given to the patient or family member face to face. It is especially important under these circumstances to determine that patients have access to support in their location. Take the example of Mrs. Saunders and her daughter, Ms. Flint. Mrs. Saunders, an 85-year-old woman living in her own home, fell, breaking her left hip. Her daughter, Ms. Flint, who lived several states away immediately came to be with her mother during surgery and the postoperative period. Mrs. Saunders appeared to be progressing well and transferred to an extended care facility for recovery and rehabilitation. Her daughter returned home, planning to return periodically to monitor her mothers progress. Shortly after Ms. Flint returned home, Mrs. Saunders unexpectedly experienced a pulmonary embolus and died. The nurse had no choice but to relay the news of Mrs. Saunders death to her daughter over the phone.

Before beginning discussion with patients, health professionals should be sure they have all the information needed, including potential resources that patients may find useful. When giving bad news, timing should be considered. The time chosen for delivering the news should be convenient for the patient and when they are relatively comfortable. Sufficient time should be allowed so that information is not presented in a rushed manner and so that there is time for patients to vent feelings and to ask questions. Patients should be given the option of having a family member or a friend present; however, if patients prefer no one else to be present, their wishes should be respected. If the patient chooses to have a friend or family member present who is unfamiliar to the health professional, the health professional should introduce him- or herself before beginning the discussion.

News should be delivered in a comfortable, relatively quiet location where there are no interruptions, and in which the patient has privacy. Presenting information to the patient in a hallway, waiting room, or the patient's hospital room where another patient is present should be avoided. If news is being given to the patient in an examining room, they should be allowed to dress before the discussion begins.

In most instances, health professionals should sit close to the patient and make sure no physical barriers, such as a desk, are separating them. This enhances health professionals' ability to monitor patient reactions and to use touch, when appropriate, for reassurance or comfort. Health professionals should be aware of their own body language while delivering the information, attempting to look as at ease as possible. Nonverbal cues should be used to convey warmth, sympathy, encouragement, or reassurance. Cues such as eye contact, rather than looking at the floor or out the window, and giving the patient full attention is crucial. Flipping through the chart, or other materials, writing notes, or checking the clock should be avoided during the discussion.

Rather than giving the news immediately at the beginning of the session it is usually helpful to begin with a statement that gives patients warning so that there is some preparation for bad news. Compare the differences in impact on Joseph, a patient returning to a clinic after being tested for HIV infection:

> *Scenario I:* The health professional walks into the room, sits down, looks at Joseph, and says, "Your test show that you are HIV positive."

> *Scenario II:* The health professional walks into the room, greets Joseph, sits down, then looks at Joseph and says, "We are here today to discuss the results of your lab tests. I'm afraid they didn't turn out as well as we had hoped. . . ."

In the first scenario, Joseph has no time to prepare emotionally for the news he is about to receive, causing him potentially to be overwhelmed. The second scenario allows Joseph time to ease into the notion that bad news is about to be given and to mobilize coping mechanisms that will make him better able to withstand the shock.

News should be delivered in a direct, nontechnical way. Although information should be honest and direct, it should also be presented in a hopeful way. Rather than saying, "You have a terminal condition and nothing can be done," a more appropriate statement may be, "Although currently there is no cure for your condition, there is much that can be done to help assure that you continue to be as comfortable as possible."

After patients have received bad news, health professionals should remain silent, allowing patients to absorb the news they have received, to ask questions, or to react. Time should be provided for exploration, expression of concerns, and review of the circumstances. Patients and their families should be allowed to express emotions freely. Reactions may consist of crying, silence, or anger. Regardless of feelings expressed, health professionals should convey a presence and accept patients' feelings. By observing patients' reactions, health professionals will be better able to know how they can best lend support. By listening to patients, health professionals can also determine how they are interpreting the news given. Patients' most immediate concerns can then be assessed and health professionals can then tailor their response to match patients' reactions. In the case of Joseph in Scenario II above, after hearing that he was HIV positive, his first statement was, "You mean I'll be dead soon?" The health professional was able to explain to Joseph that there are now a number of medications available that can help people who are HIV positive from developing symptoms of AIDS, thereby enabling them to continue to live productive lives with their diagnosis. The information given by the health professional did not provide false hope, but helped to correct misinterpretation of the information given, addressing Joseph's most immediate concern.

After receiving bad news, ample time should be provided for patients to talk and to ask questions. After responding to patients' immediate concerns after receiving bad news, health professionals should assess the extent to which patients understand the information presented and their knowledge and understanding about the condition. In this way, patient education needs are identified and any misinformation present may be corrected. Before providing additional information, health professionals should assess patients' ability to absorb information. If the patient seems overwhelmed, additional information is better given at a later time. Patients are often in a state of shock after first hearing bad news and may not be able to immediately process additional information (Eden 1994). In most instances, providing patients with additional, detailed information is better done at a later date when patients are more likely to hear and comprehend the information presented.

After being given bad news, patients may be in shock and consequently unable to carry out regular tasks safely. For example, if patients have received bad news while at an outpatient facility and they are unaccompanied and are driving themselves home, they should be asked if there is someone who could be called to drive them home or if alternative means of transportation could be arranged. Other supports and resources available to them should also be assessed.

At subsequent patient education sessions, health professionals should be open to expression of emotional experiences and help patients and families gain a sense of personal control by encouraging them to be actively involved in treatment decisions. Pacing information and presenting it gradually over several patient education sessions in clear, understandable terms helps patients to adapt and to incorporate information given. Health professionals should be prepared to offer resources as needed such as support groups or other resources such as clergy or social service.

Arrangements for follow up should be made. Additional questions may arise as patients have time to come to full realization of their diagnosis and its implications. Need and desire for additional information may also change. As patients adjust to the news, facts may need to be repeated or revised. Follow-up visits also enable health professionals to monitor patients' adjustment and provide additional assistance as the need arises.

TEACHING PATIENTS LIVING WITH LIFE-THREATENING ILLNESS

End-of-life discussions may be precipitated when patients are living with a life-threatening condition (Cherny et al. 1996). Although patients may not be in the terminal stages of disease, the nature of the condition or its expected progression may necessitate discussion about the potential for death.

The prospect of dying raises many practical issues, and patients may look to health professionals to provide information that helps them address these issues. Resolving practical matters can help patients focus on issues of living with a life-threatening condition, thus enabling them to enhance their overall quality of life.

The nature and focus of patient education in end-of-life discussions with patients with life-threatening conditions should be based on patients' individual needs and priorities. Many of the same principles used in teaching patients with other conditions also apply to teaching patients with life-threatening illness. Timing of patient education, assessing specific learning needs, evaluating supports and barriers, appraising patients' social situation and life circumstances, and considering patient's ability and willingness to follow recommendations are all crucial regardless of the patient's condition. The difference in patient teaching results from the emotionally charged potential of loss of life.

Under these circumstances, patients and their families need honest, realistic, and accurate information about the condition and general status of the patient, options for treatment, and prognosis (Shields 1998). Only with clear, concise information can patients make informed choices about treatment and care. Having straightforward information about the condition and its prognosis also enables patients to establish priorities regarding personal or relationship issues or regarding business concerns they need to put in order.

Part of establishing patient priorities is to determine patient goals, which also help determine specific treatment preferences. Some patients may have a major goal of maximizing quantity of life, while others focus on quality. In either instance, patients' definition of terms should be clarified because concepts of quality and quantity of life can be broadly and individually defined. Although it is difficult to predict patients' reactions to life-threatening illness, open discussions help alleviate fears and build a sense of collaboration and support.

Initially, after diagnosis, patients may have extreme concern for the well-being and future of their family. They may have concern about abandonment and isolation. Financial issues in the face of increasing medical bills or potential loss of income if they are no longer able to work may be a major concern. There may be concern for the completion of various work-related projects. In other instances, patients may have major concerns about pain, discomfort, or loss of function as their condition progresses.

Patient education with patients with life-threatening conditions extends beyond teaching about their condition and treatment (Laury 1987). In these circumstances, patient teaching should also be directed toward helping patients increase awareness and acceptance of their condition, helping them frame their condition as a positive, life-promoting event. The manner in which patients are given information about a life-threatening illness is crucial so that a facilitative relationship can be established with the health professional.

In addition to providing patients with factual information about their condition and treatment, discussion may also include explorations of patients' underlying values, which can help them when faced with decisions to choose or decline various treatment options. In some instances, patients may choose end-of-life options because they fear the cost of ongoing medical care or that family members will view them as a burden. Although these reasons may be valid to the patient, the health professional can encourage the patient to further discuss their feelings and options, ascertaining that they have not been pressured to make decisions that are not within their value framework.

Information about treatment options should be provided in small pieces, with frequent pauses to assess patients' understanding of the information and the context in which specific treatment decisions might apply. Patients should be helped to determine how treatment options relate to their general goals or values. Although the amount of information patients want may vary, information provided should address potential consequences and implications for selecting as well as not selecting treatment options.

PATIENT EDUCATION IN TERMINAL STAGES OF DISEASE

Personal care for patients in terminal stages of disease is an appropriate and expected part of the health professional's role (Engle 1998). Even though treatment and cure may no longer be possible, active care of patients who are terminally ill is important. Effective patient education with individuals with terminal conditions needs a broader perspective than other patient education interactions. Although helping patients manage pain and increase physical comfort are essential tasks, helping them achieve emotional comfort is equally important (Perron and Schonwetter 2001). Helping patients and families acknowledge the prospect of death gives patients the opportunity to focus attention on living the remainder of their life to the fullest extent possible. The last stages of life offer patients the opportunity to clarify priorities and values and to seek a stance most consistent with their own sense of self. Facilitation of this type of self-exploration as well as identifying practical considerations and patient priorities can help patients make informed choices, stay in control of their life as long as possible, and view death as an opportunity for growth.

Effective patient education in all situations depends on appropriate assessment of patient and family characteristics and needs and tailoring information to the individual. The same is true for patients with terminal illness. Assessment information provides a framework on which to base patient education activities and establish priorities for patient teaching. Helping patients learn to make adjustments in the last stage of life should be based on identifying patients' needs and priorities rather than those perceived by health professionals.

Health professionals should assess the patients' family system, identifying family members and specific roles they play within the family unit. Both formal and informal support networks should be identified. Information regarding previous family crisis or losses within the family and methods family members used to cope provides information that can be used to help patients and their family cope with the current situation. Identifying experiences patients and families have had with the health care system in the past can also help health professional determine attitudes that can help or hinder care in the future. For example, take the case of Mr. Schmidt, who had been hospitalized in the final stages of AIDS. Mr. Schmidt's older brother had died of AIDS several years earlier. Mr. Schmidt's mother became very demanding of the nurses, berating them for not answering his light promptly enough or not adequately straightening his bed, and finding fault no matter how much they tried. Mrs. Dewitt, the nurse, approached Mr. Schmidt's mother one evening and said, "This situation is very difficult for you, I know, especially since you have already lost one son. How has that experience impacted on how you deal with your son's current illness?" Mr. Schmidt's mother broke into tears. "When my first son was dying, everyone just ceased to care. No one checked on him. No one provided adequate care for him. He deserved more. I wasn't there to advocate for him. I won't let the same thing happen to my son now. Although we can't prevent him from dying, we can see to it that he has an appropriate death in which he is comfortable and at least treated with respect and concern."

For many people, dying an "appropriate" death means dying in a way consistent with their concept of self, maintaining values and ideals that guided them through life. Receiving a diagnosis of terminal illness places thoughts of death and dying at the forefront. Issues and concerns the patient and their family have about the patient's illness, and about death and dying, must be addressed. Patients may place priority on continuity of relationships with significant others. They may place priority on maintaining dignity and control. Many patients place priority on a death that is peaceful, relatively pain free, and free of conflict.

When patients are terminally ill, concerns take on different meaning because dying, in this instance, is imminent and real. Although patients with conditions that are not terminal may still face alterations in perceptions of self and identity, patients with terminal illness face loss of self in addition to other things they hold dear such as family, job, or experiences they will not have in the future. Issues that health professionals may consider mundane may be of utmost importance to patients and may need to be addressed before patients are able to actively participate in other patient education activities.

Spiritual components of health and illness are imbedded in all aspects of health care (Anandarajah and Hight 2001). Regardless of religious affiliation, terminal illness, especially, adds a spiritual dimension, which must be addressed and which should not be underestimated or ignored. Although spiritual dimensions of experience should not be imposed on individuals, health professionals should be open to allowing patients to express their needs. If health professionals are uncomfortable discussing spiritual topics with patients, they should at least ask if the patient would like to speak with a clergy or other professional about these issues. Whether the referral takes place, and to whom the patient is referred, should, of course, be the patient's choice. When patients express spiritual needs, it is often a comfort for them to know that their needs were acknowledged and that the health professional took steps to help them meet those needs, even if it was in the form of a referral.

Patient education with patients with terminal illness can help individuals learn to live with a terminal illness. The focus of patient education under these circumstances should be on issues the patient deems as important. A crucial part of patient education in terminal illness is identifying and confronting concerns, developing interventions to deal with those concerns, and helping patients and families learn how to cope with the diagnosis (Reichel 1999). Information needed will vary with individual patients. Some patients may need information that will help them make appropriate financial arrangements. Others may need information about burial or cremation, bequest of body or specified organs, or distribution of personal items. Patients may need information about hospice or about other services they can utilize at home. In some instances, they may need information about hospital care. In each of these instances, patient education information can be provided to the patient in the form of written material, or they may be given information about appropriate resources that can provide information they are requesting.

Patients' terminal conditions may take away their ability to control their environment as well as their ability to function effectively within it. This inability in turn can affect self-concept. Many of the values attached to self-concept are specific to the stage of development of the patient. Consequently the individual's stage of development and its impact on their perceptions and acceptance of their experience with death and dying must be considered. Patients should be helped to gain as much control as possible. Although the diagnosis or outcome cannot be changed, providing opportunities to explore their experience and options through patient education can help patients with terminal illness recognize that they still have choices and that they can control how they live in the terminal stages of their illness (Caloras et al. 2000).

Symptoms experienced by patients with terminal illness cause physical problems that require patient education to help patients achieve maximum relief from symptoms (Frederich 2001, Bruera and Byock 2000). Again, however, when teaching patients about control of symptoms, health professionals should clarify patients' values and preferences. For example, does quality of life during the terminal stages of illness mean being pain free even though level of consciousness is affected as the result; or does quality of life mean staying alert and aware despite pain that may be experienced. Does the patient measure quality of life by functional capacity and independence, or is merely sanctity of life of the utmost importance?

Helping patients gain emotional comfort can also be addressed in patient education. One aspect of loss experienced by patients with terminal illness is the sense of self. By helping patients review their past, there may be a consolidation of sense of self and a validation of their sense of being. Patients can be encouraged to write journals outlining important events, reaffirming what they have been, or to jot down current thoughts and feelings. Journal writing can provide patients with a sense of completion. It should be noted that, although this activity may be helpful for some, it may not be appropriate for all patients with terminal illness. Health professionals still must remain sensitive to the needs and priorities of the individual.

When, in the terminal stages of illness, the patient is unable to speak for him or herself, the person designated by the patient to make medical decisions should be asked about the patient's values and goals for care at end of life. Take, for example, Mrs. Carter, whose husband was in the terminal stages of cancer and in a coma. Dr. Jones approached Mrs. Carter with the following statement: "Your husband is dying. He is now unconscious so he can no longer make decisions for himself. We can insert a feeding tube into his stomach which will keep him alive longer, however, it is uncertain at this point whether it will increase his quality of life. In fact, the tube may cause additional discomfort. What do you think he would want to do?"

Family members may not fully understand, or be ready to accept, the terminal nature of the patient's condition. In some instances, family members may understand the terminal nature of the condition but not the impact or implications of maintaining or continuing treatment. There are also situations in which disagreements about end-of-life decisions arise among family members. In each of these instances, health professionals should approach the family in a nonjudgmental way and should facilitate further exploration and explanation. Take, for example, the case of Mr. Bower.

Mr. Bower, an 84-year-old widower, experienced a massive stroke and was placed on a ventilator. Dr. James called the family together to discuss the gravity of Mr. Bower's condition and the limited chance of recovery. His three children had been emotionally close to Mr. Bower, although only his eldest son lived close by and saw him frequently. Due to geographic distance, Mr. Bower's other son and daughter visited him only once a year. When discussing the situation with the family, given the status of Mr. Bower's condition, Dr. James discussed the option of removing life support. Mr. Bower's eldest son was in favor of this option, but his other children were vehemently opposed. Dr. James said: "This type of decision is a very difficult one, I know. I wonder if we could explore each of your views a bit more and see if we can identify your expectations of the consequences and implications of taking your father off life support or leaving the life support in place." By encouraging family dialogue and exploration of feelings and beliefs about consequences of their decision, Dr. James enabled family members to voice their concerns and clarify their own realities regarding the decision. By further exploring the family's beliefs, Dr. James was also able to identify misinformation or unrealistic expectations family members may have and consequently address these issues. Such was the case of Mrs. Nance.

Mrs. Nance was in the terminal stages of pancreatic cancer. Although she was unresponsive, her children insisted that they wanted the doctor to "do everything." In this situation, it might be appropriate for the physician to make a statement such as, "Your mother is dying. There is no treatment we can provide that will prevent her death. We can, however, do much for your mother by keeping her as comfortable as possible." This statement helps clarify the situation for the family, while at the same time providing comfort in the knowledge that although there are not treatment options for cure or reversal of the condition, "something" can be done.

Some family members may find it helpful to be given general guidelines for caregiving. Teaching family members specific techniques for meeting patients personal needs such as mouth care, skin care, nutrition, and elimination provides family members with a sense of confidence in providing care to the patient. Helping family members learn how they can help patients with other specific needs such as pain management, control of nausea and vomiting, or breathing difficulties can help reduce anxiety and frustration when symptoms occur. Of course, not all family members are able to accept responsibility for this type of personal care, and if this is the case, patient teaching about personal care should be limited to their wishes and capabilities.

Effective patient education with families of patients with terminal illness depends to a great extent on their response to the diagnosis itself. Families' responses throughout the dying process are determined by a number of factors, including the emotional make up of the family, the degree of family cohesion, and the role of the patient within the family structure. There may be unfinished emotional business with the patient that can alter family members' reactions to the diagnosis as well as to the patient.

Part of patient teaching should involve helping family members understand that as the patient's illness progresses, both physical and emotional needs will change. A major focus of patient teaching should include helping family members learn how they can be of help to the patient without taking away the patient's sense of independence and control. Providing families with information about resources and services available in the community can also help them feel a sense of control, by helping them learn ways specific needs can be met.

Teaching families specific things they can do to help patients manage their condition and how to maintain a relatively low-stress environment can also be helpful. Patients and family members should be encouraged to communicate so that family unity and mutual support is facilitated. Family members and the patient can be encouraged to talk openly about the diagnosis and to discuss experiences they are having. They can also be taught how to provide feedback to individuals within the family unit about specific behaviors and their impact.

Family members may begin the grief process while the patient is still alive. This type of grieving may be confusing for both the family and the patient. While family members are attending to the patient, they may also be beginning to anticipate their life without them. In some instances, family members may begin to divest emotional energy from the patient, investing it instead in preparation for life after the patient dies. Some divestment may be healthy and necessary for continued function. In instances where family members reach a state of emotional depletion, they may naturally begin to withdraw. Helping both the patient and family members understand this reaction helps to avoid misunderstanding and to facilitate future communication and understanding. Family members should be helped to understand that they too have physical, emotional, and spiritual needs and that building time for self-care is crucial. Helping families balance attending to their own needs while still offering care and support to the patient are important aspects of patient education with patients who have terminal conditions.

THE FAMILY CONFERENCE

When advance directives are not available and the patient's condition has progressed so that decisions about withholding or withdrawing medical treatment must be addressed, detailed and complex dialogue with family members is appropriate. Such discussions are usually held in the context of the family conference. Although most states have a hierarchy regarding decision making and the legal next-of-kin retains responsibility for decisions, the ultimate goal in talking with family about these decisions is to gain consensus among family members if possible (Curtis et al. 2001).

The family conference should be approached with the same care and planning as other patient education activities. The conference should occur in a private room that provides little likelihood of interruption. Who will be present at the family conference should be decided in advance. Family members attending the family conference should be prepared as to what to expect during the conference. They should be instructed that the purpose of the conference is to review the patient's status and to make decisions regarding the extent to which medical interventions should continue.

At the beginning of the family conference, the health professional should review the family's understanding of the patient's current situation. The patient's illness and treatment should be reviewed in terms the family can understand, avoiding medical jargon. Family members should be allowed to maintain hope even in a poor prognosis. This does not mean providing unrealistic or false information. Rather it means the health professional helps families to redirect their hope from cure to hope for maintaining as much comfort and dignity for the patient as possible. Discussion of the patient's values and goals should be encouraged by asking the family to speculate what the patient may want if they were able to participate in the decision-making process. Spending time with the family reminiscing about the patient can also put the family at ease and bring them comfort in the decision-making process.

During the family conference, family members should be given the opportunity to discuss their own feelings as well as spiritual, religious, or cultural needs. Feelings of the family should be acknowledged and action should be taken to address any unmet needs that have been expressed (Clary et al. 2000).

The family should be assured that even if treatment is withheld or withdrawn that the patient will not be abandoned and that they will continue to be cared for (Ackermann 2000). After the patient's current medical situation and treatment options have been discussed, information should be reinforced by putting information and decisions into perspective. Questions family members raise should be addressed and family reactions to information discussed should be explored. If family members express strong emotions, these emotions should be acknowledged and explored. At times, family members may find expression of emotion difficult. In this case, health professionals should be respectful of the difficulty the family member is experiencing. Periods of silence should be tolerated while family members struggle to express feelings and emotions.

Before completion of the family conference, information discussed should be briefly summarized. Family members should then be offered a private place where they can engage in discussion among themselves and take time to agree on a decision if a decision has not yet been reached. After family members have had sufficient time to discuss the situation, the health professional should again convene the family and explore their feelings. Any disagreements that exist between family members regarding how to proceed should be identified. Decisions made by the family should be supported by the health professional. After making a decision, family members should be encouraged to visit, touch, and talk with the patient. Most importantly, if the decision to withhold or withdraw treatment has been made, the health professional should make a point of being available and checking on the patient and family frequently.

IMPACT OF END-OF-LIFE TEACHING

Patient education about end-of-life issues involves more than information giving. When talking with the patient about issues surrounding death and dying, the emotional bond between the health professional and patient and their family transcends information exchange. Patient education about end-of-life issues can be a meaningful and significant experience, bringing both the health professional and the patient to a deeper understanding of their own values and crucial life decisions.

REFERENCES

Ackermann, R.J. 2000. Withholding and withdrawing life-sustaining treatment. *American Family Physician* 62(7):1555–1560.

Ambuel, B., Mazzone, M.F. 2001. Breaking bad news and discussing death. *Primary Care: Clinics in Office Practice* 28(2):249–267.

Anandarajah, G., Hight, E. 2001. Spirituality and medical practice: using the HOPE questions as a practical tool for spiritual assessment. *American Family Physician* 63(1):81–89.

Arenson, C.A., Novielli, K.D., Chambers, C.V., Perkel, R.L. 1996. Models of ambulatory care: the importance of advance directives in primary care. *Primary Care: Clinics in Office Practice* 23(1):67–82.

Bone, R.C. 1997. End-of-life issues: the physician's role. *Critical Care Medicine* 25(6):1083–1084.

Bruera, E., Byock, I. 2000. Management of pain and other discomfort. *Patient Care* 34(21):38–45, 49–50, 52, 55–56, 59–62, 65, 69–71.

Buckman, R., Byrock, I., Fry, V.L. 2000. Talking with patients and families. *Patient Care* 34(21):16–18, 20, 29, 33–36.

Caloras, D., Coloney, M.J., Kangas, C.A., Wegryn, R.L. 2000. The virtues of hospice. *Patient Care* 34(21):72–74, 76–78, 80–81, 85–88, 91.

Cherny, N.I., Coyle, N., Foley, K.M. 1996. Pain and palliative care: guidelines in the care of the dying cancer patient. *Hematology/Oncology Clinics of North America.* 10(1):261–286.

Clary, P.L., Ogle, K.S., Plumb, J.D., Prendergast, T.J. 2000. The role of life prolonging technology. *Patient Care* 34(21):113–116, 119–126, 129.

Covinsky, K.E., Fuller, J.D., Yaffe, K., Johnston, C.B., Hamel, M.B., Lynn, J., Teno, J.M., Philliips, R.S. 2000. Communication and decision-making in seriously ill patients: findings of the SUPPORT project. *Journal of the American Geriatrics Society* 48:S187–S193.

Curtis, J.R., Patrick, D.L., Shannon, S.E., Treece, P.D., Engelberg, R.A., Rubenfeld, G.D. 2001. The family conference as a focus to improve communication about end-of-life care in the intensive care unit: opportunities for improvement. *Critical Care Medicine* 29(2):Suppl N26–N33.

Dangler, L.A., O'Donnell, J., Gingrich, C., Bope, E.T. 1996. What do family members expect from the family physician of a deceased loved one? *Family Medicine* 28(10):694–696.

Detmar, S.B., Muller, M.J., Wever, L.D.V., Schornagel, J.H., Aaronson, N.K. 2001. Patient–physician communication during outpatient palliative treatment visits: an observational study. *Journal of the American Medical Association* 285(10):1351–1357.

Doukas, D.J., McCullough, L.B. 1991. The values history: the evaluation of the patient's values and advance directive. *Journal of Family Practice* 32:145–153.

Eden, O.B., Black, I., MacKinlay, G.A., Emery, A.E. 1994. Communication with parents of children with cancer. *Palliative Medicine* 8:105–114.

Elder, N.C. 1996. Dealing with death in patients and families. *Family Medicine* 28 (10):692–693.

Emanuel, E., Goold, S.D., Hammes, B.J., Lynn, J., Tonelli, M. 2000. A detailed examination of advance directives. *Patient Care* 34(21):92–94, 97–98, 101–102, 105–108.

Engle, V.F. 1998. Care of the living, care of the dying: reconceptualizing nursing home care. *Journal of the American Geriatrics Society* 46(9):1172–1174.

Frederich, M.E. 2001. Nonpain symptom management. *Primary Care: Clinics in Office Practice* 28(2):299–316.

Garfinkle, C.L., Block, P. 1996. Physicians' interactions with families of terminally ill patients. *Family Medicine* 28(10):702–707.

Hallenbeck, J.L. 2001. Intercultural differences and communication at the end of life. *Primary Care: Clinics in Office Practice* 28(2):401–413.

Kassirer, J.P. 1994. Incorporating patients' preferences into medical decisions. *New England Journal of Medicine* 330(26):1895–1896.

Klessig, J. 1998. Death and culture: the multicultural challenge. *Annals of Long-Term Care* 6(9):285–290.

Kvale, J., Berg, L., Groff, J.Y., Lange, G. 1999. Factors associated with residents' attitudes toward dying patients. *Family Medicine* 31(10):691–696.

Laury, G.V. 1987. Sexuality of the dying patient. *Medical Aspects of Human Sexuality* 21(6):102–105, 109.

Levenson, S.A., Feinsod, F.M. 1998. Obtaining instructions for care. *Annals of Long-Term Care* 6(9):295–300.

Lynn, J., Miles, S.H., Olick, R. 1998. Making living wills and health care proxies more useful. *Patient Care* 32(9):181–182, 185–186, 189–192.

Parkman, C.A., Calfee, B.E. 1997. Advance directives: honoring your patient's end-of-life wishes. *Nursing* April:48–53.

Perron, V., Schonwetter, R. 2001. Hospice and palliative care programs. *Primary Care: Clinics in Office Practice* 28(2):427–440.

Peteet, J.R., Abrams, H.E., Ross, D.M., Stearns, N.M. 1991. Presenting a diagnosis of cancer: patients' views. *Journal of Family Practice* 32(6):577–581.

Ptacek, J.T., Eberhardt, T.L. 1996. Breaking bad news: a review of the literature. *Journal of the American Medical Association* 276(6):496–502.

Reichel, W. 1999. End-of-life care and family practice. *American Family Physician* 59(6):1388, 1395–1396.

Safonte-Strumolo, N., Dunn, A.B. 2000. Consideration of cultural and relational issues in bereavement: the case of an Italian American family. *The Family Journal: Counseling and Therapy for Couples and Families* 8(4):334–340.

Schears, R.M. 1999. Ethical issues in emergency medicine: emergency physicians' role in end-of-life care. *Emergency Medicine Clinics of North America* 17(2):539–559.

Shields, C.E. 1998. Oncology: giving patients bad news. *Primary Care: Clinics in Office Practice* 25(2):381–390.

Siegler, E.L., Levin, B.W. 2000. Communication between older patients and their physicians: physician–older patient communication at the end of life. *Clinics in Geriatric Medicine* 16(1):175–204.

Vincent, J.L. 2001. Cultural differences in end-of-life care. *Critical Care Medicine* 29(2):Suppl: N52–N56.

Ethical Issues in Patient Education and Patient Compliance

14

All health professionals have a code of ethics by which they are to abide. Ethics is a system of values that guides health professionals in their behavior toward patients in a variety of situations. Although each profession's code of ethics provides a statement of responsibilities for members of that profession, the code alone is not adequate for every decision and action with which health professionals may be confronted. Some situations confronting health professionals in the health care setting are straightforward; however, other situations raise ethical issues that involve questions not so easily resolved.

Health professionals sometimes perceive ethical decisions made in one situation as applicable to all similar situations. However, a more appropriate description of ethical decision making is determining what is better or best in a particular situation under the given circumstances. Ethical principles do not determine absolute, eternal law. What is considered ethical in one situation may not necessarily be considered ethical in a similar situation but under different circumstances. Ethical principles provide guidelines by which health professionals can reach decisions about what should be done in a particular situation after considering all relevant factors.

ETHICAL THEORIES

Ethical theories provide a broad framework of rules and principles that serve as a foundation for judgments or courses of action. There are two major types of ethical theory: (1) teleologic and (2) deontologic.

Teleologic theory, sometimes called utilitarian theory, pertains mainly to consequences or results of action. Using this theory as a basis for ethical problem solving would mean that health professionals would consider the consequences of performing or not performing an act and base their decision on which course of action to follow or which course of action would bring the greatest good to the greatest number of people.

Consider the following example of applying teleologic theory to patient education. A health professional developed new patient education materials that he was interested in marketing to a publisher of patient education materials. Before approaching the publisher, however, the health professional was interested in testing the effectiveness of the materials with regard to enhancing patient compliance, to have a means of comparison. In so doing, the health professional had decided to give one group of patients patient education materials that were of lesser quality and that did not contain all the relevant information about their condition and the potential side effects of treatment. In determining whether this practice was ethical or not, the health professional reasoned that the action was justified because a greater number of people would benefit in the long run by knowing which material would produce the greatest results.

A problem with this approach, of course, is that it is often difficult to measure or to reach general agreement on what is the "greatest good." "Good" may be based on an individual's values, which may differ significantly from the values or perception of "good" held by others.

Another type of ethical theory, deontologic, sometimes called formalist theory, pertains to duty or obligation. In this case, health professionals would consider their own motivation when justifying an action rather than considering the consequences of the action itself.

For instance, consider the same preceding example, but with deontologic theory applied instead. In this case, the health professional would consider his motivation for giving the patients the patient education materials that had incomplete information. If, in self-evaluation, the health professional believed that the real reason he was giving the patients the inferior materials was not to form a valid comparison, but rather to be assured that his materials would look better, making it more likely that the publisher would accept the brochure, thus resulting in financial profit for him, he may determine that the action is unethical.

ETHICAL PRINCIPLES
Autonomy

Autonomy is the degree to which individuals are allowed to make their own choices and choose their own destiny. To be autonomous, people must be self-governing, having the ability to exercise control over their own actions and circumstances. This means that to be autonomous in decision making, individuals must make decisions voluntarily without coercion and without undue influence. Autonomy is, however, based on a presumption of the individual's competence to understand information needed to help him or her make decisions and on the individual's ability to understand fully the consequences of the decisions.

In patient education and patient compliance, the principle of autonomy is used when health professionals allow patients to make their own choices about which instructions they will follow and the extent to which they will follow them. Health professionals are, at times, reluctant to afford patients autonomy, believing that patients do not have the full range of knowledge that would allow them to make reasonable decisions. In other instances, health professionals allow their own values to impose upon those of patients in deciding what is best. There are limitations to autonomy. No principle is absolute. When allowing patient autonomy would threaten the autonomy or well-being of others, patient autonomy does not take precedence. Take, for example, an individual who has been diagnosed with active tuberculosis but refuses to take the medication needed to treat the disease. To allow the patient complete autonomy in this decision and not attempt to influence him or her to take the medication would not be responsible on the part of the health professional, since actions of not following the treatment protocol could impinge on the health or well-being of others.

Beneficence

Most health professionals hope to do what is ultimately best for the patient to further enhance the patient's welfare or well-being. In holding this view, the health professional is guided in promoting the patient's best interest by preventing harm.

Beneficence is in conflict with autonomy, and like autonomy, it is not absolute. Beneficence is ethically applied if, in so doing, the individual generally believes that what is done will cause more benefit than harm. It is not justified, however, if the individual applying the principle of beneficence has an ulterior motive, such as his or her own gain, or benefit that would not be experienced by the patient but by others. Although beneficence, when applied appropriately, can be noble, it must be applied with caution so as not to infringe on the patient's rights.

Nonmaleficence

Nonmaleficence can be defined simply as "do no harm." Although it may be difficult to see how providing patient education information could ostensibly harm an individual, it could, if in so doing, the information encouraged the patient to engage in behavior that was ultimately harmful, or if in withholding information from a patient, he or she was denied information that could have prevented harm.

Health professionals would not, of course, deliberately give patients information or withhold information knowingly that would cause patients harm. However, when determining if or to what extent health professionals should attempt to coerce patients to follow treatment recommendations, or to what extent information should be withheld or emphasized for this purpose, awareness of this principle is important.

Take the case of Mrs. Raines, admitted to the hospital because of chest pain. Mrs. Raines underwent a series of tests indicating no permanent myocardial damage, but tests did demonstrate compromise of oxygen to her heart upon exercise. Believing that a more thorough evaluation of her coronary arteries and cardiac function should be obtained, the physician recommended that she undergo cardiac catheterization. The nurse spent considerable time explaining the procedure to Mrs. Raines, including risks and benefits. Mrs. Raines became quite frightened at the information and declined to have the procedure done. The physician and nurse continued to talk with her, insisting there was nothing to fear from the procedure, but also alluding to a scenario that unless she had her condition evaluated so she could be properly treated, she could put herself at considerable risk of sudden death. The doctor also talked with Mrs. Raines' family members, encouraging them to influence her to have the procedure done, emphasizing that not doing so could have grave consequences. Finally, Mrs. Raines consented to the procedure, only to suffer a cardiac arrest from which she could not be resuscitated during the procedure.

When encouraging patients to follow recommendations, health professionals must keep in mind that they have no way of knowing all the potential risks of treatment or whether side effects or risks will occur if the recommendations are followed. Therefore, factual, truthful information that enables patients to be aware of all potential risks, and consequently to weigh risks and benefits based on their own values, helps to ensure that the principle of nonmaleficence is not violated.

Although the basic assumption of nonmaleficence underlies all patient education activities, it is not often made explicit. Giving information is at times taken for granted as an innocuous activity that has the potential for influencing behavior and enhancing well-being but has little potential for causing harm. As illustrated in the case above, patient education has the potential to do both.

Justice

Justice is a principle that implies fairness and consistency. In other words, justice implies equality in all cases. More broadly, justice may be viewed in terms of how decisions should be made when the interest of one person or group competes with the interest of another person or group. Whatever decision is made, the principle mandates that individuals should be treated impartially and not in a capricious manner. An example of application of this principle to patient education may be found in a situation in which there are limited resources, so patient education is not available for all patients. In this situation, of course, a decision about which patients will receive patient education would need to be made. If, in making the decision, the health professional based his or her reasoning on patients' ethnic or religious background alone, the principle of justice would be violated, and the process used by the health professional to make the decision would be considered unethical. If, however, the health professional made the decision based on a process in which there were equal criteria applied to determine distribution of patient education, the principle of justice would be appropriately applied.

Confidentiality

Confidentiality relates to the concept of privacy. Most health professionals understand that information gained from the patient is to be considered confidential and not to be shared with others without the patient's expressed consent. In the case of patient education, however, this principle may at times be overlooked. Take, for example, the case of Mrs. Wells, who had recently referred her husband for Alzheimer's screening at a local medical facility. As part of the screening protocol, patients and families were asked to participate in a patient education program in which they learned about Alzheimer's disease. A few weeks after they had participated in the patient education session, Mr. and Mrs. Wells returned to the medical facility to receive results of the screening that Mr. Wells had undergone. The nurse, Ms. Lee, who had conducted the patient teaching session, saw Mr. and Mrs. Wells in the waiting room and approached them, asking for feedback regarding the patient education program on Alzheimer's disease they had attended. Mrs. Wells became visibly upset and later complained to Ms. Lee's supervisor for what she considered to be a breech of patient confidentiality. Mrs. Wells had felt very ill at ease taking her husband for Alzheimer's screening, fearing that the possibility of such a diagnosis may have some social stigma for them in their community. One of Mrs. Wells' neighbors had been in the waiting room. Overhearing Ms. Lee's comment, she later began questioning Mrs. Wells about why she had attended the patient education session about Alzheimer's disease. What Ms. Lee had considered a harmless comment, Mrs. Wells considered to be a breech of confidentiality, which caused her considerable discomfort.

VALUES

Health professionals' assumptions about the nature of patient education are based to a great extent on their own values. These values in turn have a direct impact on how they conduct patient education. This includes goals considered to be important, techniques and methods used, and the degree of responsibility shared by both health professional and patient.

The question of values permeates patient education. Health professionals' values inevitably affect the patient education process. Health professionals should be clear about their own values and understand how their values influence patient education. Being aware of his or her own values does not, however, mean that the health professional should attempt to persuade a patient with different values to accept the values that the health professional purports.

Not all health professionals involved in patient education would accept this view. Some health professionals believe that their role in patient education is to exert influence on patients to adopt the values that they believe are correct. These health professionals tend to direct patients toward attitudes and behaviors that the health professionals judge to be best. There is a delicate balance between imposing one's values on patients and being so concerned about infringing on patient autonomy that the health professional fails to be effective in the patient education process.

Patient education is not a form of indoctrination or a way to make patients conform to what the health professional believes to be an acceptable form of behavior. No health professional has absolute wisdom regarding what is best for the patients he or she serves. Health professionals have no way of knowing absolutely how following all the recommendations given will affect the patient's life and the extent to which following recommendations may be helpful or harmful.

However, patients do learn in both direct and indirect ways. If health professionals remain open to patients' values that may be different from their own, presenting objective information that has basis in fact, an atmosphere of respect and trust is created. In so doing, health professionals not only demonstrate respect for patients' autonomy while also practicing beneficence, but also increase the possibility that patients will, through informed choice, choose the behavior that is in their own best interest.

Health professionals who, on the other hand, attempt to be purely objective without introducing their own personality may appear to be giving information in a mechanical, routine way, which can diminish patients' sense of trust and feeling that the health professional has direct interest in them as individuals or in their well-being. In such instances, the patient teaching will be less than effective. Patients need more involvement from their health professional than merely information transfer. They often want to know the opinion of the health professional in order to test their own thinking. Since trust is an important factor in patient education, it is important that health professionals be honest but tactful about their own values when they are relevant to questions that arise. If health professionals do relate their values to the patient, they should always make it clear they are presenting their personal opinion, based on their own values and circumstances that may be totally different from those of the patient and that may have entirely different consequences.

Health professionals convey values to patients in a number of ways other than verbally. In the patient education interaction, whether intended or not, health professionals are continually giving patients positive and negative reinforcement with behavior as well as words. A frown, grimace, or look of approval in response to a patient's statement or behavior all communicate something about the health professional's values. Consequently, health professionals should be aware of their own values and how those are demonstrated to patients both covertly and overtly.

It must be remembered that values are often culturally inherited and determined. This may include religious beliefs and values imbedded within the cultural milieu. Therefore, what one individual considers ethically correct based on his or her own standards or values may not apply universally to all other individuals. Likewise, overreliance on cultural and/or religious principles alone to determine an ethical course of action is not always sufficient to reach an ethical decision acceptable or applicable to all individuals. The same cultural traditions or religious beliefs may not be held by all parties. Consequently, rather than using personal, cultural, or religious values alone, a more reasonable approach to ethical decision making may be to rely on commonly shared principles, rather than attempting to force one's view on a particular situation in which a common view is not shared by all.

Differences in religious values, in particular, between patient and health professional can be a barrier to effective patient education, especially when these values affect health care. It is important for health professionals to examine their own religious values and be sensitive to how they influence the way they teach patients. If health professionals have no religious affiliation or are hostile to organized religion, they should be aware of how their own views may affect patient teaching of patients who hold strong commitments to the beliefs of certain religions. Religious beliefs and practices affect many dimensions of personal life as well as health and health care. It is important that health professionals maintain awareness of the extent to which they understand their patients' religious beliefs and their meanings, and if different from their own, how this affects their relationships with patients during patient teaching.

Take, for example, Mrs. Brown, a migrant worker who came to a prenatal teaching session that the nurse, Mr. York, was conducting with her on an individual basis. Mrs. Brown was expecting her ninth child. Both Mr. and Mrs. Brown were obviously excited about the pregnancy in anticipation that the baby may be a boy, given that six of their eight children were girls. Mr. York knew that the financial situation of the family was poor, although the children appeared well nourished and well cared for. During the teaching session, Mr. York brought up the issue of birth control and the possibility of sterilization after the birth of the baby. When Mrs. Brown seemed reluctant to accept the idea, Mr. York became more coercive in his presentation, implying that under the circumstances, to have more children would be irresponsible. Mrs. Brown looked shocked and attempted to explain that she and her husband believed strongly that God would provide for any children that would be born. She said they believed that to do anything to prevent pregnancy would be interfering with nature and a demonstration of lack of trust in God.

Mr. York shook his head in despair and said coldly, "I see." He put away the teaching material and said to Mrs. Brown, "Then I guess that will be all. You obviously are not prepared to listen to reason. I need to devote my time to patients I can help." Mrs. Brown, although not saying anything, left with sadness, reluctant to bring up other issues with Mr. York in the future.

By Mr. York's actions, he had essentially influenced Mrs. Brown's behavior, but not necessarily in a positive way. Health professionals must determine the extent to which they can remain true to themselves and at the same time allow patients freedom to select their own course of action, even if it differs sharply from the action the health professionals would choose. Likewise, health professionals might need to determine when their values are in conflict with those of the patient to such a degree that referral to another health professional should be made. The most difficult aspect may be the difference between giving patients information in a way that will help them make their own informed choices and giving it in a way to influence them subtly to accept the health professional's values.

Health professionals who have liberal values may find themselves working with patients who have more traditional values or vice versa. By questioning these values or imposing their own, health professionals do not show respect for patients' beliefs and consequently lose credibility. In some instances, health professionals may have a strong commitment to values they do not even question, promoting their views at the expense of providing unbiased information that would help patients to reach their own informed choices. Health professionals should be clear about their own values and how these affect the patient education process.

Values may also be related to personal characteristics of individuals. Health professionals should be aware of their own biases and prejudices. For instance, the health professional may have a bias about individuals who are elderly, who are from different racial or ethnic groups, who are physically disabled, who have a criminal record, who abuse substances, or who are obese. Any of these biases, whether positive or negative, can affect the content of or manner in which patient education information is presented. Take, for example, the situation described below.

Mr. Slavinsky was a 72-year-old man scheduled for an appointment in the form of a consult with Dr. Penn. When calling for the appointment, Mr. Slavinsky had been reluctant to tell the appointment clerk the purpose of the visit, saying only that it was "a personal matter." At the office visit, Mr. Slavinsky began by saying that he had not felt well lately and that he had been tired with a slight cough. Dr. Penn examined Mr. Slavinsky briefly and concluded that she could find nothing wrong. Mr. Slavinsky said shyly, "I've been hearing a lot about AIDS lately and I just thought I should get checked out. I don't know very much about it." Dr. Penn smiled and said, "Oh, I don't think you have to worry about that at your age. You haven't had any blood transfusions, so it's unlikely that you would even have been exposed to the virus that causes AIDS."

When Mr. Slavinsky became more insistent about receiving information, Dr. Penn said gently, "Mr. Slavinsky, we have a very busy practice here. Although I would like to have the time to talk with patients about all kinds of things, I have to limit my time to giving them information that is most relevant for them realistically. At your age, you should be more concerned about keeping your blood pressure under control."

Dr. Penn not only made some assumptions about Mr. Slavinsky that she did not attempt to explore for their validity, she also imposed her own values on Mr. Slavinsky based on her bias regarding age, and not on Mr. Slavinsky as an individual.

There are many value-laden patient education situations. In all instances, it is important that health professionals be clear about their own values and how they influence patient teaching. Values can affect not only the way health professionals conduct patient education, but in the end, how effective patient education interactions will be.

IDENTIFYING ETHICAL ISSUES IN PATIENT EDUCATION AND PATIENT COMPLIANCE

Not every patient education situation has ethical ramifications; however, it is important that health professionals be aware of potential ethical problems related to both patient education and patient compliance. As health care becomes more complex, so do ethical issues related to patient education and patient compliance. Advances in technology in medical care as well as economic issues have brought about significant changes in the health care delivery system and subsequently in the amount of responsibility patients are expected to assume for their own health and health care. Patients now are often discharged from the hospital earlier and expected to manage more complicated treatment regimens at home. Likewise, as more is learned about the role of lifestyle in the development of chronic disease, prevention issues have become more prevalent. Most often, ethical issues in this regard are related to situations in which health professionals and patients have conflicting views or interests or in which the consequences of decisions made will have impact on others.

Theoretically, the purpose of giving patient education information is to enable patients to engage in some behavior change. The behavior change may involve living a healthier lifestyle to prevent disease or complications from occurring, or it may involve managing a disease or condition by following a specific treatment regimen.

The underlying assumption of patient education is that the goal of both health professional and patient is to help the patient to attain his or her maximum degree of health. Much of what constitutes health, however, and how that goal is attained is subjective. The patient and health professional may have differing views. Take the example of Mr. Lopez.

Mr. Lopez was a serious jogger, running several miles every day. In addition to jogging for health reasons, jogging also constituted a major portion of his social life, since he jogged with friends every morning and was involved with a jogging club, which met for jogging followed by brunch every Sunday morning. During an examination, Dr. Diego instructed Mr. Lopez that he must relinquish jogging because continuing it would only further injure his knee, which had been injured previously. Mr. Lopez, however, continued to jog, a choice made based on his own priority, believing that the other physical and psychological benefits be received from jogging made the risk of continuing to jog worth the benefit, despite Dr. Diego's instructions. Dr. Diego's view was, of course, much different, believing that the increasing damage from jogging would be a future impingement on Mr. Lopez's well-being, having the potential to cause disability requiring more aggressive treatment.

Looking at the situation described above from a patient compliance perspective, it would appear that the patient education intervention was ineffective, given that Mr. Lopez did not change behavior and therefore might be labeled as noncompliant. Although this situation does not present an ethical dilemma per se, it might have if, for instance, Dr. Diego had exaggerated his description about the degree of risk involved if Mr. Lopez continued to jog, or if Dr. Diego had taken other steps to coerce Mr. Lopez into changing his behavior to coincide with his point of view.

Another ethical implication when conducting patient education involves the amount of personal bias the health professional interjects into the patient education interaction. Bias of the health professional is often reflected by what information is given; which instructions are stressed; and what, if any, alternatives are discussed. In the above situation, after learning Mr. Lopez's values and, consequently, that he would continue to jog, Dr. Diego may have given Mr. Lopez additional information relating to how he could minimize the chance of further injury.

Another ethical implication relates to the degree to which specific techniques are used by the health professional with the specific goal of increasing patient compliance. Patient education, even if successful in terms of compliance, cannot ensure the patient's well-being. Not only is the health professional's ability to predict outcomes not exact, nor is any treatment always 100 percent effective, well-being itself is often subjective. Even if the health professional perceives the patient's well-being to be improved, the patient may not share this view. When the health professional imposes his or her values on the patient with little respect or attention to the patient's own subjective preference, although increasing compliance, the health professional may actually decrease the patient's quality of life rather than improving it. Such was the case of Mr. Ford.

Mr. Ford was an 84-year-old patient who still was very active. He had undergone exploratory surgery because of abdominal pain. The surgery revealed a malignancy, which was removed. There was little evidence of metastasis, but chemotherapy was strongly recommended. The recommendation for chemotherapy was discussed with Mr. Ford by the physician. Mr. Ford seemed somewhat resistant to undergoing treatment, stating that he had concerns that the medicine used in the treatment might make him worse. The nurse made arrangements for Mr. Ford and his family to receive detailed patient teaching about chemotherapy. In the teaching sessions, although both the physician and nurse discussed the possibility of side effects, they minimized side effects' occurrence and the discomfort that might result if they were to occur, believing that the extended life they thought chemotherapy could afford Mr. Ford would be well worth any side effects and subsequent discomfort he may experience. When Mr. Ford continued to be reluctant to have chemotherapy, the physician stated that he would then be forced to withdraw from the case, because if Mr. Ford would not cooperate with his recommendations, he could be of no further help. Feeling frightened of losing a physician he had grown to know and trust, Mr. Ford agreed to the treatment.

Unfortunately, with the first treatment, Mr. Ford experienced more of the side effects than the physician or nurse had anticipated. Mr. Ford, had severe nausea, hair loss, and general malaise. When the physician and nurse talked with him later about scheduling the second series of chemotherapy, they were surprised to hear him state with conviction that he refused to undergo any more treatments. The nurse and physician examined ways in which they could convince Mr. Ford of the necessity of continuing chemotherapy, emphasizing how important the treatment was to his well-being and longevity. They assured him that the discomfort would subside after treatment was completed.

Continual attempts to get Mr. Ford to change his mind were unsuccessful. Mr. Ford finally said the following:

> You don't understand that when you reach my age, every day becomes very precious. I've wasted some of my precious days being sick from the treatments. I want to live out the rest of my days in as much peace as possible. I want to enjoy my grandchildren. I don't want them to remember me like this. Besides, how can you be sure that the treatment will extend my life? Even if it does, at my age, I could just as easily die tomorrow of something else. Then my last days would have been wasted. Not everyone may place the same value on long life as you do.

The physician and nurse had assumed that Mr. Ford had the same values and priorities they held. Their assumption of well-being and health was not shared by Mr. Ford. In the case of Mr. Ford, he was not allowed to function as an autonomous person in his decision about whether or not he would undergo chemotherapy. He was not given complete information about the potential side effects of chemotherapy, which he could then use in making his decision. The threat by the physician to withdraw from the case applied coercion, which in turn influenced Mr. Ford's decision. The physician and nurse both imposed their values regarding the extension of life on Mr. Ford, even though they were both acting out of beneficence, believing that having chemotherapy was ultimately in Mr. Ford's best interest. As illustrated in this case, however, it turned out not to be true.

Although health professionals may have difficulty understanding patients' views, ultimately, each patient has the right to make his or her own decisions. It is frequently difficult for health professionals dedicated to the idea of effective patient education to accept patients' basic rights and responsibilities for determining their own course of action related to health instructions. The zealous professional may believe that health advice given is naturally beneficial to the patient. Professionals may believe they know what is best for the patient and consequently have the responsibility to influence the patient into following that course of action.

This view contains several assumptions. First, such a view assumes that the diagnosis is correct and that the treatment prescribed is appropriate. Although certainly this is true for the majority of patients, it is also true that there have been instances in which patients were misdiagnosed and/or received the wrong treatment. If patient education information is given and steps taken to pressure the patient into following the recommendations, but the diagnosis and/or treatment is inaccurate, the results could be harmful if not disastrous. Such is the case of Mrs. Jackson, described below.

Mrs. Jackson received a prescription for Inderal for her heart condition. She had the prescription filled at her local pharmacy, but at follow-up with her physician, she admitted that she had not taken the medication as directed. Mrs. Jackson complained that the medication made her "feel strange." Rather than questioning Mrs. Jackson more closely about her symptoms, both the physician and nurse began assessing ways they could motivate Mrs. Jackson to follow her medication regimen more closely. The nurse conducted additional patient education, stressing why taking the medication was important and emphasizing possible consequences of not taking the medication as directed. During the teaching session, the nurse became quite forceful in her attempt to convince Mrs. Jackson to comply with the instructions she had been given.

Unfortunately, neither the physician or nurse had listened closely when Mrs. Jackson had tried to explain why she was not taking the medication as directed. Neither the physician or nurse had explored her symptoms of "feeling strange" after taking the medication, nor had either of them actually examined the medication that Mrs. Jackson was taking. Had they done so, they would have noted that Mrs. Jackson had actually been given the wrong medication at the pharmacy. Instead of Inderal, she had actually received an oral antihyperglycemic agent. The mistake was finally discovered when Mrs. Jackson was brought to the emergency department with hypoglycemia.

This case illustrates not only the importance of not coercing patients into following instructions, but also the importance of taking time to interact and listen to what the patient says. Although patients may not always be able to explain feelings or symptoms in sophisticated terms, they do have important information to give if the health professional takes the time to listen.

Another assumption underlying the view that health professionals have the responsibility to coerce patients into following instructions is the belief that the health professional is the expert in the situation. This view does not acknowledge that the patient also has expertise that could make a valuable contribution to the situation, and could, in fact, help make the patient education outcomes more effective. Although the health professional may be an expert in medical or health-related matters, the patient is the expert in his or her own feelings, symptoms, values, and circumstances.

The same advice may not be appropriate or in the best interest of all patients. Giving standardized advice and information without considering the patient as an individual is to make the process of patient teaching a rigid, technical exercise rather than a process in which patients are helped to internalize recommendations made and apply them in their own best interest.

The two examples of Mr. Ford and Mrs. Jackson may seem extreme; however, similar principles apply no matter what type of patient education information is to be given. Effective patient education is not so much a matter of persuading patients to do what the health professional wants them to do but rather a process in which possible courses of action and consequences of each course of action are communicated to the patient. Patient education thus becomes a matter of outlining facts so that patients and health professionals can work together to devise a plan that will be most beneficial to the patients. Although some patients may be reluctant to accept this type of responsibility in decision making, the health professional has the responsibility to leave the option open and to consider patients' individual needs when giving instruction.

Rather than having the responsibility to promote patient compliance through patient education, health professionals have the responsibility to communicate effectively with patients, making sure that the advice and recommendations they receive are based on fact rather than prejudice. Too often when patients fail to comply with recommendations, they are viewed as uncooperative, difficult, or not fully understanding of the consequences of their actions. Health professionals have the responsibility for presenting the full range of information and options, and for ensuring that patients have the opportunity for self-determination in matters related to their own health and health care. Given this approach, health professionals then have the duty to assist patients in carrying out the mutually determined instructions in order to promote patients' welfare.

The mutual participation approach to patient education assumes that effective outcomes are the shared responsibility of patients and health professionals. The focus of this book is to help health professionals develop skills by which patients' responsibility can be enhanced. In many patient education situations, patients are vulnerable and distressed by their illnesses, symptoms, or the impact of their condition on their lives. Health professionals are in a position to help them deal with these issues and to attain maximum benefit from instructions given. This is accomplished by offering not only accurate information but also support and guidance based on the individual patient's needs.

A truly ethical approach to patient education, then, demands mutual participation by both patient and health professional to attain the most beneficial outcomes. To do so, however, health professionals should have an understanding of basic ethical principles used as a basis for ethical decision making. Problems may relate to how much or what type of information patients should be given or to what extent strategies should be implemented to increase patient compliance.

A number of specific problems and questions can arise. The first relates to the amount of patient education information the patient should receive. Does the patient have the right to complete information, or are there instances when the health professional has the right to determine how much and what type of information the patient should be given? For example, if the health professional believed that giving the patient complete information about remote side effects or risks of a certain treatment would cause the patient to not follow the recommendations, and thus not receive the potential therapeutic benefits, is the health professional justified in withholding that information from the patient in his or her own best interest? Take the example of Ms. Queen.

Ms. Queen had made an appointment with Dr. Abernathy for health care advice regarding an overseas trip she was to take. The area she was to visit had a high prevalence of malaria. Dr. Abernathy had cared for a number of patients with malaria and concluded that taking medication prophylactically is crucial. Although the medication he chose to prescribe for preventing malaria had some potentially serious side effects, Dr. Abernathy concluded that having malaria would be a greater risk than the side effects, which may or may not occur. Consequently, he advised Ms. Queen to take the medication but did not share with her the serious nature of potential side effects. Dr. Abernathy's assumption, was, of course, that knowledge of potential side effects may influence Ms. Queen's decision of whether or not to take the medication, so he made the decision to withhold information. Was Dr. Abernathy justified in withholding information from Ms. Queen, or in so doing did he violate her right to self-determination? Under what circumstances would withholding information be justified?

Another issue relates to situations where information contains half-truths or untruths judged by the health professional to be in the patient's best interest. Is telling a "therapeutic lie" ever justified, whether that involves withholding the truth, giving an incomplete truth, or outright lying? Take, for example, the case of Mr. Dubois, who had insulin-dependent diabetes. Dr. Little had spent considerable time giving Mr. Dubois information about his condition and treatment, and was pleased at the extent to which Mr. Dubois's blood sugar seemed to be under control. One day at an office visit, Mr. Dubois said the following:

> Although I don't find following the diet and insulin protocol easy, I'll continue it as long as I know it makes a difference. I know the complications of diabetes can be serious, and I'd do anything to prevent them. But if I thought that I might develop complications anyway, I sure would have to think twice about how carefully I would continue to follow the protocol. Will good compliance ensure that I won't develop complications?

Although Dr. Little recognized that there are no guarantees that complications would not develop despite good compliance and blood sugar control, he was also aware of the risks of not maintaining good control. Based on this judgment, he turned to Mr. Dubois and said, "You just keep doing as well as you are, and you'll do fine." Dr. Little decided if Mr. Dubois knew about the potential of complications despite good compliance, he may fail to follow the diet and insulin protocol as carefully and thereby jeopardize his well-being. Consequently. Dr.

Little elected to withhold information from Mr. Dubois. In so doing, was Dr. Little infringing on Mr. Dubois's right to know, or was his action justified to preserve Mr. Dubois's well-being?

Does, on the other hand, the patient have the right not to know? Should patients be coerced into hearing information they do not want to hear? There are instances in which patients may not want information about their condition or treatment. In these instances, do health professionals have the duty to give the patient information anyway, or should they respect the patient's right to refuse information? Take the example of Mrs. Bowland, who had been diagnosed with pancreatic cancer. Although Mrs. Bowland was given full information about her condition, possible palliative treatments, and the gravity of her prognosis, and appeared to understand the seriousness of her condition, she continued to remain hopeful that she would "beat the odds" and continued to make plans for the future. In this situation, when there appeared to be little indication that the condition could be treated or that in so doing life would be extended, to what extent should the health professional be "insistent" that the patient recognize the implications of her condition for the future? If there is a situation in which the patient must be given information he or she does not want to hear, the health professional should refrain from tactless truth, giving information with gentleness and sensitivity. Projected outcomes should only be given as they can be predicted accurately.

Another issue involves the extent to which the health professional is obligated to share all treatment alternatives with the patient. Does the health professional have the duty and responsibility to give the patient information about alternative forms of treatment, even though the health professional might not favor them? Is there more than one course of action or treatment that may be recommended? Can the health professional be absolutely sure that the course of treatment he or she prefers over the one the patient prefers is actually in the patient's best interest? Obviously, when considering treatment alternatives, the health professional has the responsibility to endorse only those treatments that are medically sound. For example, a patient with rheumatoid arthritis who proposes being treated with injections of snake venom rather than the nonsteroidal anti-inflammatory drugs (NSAIDs) the health professional had recommended may need additional counseling regarding treatment choice. In some instances, there are alternative choices of treatment that may be reasonable and that may be more palatable to the patient than those the health professional has recommended. In these instances, the health professional should keep an open mind and at least consider that there are other treatment alternatives.

The final issue of concern involves the degree to which health professionals implement strategies to increase patient compliance. Is the role of patient education to convince patients to acquiesce to health professionals' beliefs about the best course of action, or is the purpose of patient education to enable patients to make their own informed decisions based on factual information and their own values and priorities? Although health professionals have the responsibility to offer information, reinforcement, and strategies that can assist patients in following treatment directives, when these approaches become coercive with the expressed purpose of coercion, the ethical justification of such actions are questionable.

Additional ethical questions arise around the issue of who should be involved in decisions regarding what and how much information patients should be given. Are there instances when individuals close to the patient, who fear that information may cause the patient undue anxiety or have other deleterious effects, have the right to request that information be withheld? How do patient factors such as severe pain, limited intellectual capacity, or emotional strain affect the amount or type of information given or strategies used to affect patient compliance with treatment recommendations?

There are no absolute answers for any of these questions. Health professionals must judge each situation individually, considering the specific circumstances in that particular situation. Although some may argue that this means that health professionals could use any rationale to justify any action, for the most part, individuals should be guided by a set of principles on which to base moral judgments. In so doing, however, health professionals must also be honest about their own motives and bases for their decisions, realizing that no one is infallible, nor any decision always right in all circumstances.

In addition, patient education generally takes place in some type of institution, whether inpatient or outpatient. Each of these types of settings also has constraints or regulations that may influence what type of decisions and how certain decisions are made. These institutional constraints may go beyond the control of the health professional conducting patient education. The goal of ethical decision making for health professionals in these settings is to remain true to one's own ethical standards and values while working within the limits of the institution, but maintaining some degree of freedom within those limits both for themselves and for the patients they teach.

THE HEALTH PROFESSIONAL/PATIENT RELATIONSHIP

Effective patient education is built on a partnership between patient and health professional. Although a partnership implies equality, the relationship between patient and health professional is not equal, by nature of the relationship. Patients enter the relationship with greater vulnerability. Health professionals must remain mindful that in the context of the professional relationship, not only is there the potential to do good but also the potential to do harm, even if unintentional. Demonstrating empathy, compassion, and respect for the patient should remain within the professional relationship so that the health professional, while being an advocate for the patient, also maintains appropriate boundaries and does not become over-involved. Health professionals have a legal and ethical responsibility to provide information and base decisions on patients' interests and needs, not on their own. This means that health professionals have a duty to approach patients in an unbiased, fair, and honest manner. Examples of ethical breaches of the professional relationship would include actions such as cultivating patient dependency, treating patients in a paternalistic way, providing patients with limited information that promotes the health professional's views, or terminating services if the patient fails to comply with recommendations.

Take, for example, the case of Mr. Norton who had been a patient of Dr. Nash for 20 years. When Mr. Norton was being seen for his annual physical exam, Dr. Nash noted that Mr. Norton, who had just turned 50, had never had screening for colorectal cancer. Dr. Nash believed strongly in prevention and believed flexible sigmoidoscopy to be the most effective type of screening for colorectal cancer. He began to talk with Mr. Norton about the importance of the screening exam.

> *Dr. Nash:* Now that you've had your 50th birthday you'll need to be screened for colorectal cancer. I know you have no family history of colorectal cancer, but it's good for everyone over 50 to be screened. I would like to schedule you for a flexible sigmoidoscopy.

> *Mr. Norton:* Well, I'm not too worried about colon cancer. I've never had any problems and I'm not at high risk. I think I would like to wait for a while.

> *Dr. Nash:* Do you know that colorectal cancer has one of the highest incidence rates of all cancers, with well over 100,000 people being newly diagnosed each year? Last year, almost 60,000 people died of colorectal cancer. The sad thing is that if it's found early it is highly curable. I really believe you need to be screened.

> *Mr. Norton:* That sounds like a lot of people. I'm still not sure at this point that I want to go through a screening though. I've heard that sigmoidoscopy can be really uncomfortable. If you insist that I be screened maybe instead I could have one of those fecal occult blood tests if you think I really need to be screened.

> *Dr. Nash:* The occult screening isn't nearly as effective, and there is a lot of preparation involved. With flexible sigmoidoscopy we can actually visualize the intestine and see small growths that may be precancerous and wouldn't even been found on an occult blood test. The flexible sigmoidoscopy only has to be done every few years or so, only takes about 20 minutes, and is safe. You should only have minimal discomfort. Isn't that worth it when you consider it could save your life? I've known you for a long time. I would hate to see you develop a disease that could have been so easily prevented.

After more discussion, Dr. Nash finally convinced Mr. Norton to have the test. Unfortunately, Mr. Norton experienced intestinal perforation during the test and developed peritonitis.

Dr. Nash, although well intentioned, used his power in the relationship to pressure Mr. Nash into having a procedure that he was reluctant to have performed and one that ended with unforeseen harmful consequences. In the case of Dr. Nash and Mr. Norton, there was conflict over the definition of the problem, the goals, and the priorities in treatment. Had Dr. Nash worked within the framework of partnership within the relationship and not exerted the power of his position, the two might have come to some agreement or compromise that would have proven satisfactory to both and avoided what became a disastrous end.

ETHICAL ISSUES IN RESEARCH IN PATIENT EDUCATION AND PATIENT COMPLIANCE

Although research in patient education and patient compliance is important, the health professional conducting it has the obligation to protect the rights and dignity of patients participating. Health professionals should not assume that the research they are conducting is so innocuous that it could cause no potential harm, nor should they attempt to coerce patients into participation. Likewise, health professionals should not assume that the importance of the research they are conducting justifies violating the rights of patients.

Most institutional settings have a human subjects research review board, which consists of people whose responsibility it is to review research projects involving human subjects before they are conducted in order to ensure that the research protocol does not violate patient rights or does not present a hazard or danger to patient well-being. When conducting research, the health professional is responsible for ensuring that the research is conducted ethically. One of the first responsibilities is to make sure that patients are fully informed of all features of the research that might influence their willingness to participate. This means that except under very special circumstances, information regarding features of the study cannot be withheld. Patients should be given complete information so that they can make a free choice about whether or not they want to participate. Patients should not be included in a study without their knowledge, and they must have complete information about the study. For example, a health professional who is interested in monitoring the effect patient education about epilepsy has on patients' compliance rates of taking antiepileptic medication cannot have the patient return for weekly blood levels at the patient's expense if the blood work is only for research purposes and if the patient has not been informed and has not agreed to pay for the lab work.

Patients participating in any research project must also be ensured the freedom to discontinue their participation at any time. It is particularly important to be sensitive to this issue since patients may feel that if they decline to participate or discontinue their participation, their future health care would in some way be threatened. Patients must understand that failure to participate or withdrawal from the study in which they are participating will not influence the quality or quantity of health care they receive at the facility in the future.

Complete disclosure can be a problem when conducting patient compliance research. Informing patients of the complete research protocol may very well affect the results of the study so that conclusions drawn cannot be considered valid. If, for example, patients know that the degree to which they follow recommendations is being studied, any behavior change observed may actually be a function of the patients' being monitored, rather than the strategy designed to improve patient compliance. To draw a conclusion that the intervention itself changed compliance behavior would, under these circumstances, be inaccurate, unless the intervention to increase compliance was merely telling patients that their compliance behavior would be monitored.

In situations when fully informing the patient might influence results, alternatives should be considered. If deception or incomplete information about the nature of the study is used, health professionals have the responsibility to inform patients at the completion of the study and to reveal the conditions of the study and the true intent of the study, so that any misconceptions are dispelled. It is important for health professionals to conduct this debriefing in a sensitive manner, since in some instances, patients may feel that their trust has been violated or may become angry or embarrassed when they find they were deceived. Before deception or incomplete information about the study is considered, health professionals should carefully consider and weigh the possibility of harm or risk to patients and the justification of the research protocol under those circumstances.

In all instances, patient confidentiality should be maintained. Steps should be taken to protect patient identity and to maintain patient anonymity. This includes review of patient records. If, as part of data gathering, information from patients' records prior to or after the patient education intervention is necessary, patients should be made aware of this fact and should be told who will have access to the chart and any other subsequent information.

ETHICAL PATIENT EDUCATION PRACTICES

Patient education and especially patient compliance can be value-laden concepts. Patient education information, depending on the content and manner presented, can introject bias of the health professional, which may infringe on patients' ability to make their own free choices about the degree to which they will follow the advice given. Implicit in patient education is the assumption that information health professionals give to patients is what the patients need to know for their own benefit. Health professionals must be mindful, however, of patients' rights to determine what constitutes benefit for them. The term *compliance* itself implies a certain degree of authority on the part of the health professional and cooperation on the part of the patient with recommendations or information that has been given. The health professional must keep in mind that if compliance is to be an outcome measure of effective patient education, the most successful outcome will be based on patient participation in decision making and collaboration between patient and health professional in making those decisions. Likewise, although research is important to both patient education and patient compliance, health professionals must be ever mindful that patients' rights must be protected. Whether conducting patient education, or research about patient education or patient compliance, the health professional should keep in mind the following concepts:

1. Information provided should be accurate and should reflect the most current theory or view.

2. Information provided, if followed, should cause the patient more good than harm.

3. Information should be presented in a factual way, without distortion or exaggeration of facts and without falsification.

4. The patient's decision to follow recommendations should be based on factual evidence rather than on the bias of the health professional that has been inadvertently introduced.

5. Patients' values, beliefs, resources, and barriers regarding following recommendations should be identified and addressed.

6. Any intervention designed to assist patients to follow recommendations should not be coercive.

7. Any research conducted with patients should protect patients' right of freedom to choose to participate and should be based on informed choice.

8. Patient confidentiality should be protected.

Informed Consent 15

Previous chapters discussed negotiation between patients and health professionals as it relates to patient education and, ultimately, decision making about recommendations patients will carry out. The concept of negotiation in patient education emphasizes that, to be effective, health professionals must talk *with* patients rather than *at* them. Negotiation in the context of patient education involves a relationship between patient and health professional in which there is a genuine effort by the health professional to provide information that is relevant to the patient to clarify uncertainties, to identify problems, and to work together to arrive at a mutually satisfactory course of action based on the information at hand.

It would appear that this type of shared decision making is ideal for an effective patient–health professional relationship and that certainly such an approach upholds the ethical principles of autonomy and beneficence discussed in the previous chapter. Although informing the patient about care and treatment is certainly ethically desirable, it is also legally incumbent upon the health professional in the form of informed consent. Beginning in the early 1900s, the courts asserted that based on the principle of self-determination, patients have the legal right to make decisions regarding their medical care. Historically, informed consent has been the major responsibility of the physician, the law having been developed in the context of claims against physicians who neglected to inform their patients adequately before initiating treatment. As other health professionals assume increasing responsibility as independent providers of care, however, the legal requirements of informed consent will apply to them as well. The legal doctrine of informed consent requires the health professional not only to obtain consent from patients before treatment is initiated but also to engage in a meaningful exchange of information and discussion with patients so that their consent is actually "informed."

THE MEANING OF INFORMED CONSENT

Informed consent, although a legal doctrine, also involves fundamental values. Informed consent is based on respect for individuals, their right and ability to determine their own goals based on their own values and to decide how they will achieve the goals they have established.

The concept of informed consent is viewed in the context of the relationship between patient and health professional in which the health professional provides patients with enough information to make intelligent, informed judgments. In addition to being based on patients' right of self-determination, informed consent is strongly rooted in the value of active participation by patients in their own health care.

The legal aspects of informed consent are related to the concept of battery, which is essentially the intentional touching of another person without authorization. In other words, theoretically, before patients submit to a treatment, procedure, or examination, they must give their consent or authorization for the action in question to be performed. Unfortunately, in the past, this type of consent was often based more on patients' trust and faith in the health professional than on the quality of information they had been given on which to base their decisions.

During the past years, there has been increasing interest not only in obtaining patient authorization before performing various procedures but also in the quality of the information given by the health professional, which underlies the patient's informed consent. There is general consensus that informed consent is a process involving more than merely obtaining the patient's signature on an informed consent form. The patient's signature only serves as an indication that this process has taken place. It cannot be equated with the process. For the process to be valid, information given to the patient must be adequate, the patient must understand the information, and the decision to agree to the treatment or intervention must be voluntary. Health professionals are, therefore, held responsible not only for what they do to the patient but for what they say to the patient as well. Information given to patients by health professionals must be clear, accurate, and in terms the patient can understand. This responsibility can be extended to information given to the patient by the health professional in the form of written patient education materials as well. If information contained in written materials is inaccurate or insufficient, and as a result of receiving the material and following the advice given in it the patient suffers harm, the health professional could be held responsible. As an example, consider the case of Mr. Samuel.

Mr. Samuel was a 64-year-old patient who had been admitted to the hospital because of circulatory problems in his lower extremities due to arteriosclerosis.

He was well educated and widely read. His physician felt that an arteriogram of the lower extremities was indicated in order to explore the extent of the circulatory problem. The procedure was discussed with Mr. Samuel, and the nurse was asked to give Mr. Samuel the patient education booklet on arteriograms, which had been prepared by the hospital patient education staff.

The nurse gave Mr. Samuel the booklet, leaving him alone for some time while he read over the information it contained. The booklet specifically outlined what the arteriogram is, what the procedure consists of, and what it can show. Upon returning, the nurse asked Mr. Samuel if he had any questions and again highlighted certain information contained in the book. Mr. Samuel subsequently signed the consent form to have the procedure performed. The booklet unfortunately neglected to mention possible risks associated with the procedure, and in fact stated that the procedure was a safe and efficient way of gaining the type of information needed to help physicians in further diagnosis and treatment. Neither the physician nor the nurse mentioned the possible risk of the procedure to Mr. Samuel.

If, as a result of the procedure, Mr. Samuel suffered some form of complication resulting in harm to him, it is quite likely that he could question the extent to which his consent to the procedure was actually "informed," since he had not been told about the risks involved. Neither the physician nor the nurse could assume that Mr. Samuel was already knowledgeable about arteriograms and the possibility of risk simply because of his apparent sophistication and educational level. In addition, the physician could not assume that the nurse would discuss possible risk of the procedure with Mr. Samuel. Also, unless the physician had reviewed the education material given Mr. Samuel, there is no way the physician could make a judgment about its accuracy and completeness.

Before patients can make a reasonable informed consent, they must understand not only the procedure to which they are consenting but also any risks involved, as well as alternatives that might be available. Informed consent, then, hinges not only on the accuracy and clarity of the information given to patients but also on patients having enough information to make an informed decision.

Although the issue of informed consent has received increased attention and support, many health professionals, as well as patients, continue to have misperceptions as to what informed consent actually is. In a classic study conducted by the President's Commission for the Study of Ethical Problems in Medicine and Biomedical and Behavioral Research, a group of patients and physicians were asked what the term *informed consent* meant to them (President's Commission for the Study of Ethical Problems in Medicine and Biomedical and Behavioral Research 1982). Twenty-one percent of the public said they did not know what the term *informed consent* meant. The majority of the rest of the public samples defined *informed consent* in terms of being informed or agreeing to treatment, but usually agreement to treatment was put in the context of whatever the health professional, in this case the physician, thought best. Only 11 percent of the public asked about their conception of the term *informed consent* mentioned that it involved knowledge of risk or alternatives.

In the physician group, most of those asked stated that *informed consent* consisted of generally informing patients about their condition and treatment. Only 34 percent included patient understanding of the information given as a part of informed consent, and even fewer mentioned patient understanding of treatment risks as part of the concept. Few physicians mentioned treatment alternatives or that informed consent involved patient choice or preference about treatment.

To be valid, patients' consent must be informed. The meaning of informed consent has been developed over the years through individual cases brought before the courts. Consequently, the term is much more broadly defined now than initially, when it was concerned mainly with a patient's authorization to have a procedure performed. In general, information required to make a consent informed currently consists of:

- the patient's diagnosis
- explanation of the proposed treatment and its purpose
- any risks or consequences of the proposed treatment
- probability that the proposed treatment will be successful
- treatment alternatives available
- consequences of not receiving the proposed treatment

All information must also be given to patients in terms they can understand. An awareness of the meaning of informed consent is extremely important for all health professionals and especially for those involved in patient education. Through their own awareness of its meaning, health professionals may also serve as patient advocates in educating them to the information informed consent requires. Without a clear understanding of what informed consent involves, neither patients nor health professionals can use it to its optimal intent.

THE FUNCTION OF INFORMED CONSENT

The primary purpose of informed consent is the protection of individual autonomy. Autonomy is a form of personal freedom of action in which patients determine their own course of action according to a plan they themselves have chosen. No matter what the health professional thinks may be best for the patient, informed consent puts patients in a position that promotes and protects their right to make decisions concerning their own welfare. Informed consent protects patients from being placed in a position where decisions are based on values and views of the health professional rather than their own. Through informed consent, patients are given information about the procedure itself, as well as the risk and consequences of having or not having the procedure performed. If patients have obtained all the information they feel necessary to make a decision, then they are theoretically protected from submitting to procedures that, according to their own value structure, they may not feel are in their best interests.

Although the function of informed consent seems fairly straightforward, there has been much confusion over the nature and scope of information actually to be disclosed and discussed. For instance, to guarantee patient autonomy and rational decision making, how much detail of the procedure and associated risk must be given? Many health professionals argue correctly that most patients do not want to know every detail of every procedure, and that giving patients too much information could actually harm them by discouraging them from consenting to the procedure at hand. Consider, for example, the situation if Dr. Yang—when conducting preoperative teaching before having the patient sign the informed consent form—engaged in the following dialogue:

> Mr. Hall, tomorrow morning before surgery you will first receive an injection of Demerol, which is a narcotic that will help you to relax and decrease your anxiety level. The Demerol will be mixed with another drug called atropine, which will dry up the secretions of your mucous membrane. This is important because when you go into surgery, we will insert a tube down your throat called an airway that will keep your air passages open and that will allow us to give you the anesthetic. If your mouth is full of saliva, then you could choke when we put the tube in. The tube will be attached to a respirator, which will help you breathe. This is important because we will also inject you with a drug that is actually a poison called curare, which will completely paralyze all your muscles from head to toe. This obviously includes your chest muscles. Since you won't be able to breathe on your own as a result and there must be air exchange in order to keep you alive, the respirator will breathe for you. In the unlikely event that there is a power shortage during surgery, which would cause the respirator to fail, the hospital has an emergency generator that will be used to maintain the respirator's function. Also rarely, but on occasion, people for some reason react to the anesthetic and their hearts may stop. The surgery team is ready for such emergencies and, in the rare event that this happens, would be ready to resuscitate immediately, meaning that they would attempt to restore your heart to begin beating again on its own.

Obviously, if Dr. Yang went into this much detail, in all likelihood, the patient may well decide to leave the hospital. Although perhaps an extreme example, this explanation or others that include excessive detail may be considered "information dumping" rather than giving patients information to help them make an informed decision about whether or not to authorize the procedure, and whether or not they feel the procedure would be in their best interests. Conflict arises, obviously, in determining where the line is drawn to denote that the health professional is withholding details that are necessary to the patient's decision-making process. When is withholding information justified, and when is withholding information an infringement on patient autonomy?

HOW MUCH INFORMATION TO DISCLOSE

The first requirement of informed consent is that the information given must be adequate so the patient has sufficient information on which to base consent. How much information is adequate? In general, adequacy of information is determined by three standards:

1. the professional community standard
2. the reasonable person standard
3. the subjective standard

The professional community standard is based on what is generally considered customary information in a given community. This standard can apply to local, regional, or national levels, depending on the circumstances. For example, if a health professional were obtaining an informed consent from a human immunodeficiency virus (HIV)-positive patient about to receive a new drug for treatment, it might generally be expected that the majority of health professionals disclose the potential risks in taking the medication before the patient agrees to the treatment. Consequently, failure to do so may be considered negligence on the part of the health professional based on this professional community standard as it pertains to informed consent.

The second standard, the reasonable person standard, is more patient-centered than the professional community standard. It is based on the premise that information given should be sufficient and given in such a way that a reasonable person, meaning one who is competent and capable of systematic reasoning in reaching decisions about his or her treatment, could make an informed choice.

The subjective standard takes into account the personal needs and values of the patient so that the amount of information and the time it is disclosed are based on the patient's personal circumstances and need to know. This means that information may be disclosed at a pace suitable for the patient rather than all at once or before the patient is ready to accept it.

The issue of what and how much information the patient should be given is one not easily resolved. Although a consent cannot be legally effective unless it is informed, it is also impractical and probably impossible to give the patient all information that is relevant to the proposed treatment or procedure. The patient may be unable to comprehend much of the detail or may not be prepared psychologically to handle all of it. Giving every minute detail of every procedure may be so time-consuming that the effectiveness of any communication between patient and health professional would be lost. Giving a mass of facts to patients in a blunt, insensitive way can be more destructive than helpful to the process of promoting the patient's ability to make an informed decision.

The adequacy of the amount of information given to patients has frequently been determined when a patient who suffered some harm as a result of a procedure has brought the issue to court. A landmark Kansas case in 1960 set a standard for disclosure of information to be given in informed consent (Natanson

v. Kline 1960). It stated basically that the health professional—in this case, the physician—has the obligation to give the patient whatever information most other health professionals (physicians) would provide under the same circumstances. In this view, then, much of the decision as to what and how much information should be given patients to make their consent informed was left up to the judgment of the health professional.

After the Kansas case, courts tended to base the standard for how much information needed to be disclosed for patient consent to be informed on what the medical community considered appropriate. Another landmark case, however, brought about a different rule that focused more on the patient's point of view. The new case based standards of information for informed consent on the needs of the average, reasonable patient, rather than on the medical community's standard practice of information giving (Canterbury v. Spence 1972).

The question, then, remains: How much information should a "reasonable" patient be given? In making this determination, it is important to remember the function of informed consent. The health professional should discuss facts and uncertainties with patients that would help them gain a working understanding of their condition, treatment, alternatives, and possible consequences of agreeing or not agreeing to treatment, so that they can make a decision that best suits their own needs and values. Overly detailed information may, in fact, confuse and interfere with the patient's decision-making process.

This would imply, then, that in determining what type and how much information to give the patient, the health professional must be able to assess the individual and tailor the presentation of information to the individual according to his or her particular needs. This means that the health professional must gear information giving to a tactful discussion of facts, being sensitive to the individual's needs, intellectual capability, and emotional state at the time; and presenting information in terms that the patient can understand. Although the patient's questions and concerns about the proposed treatment or procedure must be addressed, the health professional cannot depend on the patient's questions to indicate how much he or she wants to know. The patient may not know what to ask or may be too intimidated to ask questions or state concerns. The stress of the condition or illness itself may preclude the patient's thinking of questions that may otherwise seem obvious.

It is therefore the responsibility of the health professional to give patients accurate and complete information about their condition, treatment, or procedure and to inform them of what is at stake if a variety of different actions are taken. Benefits gained from accepting or not accepting treatment must be assessed in terms of the patient's own values. The professional therefore should be careful not to leave out information about an alternative the patient may see as beneficial even if the health professional disagrees.

Such was the case of Ms. Caldwell, a 25-year-old woman who had discovered a lump in her breast. Upon consultation, her physician also noted some leakage of blood-tinged fluid from the nipple of her breast. The physician recommended that the mass be biopsied, but also informed Ms. Caldwell that, because of the leakage of fluid, there was a greater possibility that the lump was malignant and that more radical surgery might be needed. The physician explained the procedure of biopsy and frozen section, recommending that if a malignancy was found, a radical procedure be performed immediately rather than having Ms. Caldwell return for surgery a few days after the biopsy. Ms. Caldwell received a thorough explanation of what the surgery entailed, what risks were involved, and the consequences of having a malignancy untreated. Although shocked and upset by the news, Ms. Caldwell prepared to enter the hospital a few days later, at which time, after receiving further information, she signed the consent for a mastectomy immediately following the biopsy should a malignancy be found.

A frozen section of the biopsy confirmed the diagnosis of malignancy, and the mastectomy was performed. Ms. Caldwell's postoperative recovery was uneventful, and all appeared to be going well. Two months after her surgery, however, she returned to the physician's office, charging that she had not been given full information when she agreed to have the major surgery performed. She had recently read of the possibility of having a "lumpectomy" in which only the mass and not the entire breast is removed. After consulting with friends, she found that several of them reported knowing individuals who had had this procedure and were apparently doing well.

The physician stated that the procedure had not been extensively proven as an effective cure for breast cancer and that, given the patient's age, it appeared that the most effective means of saving her life was the mastectomy. Ms. Caldwell did not share the physician's opinion. Her decision had been made at a time of personal stress in which she felt very vulnerable, not even thinking to ask whether there were alternatives to the mastectomy. She felt that had options been presented to her, she would not have agreed to have the mastectomy.

Ms. Caldwell's case illustrates a couple of issues. First, although she received complete information about the procedure and the risks involved, the physician did not provide her with information regarding available alternatives. The physician's judgment not to disclose the information about the lumpectomy was based on the belief that the lumpectomy was not the most efficient way of treating breast cancer. Although at the time there may not have been enough evidence to suggest that the lumpectomy was more effective than mastectomy in treating breast cancer, there also was not enough information to suggest that it may not be more effective in some cases.

The physician's judgment was also based on the assumption that Ms. Caldwell would consider life to take precedence over amputation of her breast. Even if the mastectomy were to be more effective in treating Ms. Caldwell's malignancy, it cannot be assumed that she would consider longevity made possible by this surgery to be in her best interests.

Second, Ms. Caldwell did not ask about alternatives because she was not yet aware of them. In addition, because of the stress of the news she had received, she may not have been thinking clearly enough to request information about alternatives. Withholding information about the lumpectomy was probably not, in this case, in Ms. Caldwell's best interest.

The court recognizes instances in which giving the patient all the information is not desirable or in the patient's best interest. If information is from a medical point of view that is detrimental to the patient, disclosure would obviously be contraindicated. For example, the health professional may choose to withhold information from patients who are so physically ill or emotionally distraught that giving them certain information would complicate or hinder their care or cause them harm physically or emotionally. Such might be the case for a patient who has suffered a severe heart attack, is in a weakened and debilitated state, and also is suddenly diagnosed as having leukemia. Another possible example is a case in which the patient is so emotionally unstable that there is concern that knowledge of the diagnosis would cause the patient to commit suicide. Such exceptions to informing the patient are called *therapeutic privilege.*

Therapeutic privilege, however, is just that—a privilege that should not be misused. If the health professional purposefully withholds information from a patient because of fear that, with full information, the patient would not accept the treatment the professional feels is needed, the intent of therapeutic privilege has been violated. Such is the case of a person who, after having an abnormal stress test, is told that a cardiac catheterization is indicated. Fearful that the patient would refuse to have the catheterization if risks of the procedure were outlined, the health professional may not address the risks involved or may at least minimize them. This failure to disclose information is a violation of the intent of therapeutic privilege, because the purpose of withholding information was not to protect the patient from harm but rather to coerce him or her into a procedure deemed to be in the patient's best interest by the health professional. Withholding information for this reason prevents patients from making a truly informed consent about whether or not to undergo the procedure.

In cases where therapeutic privilege is exercised, health professionals should document that the patient's susceptibility to harm from receiving the information is above the norm. Factual evidence to support the health professional's use of therapeutic privilege is crucial. In addition, professionals may want to seek a second opinion confirming their observation. This second opinion should also be documented on the patient's chart.

Therapeutic privilege also applies to those patients who make it clear to the health professional that they do not want to know certain information, thus waiving their right to information specified. In this case, it is also important that the patient's request is documented. Such may be the case of a patient who does not wish to know if the condition is terminal. In these instances, however, if the patient later asks directly whether or not the illness is terminal, a truthful answer is mandated. Even in these circumstances, it should be noted that tact should prevail. Truth can, even in these instances, be presented in such a way as not to destroy the patient's hope.

CONSENT—IMPLIED OR EXPLICIT

Disclosing information to patients that allows them to make decisions about their own health care is the basis of patient education as well as the basis of the legal doctrine of informed consent. It is hardly feasible, however, that health professionals will obtain written or even verbal consent from patients every time they interact with them. Obviously, patients do not give written consent every time they visit a physician's office or receive an injection in the hospital.

Patients' consent may be either implied or explicit. Implied consent is that form of consent that seems apparent from the patient's actions. In other words, when a patient makes an appointment to be seen by a physician for a specific physical problem, it maybe assumed that he or she is authorizing the physician to do an examination to diagnose the nature of the symptoms. No specific written or oral consent is necessary. The underlying principle is that if patients voluntarily seek medical advice regarding symptoms they are experiencing, they apparently know that to diagnose and treat their symptoms, some type of information gathering or examination will be necessary.

A limitation of implied consent is that patients must be aware of what their particular action of seeking help from the physician means in the context of the situation. The patient is, therefore, giving implied consent only for the procedure that may reasonably be expected under the circumstances. Any additional treatment or procedure that is not obvious at the time the patient submitted to the original examination or procedure is not warranted without further consent. For instance, a patient who comes to the physician because of an earache may reasonably expect the physician to examine the ear. A myringotomy, however, should not be performed without giving the patient additional explanation.

Implied consent is used when procedures are noninvasive, routine, or without significant risk. Implied consent is also used when the patient has the ability to withdraw voluntarily from the procedure or circumstance. For instance, it is expected that a patient seeking advice from a physician because of an earache may expect to receive some sort of medication to treat the ear. Given that the patient receives adequate information about the treatment prescribed, he or she is able to choose whether to have the prescription filled and the degree to which the regimen will be followed. Patients would not be expected to sign a consent form stating that they understand the treatment regimen prescribed and have been informed of subsequent risks.

It stands to reason, however, that any time a procedure that imposes additional risk is to be performed, the patient must be made aware of the risks inherent in the procedure as well as alternatives that may be available. This type of procedure requires more than an assumption that, based on patients' actions, they agree to submit to the procedure. These circumstances require that the patient give express consent, meaning that the consent to the procedure is either verbal or written. This type of consent should be obtained whenever (1) a procedure is invasive; (2) anesthesia is used; (3) a nonsurgical procedure is to be performed in which there is more than slight risk to the patient, such as an arteriogram; (4) a procedure involving radiation, cobalt, or electric shock is to be performed; or (5) the procedure or treatment to which the patient is to be exposed is experimental.

In general, patients' consent is limited to the procedures described to them when their consent was given. At times, however, health professionals do not know which additional procedures may be needed until after the original procedure is performed. Under these circumstances, generally, another consent from the patient or someone authorized to give consent on the patient's behalf must be obtained. For example, if the patient has given consent to have an appendectomy, but during surgery it is discovered that the patient also has a malignancy of the colon that would require removal of the bowel and subsequent colostomy, another consent for the additional procedure would need to be obtained from the patient or another authorized person.

Some general exceptions to this rule may apply if the patient consents to reasonable steps to correct a condition, leaving the exact choice of procedure to the health professional. An example might be the case of a person undergoing surgery for cancer in which the extensiveness of the malignancy is not known; therefore, the exact procedure needed to remedy the condition may also not be known. Under these circumstances, the patient's informed consent may reflect not only knowledge of the proposed procedure to be performed but an acknowledgment that, depending upon the circumstances, additional reasonable procedures may need to be performed as well.

Another exception is in cases where it is not feasible to obtain additional consent from a patient to perform a procedure other than the one originally designated. Such would be the case if during surgery an emergency procedure that had not been anticipated were needed.

Patients have the right, when giving informed consent, to specify whether there are particular procedures they do not wish to have performed. As an example, Mr. Arnold had a barium enema because of vague complaints and constipation. As a result of the enema, a mass was discovered that appeared in all probability to be cancer. The physician discussed alternatives with Mr. Arnold, as well as the surgical procedure itself, indicating that as part of the surgery, a colostomy would probably be indicated. Mr. Arnold consented to the surgery but added specifically that under no circumstances did he want the colostomy. Having made sure that Mr. Arnold fully understood the implications of his decision, the physician was obligated to respect Mr. Arnold's decision and perform the surgery, but without the colostomy.

Patients also have the right to know who will perform their procedure or treatment before their authorization to have the procedure or treatment performed is given. If, for example, Mrs. Dean. gives her expressed consent that Dr.

Flynn will perform her gallbladder surgery, she has a right to expect that Dr. Flynn will indeed be the surgeon. Dr. Flynn is not at liberty at the last minute, and without Mrs. Dean's prior consent and knowledge, to ask one of his colleagues to perform the surgery in his stead.

Basically, the patient's expressed verbal or written consent should be based on as accurate a perception as possible of exactly what is expected to occur. The responsibility of the health professional in obtaining informed consent is to make sure the patient's understanding of what is expected is as clear as possible.

WHO OBTAINS CONSENT

The question of who is responsible for obtaining informed consent frequently arises. As mentioned earlier, as health professionals in other disciplines obtain greater independence and responsibility, the concept of informed consent as it relates to those health professionals may be broadened. At this time, however, in most instances, it is the physician performing the procedure who ultimately has the obligation and responsibility to obtain the patient's consent after sufficient information has been given. This is based on the principle that only the person performing the procedure or ordering the treatment has the expertise needed to be able to give the patient an explanation sufficient to allow him or her to make an informed decision. This expertise of information includes not only the procedure itself and its purpose but also risks, consequences, and available alternatives.

Therefore, although other health professionals may be involved in teaching about various procedures before they are performed, the physician carrying out the procedure is responsible for giving the patient a sufficient explanation of the procedure in understandable terms before the consent can be considered valid. The responsibility for obtaining informed consent cannot be delegated by the physician, although a nurse may be asked to get the consent form signed after the physician has given the patient information. The nurse, although perhaps involved in additional teaching of the patient about the procedure, cannot, however, assume the responsibility for determining that the patient knows all the risks and alternatives inherent in the procedure. A nurse who has been asked to get the consent form signed or to witness the patient's signing of the form should remember that he or she is only a witness, not the person who ultimately determines that the patient's consent has been informed.

Although the nurse is not legally responsible for obtaining informed consent, he or she is responsible for notifying the physician immediately if observations indicate that the patient does not understand the procedure or that the consent is not truly informed. If the patient confides to the nurse that he or she did not actually understand the physician's explanation or that a change of mind is occurring about having the procedure done, it is imperative that the nurse notify the physician as well as document the observation in the patient's record. In instances when the patient does not clearly understand the nature of the procedure or all its risks or consequences, it is not the duty of the nurse to clarify the information but rather to reassure the patient that the physician will be notified of his or her concerns.

The nurse is also responsible for monitoring the patient's condition. If the patient's condition changes so as to produce additional risk should the procedure be carried out, the nurse has the responsibility of notifying the physician and documenting his or her observations. Such might be the case with the patient who develops a fever the night before surgery or one whose blood pressure drops significantly after the administration of preoperative medication.

The role of other health professionals with regard to informed consent is not clearly outlined. It seems only reasonable, however, that any health professional who notes confusion or concern on the part of a patient with regard to a particular procedure or treatment has the responsibility of notifying those responsible for the patient's care of that observation so that proper steps can be taken to ensure that the patient's consent to a procedure has been informed.

ASSESSING PATIENTS' ABILITY TO GIVE CONSENT

As previously noted, competence is a legal concept. Because of increased litigation, issues of competence when obtaining informed consent have gained increasing attention. When obtaining informed consent, the health professional must be able to evaluate whether or not the patient has the ability to make an informed decision. The initial assessment may be conducted by the health professional; however, if in conducting the assessment the patient's competence is called into question, the health professional may wish to seek the assistance of someone well versed in mental status evaluations and competence determinations.

The first step in assessing patients' ability to give informed consent is to determine that they are alert and aware enough to receive the information presented. Obviously, if the patient is unconscious; delirious; or experiencing severe dementia, florid psychosis, or severe mental retardation, he or she may not be capable of rational decision making or giving truly informed consent. In instances when the patient's mental status is in question, a brief mental status examination that evaluates the individual's orientation, memory, attention, and concentration can be a useful initial screening of the patient's ability to comprehend information to be presented.

In some instances, although patients may have full cognitive ability, severe anxiety or depression may interfere with their ability to make a rational decision. In these instances, the health professional may want to obtain assistance from other professionals trained in treating the underlying emotional problem. When time is crucial, the health professional may need to consult with other professionals regarding when, how, and by whom informed consent may best be obtained.

When assessing the patient's ability to make an informed decision, the health professional must also make sure that all information was clearly communicated to the patient. In some instances, the patient's inability to relate specific aspects of the information may be the result of poor communication on the part of the individual giving the information rather than on the patient's inability to comprehend it. If the health professional is assured that the information has been presented completely and clearly, one of the best ways to assess patients' understanding of the information is to ask them to repeat what they heard in their own words. Likewise, when evaluating whether or not patients are able to make an informed choice, it is important to determine if the decision was made according to logical reasoning. If, for example, patients give a reason such as, "If I don't follow your advice, all the doctors and nurses will be mad, and I will have no one to take care of me" or, "I made the decision after the man on the television told me to do it," it would not appear that the decision was based on logical evaluation of the information they had been presented, and their ability to make a truly informed decision should probably be questioned.

Health professionals should remember that patients' refusal to accept the recommendation or treatment does not necessarily mean they are incompetent or unable to give informed consent. More important than the decision is the process by which it was made, a process underscored by patients' understanding of the information, risks and benefits, options and alternatives, and consequences of decisions that are open to them.

CONCEPTS OF COMPETENCE FOR INFORMED CONSENT

Patients who are competent have the right to decide whether or not they will follow medical advice and treatment recommendations. When patients are unable to make such decisions, competence is often called into question. Competence is at times also called into question when patients refuse to consent to recommendations, especially when these recommendations are thought by health professionals to be life saving or important to patient well-being. A major issue then becomes this: When and how is a patient deemed to be incompetent to make an informed choice, and when is refusal to accept treatment an exercise in the patient's own right to self-determination?

Competence is a legal concept that can be formally determined only through legal proceedings. Often, health professionals make decisions regarding patients' competence to make an informed choice on their own, based on assumptions that may or may not be valid. Competence must be assessed in the context of the specific situation. Competence to make an informed decision about treatment or care may not necessarily be correlated with competence for decisions about other matters. For example, an individual with a psychiatric diagnosis may be incompetent to manage his or her own financial matters but may be quite capable of refusing medication that causes untoward side effects. An individual with mild dementia may be incapable of driving a car but may be quite capable of refusing an invasive diagnostic procedure.

The term *competence* refers to patients' ability to make rational, informed decisions. There are some instances, of course, when it is clear that the patient is unable to make a truly informed decision. In some instances, however, patients' competence is called into question not because of systematic assessment of their decision-making ability, but merely because the decision they have made does not correspond with the decision the health professional believes is best.

There are several key elements involved in competence that determine whether the patient is truly able to give informed consent. First is the patient's ability to understand the information presented. This means not only the ability to remember the information but also the ability to understand the meaning of what is told and the patient's role in the decision.

Second, patients must be able to communicate their choices. In other words, even if patients are able to understand the information presented, if they are unable to indicate a choice or maintain a consistent choice, competence may be called into question. This does not mean that if patients have reasonable justification, they cannot change their minds.

Third, patients must be able to understand the situation and the consequences of various choices with which they are presented. For example, some patients may have the ability to regurgitate information they have been presented and outline choices as well as risks and benefits without having full understanding of what the implications of the information and consequently their choices would have. Patients must have the ability, realistically, to assess each option and the consequences of that option and take into account their own values when weighing the risks and benefits of each option.

Last, patients must demonstrate the ability to reach a decision by some logical process. In other words, patients must demonstrate the ability to weigh risks and benefits according to their own values and according to some reasoning process, so that they are able to give some reasonable justification for the decision they make.

CONSENT FROM SPECIAL PATIENTS

Informed consent is based on the patient's ability to understand procedures, consequences, and risks and then to make a decision of whether or not to submit to the procedure after receiving all relevant information. It goes without saying, of course, that although most patients may have the capacity to make their own informed decisions, some patients present special difficulties when obtaining consent. Examples of special groups of patients are minors, those persons who are mentally ill or mentally incompetent, or those who are under the influence of drugs or alcohol. These special groups, in general, require special consideration and generally require the consent of someone other than themselves for a procedure to be performed.

Laws differ from state to state regarding the minor's ability to give consent to a variety of procedures. In most instances, the health professional should seek to obtain consent from parents or another person authorized to give substitute consent. Emergency procedures that are necessary to prevent loss of life or permanent impairment may be considered exceptions to this rule, although there must also be sufficient documentation to prove that an emergency situation does indeed exist.

In some states, the ability of minors to give consent is based on their age, maturity, and ability to understand the consequences of their decision. Some states recognize minors as capable of giving valid consent as if they were adults if they have taken on the roles and responsibilities of adults. In this case, they are considered emancipated. Factors used to indicate that a minor is emancipated include lack of dependency on parents for support, proof of marriage, or, in some instances, having become a parent.

In some instances, an individual other than the patient may be responsible for giving informed consent. These circumstances include instances in which the person to be treated is unconscious; is under the influence of substances that affect reason, such as drugs or alcohol; or has been declared mentally incompetent by a court because of mental illness, mental retardation, or mental deterioration due to organic processes or injury. In these cases, consent may be obtained from the next of kin or from another person authorized to act in behalf of the patient. Exceptions, as with minors, generally apply in emergency treatment, when the individual's welfare or safety is at risk and substitute consent from an authorized individual cannot be obtained.

If the patient has been declared legally incompetent and a legal guardian has been appointed, then the guardian is authorized to give consent for the patient. When the patient is not legally declared incompetent but is not able to make informed decisions, as in the case of an individual who is unconscious, for example, the situation may not be as clear-cut. In general, under these circumstances, the nearest relative may give consent. If the patient has a spouse, then the spouse would be authorized to give consent for the individual. It should be recognized, however, that the right of one spouse to give consent for the other extends only in those circumstances when consent may not be deferred until the patient can give consent.

Under some circumstances, consent of a spouse may be an issue even when the patient is capable of making an informed decision. Such is the case when procedures may affect the marital relationship, such as in instances of sterilization or abortion. Although laws may vary from state to state, in general, if the spouse is competent, the power to consent to procedures still rests with the spouse on whom the procedure is to be performed.

It should be noted that different states have different laws about informed consent of special populations. Health professionals should check on the regulations of their individual states and keep abreast of changes that occur periodically with new court rulings.

USE OF CONSENT FORMS

When the patient gives consent to have a procedure performed, there must be some means of documenting that the patient was given adequate information on which to base the decision and that he or she did give consent. Although verbal consent may be just as binding, such consents may be difficult to prove if the matter is ever brought to court. With an increasing number of lawsuits brought against health professionals, there has been increased use of written forms to document patients' consent.

It should be emphasized that an informed consent form is *only* a means of documentation and in no way takes the place of interpersonal communication in explaining a procedure to a patient. Even a form that is written in great detail in the simplest of terms is useless if the patient does not understand it, cannot read it, or is not given the opportunity to ask questions.

In the past, consent forms were broad in nature rather than addressing the specifics of individual procedures. Such broad statements as "I hereby consent to surgery and to have whatever organs which are diseased or deemed by the surgeon in need of removal to be excised," although leaving considerable latitude to the physician in carrying out surgery, are also extremely ambiguous in terms of the patient and what he or she can expect as a result of surgery. There is no evidence that the patient has been told the possible consequences or risks of surgery or has even been given the option to specify which organs he or she may object to having removed.

Again, it must be emphasized that the consent form must document that the patient's consent has been informed. For the patient to give informed consent, he or she must be given information about diagnosis, the procedure and purpose of the treatment or procedure proposed, risks and consequences of having or not having the proposed treatment or procedure, and alternatives that may be available. All information must be given to patients in terms they understand. Therefore, if the informed consent form does not reflect that adequate information has been given to the patient and that he or she fully understands the explanation, the form cannot be considered valid documentation of informed consent. Even if adequate explanation has been given, a form that contains less than sufficient information or that contains information in technical terms does little to fulfill its purpose.

Although the consent form does not take the place of clear communication with the patient about procedures or treatments that have been recommended, to be effective, the form must reflect the verbal explanation the patient has received.

COMMUNICATION IN INFORMED CONSENT

Informed consent, although a legal duty of the health professional, involves much more than a duty. Informed consent becomes a vital part of the relationship between patient and health professional in which facts, concerns, and alternatives are openly discussed, and through which the patient actively participates in the decision-making process about his or her care.

Some health professionals continue to argue that fully informing the patient of risks that may be inherent in the procedure or treatment needlessly provokes anxiety, in some instances causing sufficient stress to do patients harm. Although knowledge of risks may be somewhat upsetting, there is no evidence that significant harm is caused to patients who receive information.

Another fear health professionals commonly hold is that by giving patients full information about the risks and consequences of a treatment or procedure, they will be more likely to be noncompliant. However, this too does not seem to be the case. Neither does it appear that patients who are warned of possible side effects are more likely to develop them.

The key to effective informed consent, like other forms of patient education, is effective communication between patient and health professional in which individual patient needs and concerns are identified and addressed. This requires information exchange between patient and professional in which there is a continuing flow of two-way communication.

Through the two-way process of communication, health professionals are able to give patients information best suited to their individual needs to help them make a rational decision based on what benefits can be expected from the procedure compared to the risks and what other options might be available. Obviously, to inform the patient, some technical aspects of the procedure must be discussed. The technical aspects of the procedure should, however, be free of jargon and put in terms the patient can understand.

Patients vary in their degree of understanding of terminology and technical terms. Words have different meanings to various individuals. Although health professionals may try to be extremely clear and honest in explanations, they may still fail to convey information in a way that leads patients to an actual understanding of their condition or treatment. To be confident of patients' understanding of the information, health professionals may ask patients to interpret the explanation given. In this way, the health professional can be assured that the information was received the way it was intended, and that the patient has all the facts necessary to make an informed decision.

Although it is important to give patients sufficient information to make an informed decision, giving them too much information can be cumbersome and time-consuming, and can actually impede their decision-making process. Only information pertinent to the patient's decision making need be given. Not every inconsequential detail that may confuse more than enhance the patient's ability to make a decision need be included. It is at times difficult for the health professional to determine how much detail is enough and how much, too much. This is easier to determine if the professional considers the purpose of informed consent and that, to give rational consent, the patient must be reasonably informed of benefits, consequences, risks, and alternatives. For example, if the patient is receiving an explanation about upcoming surgery, in addition to giving information about the specific procedure to be performed, the health professional may also note that all surgery contains a certain degree of risk. Not every possible risk or complication of surgery, in general, need be addressed as long as the patient recognizes the serious nature of surgery and the risks that are more likely to pose a potential problem in a particular case.

When giving information to the patient in preparation for a procedure that requires consent, it is important for health professionals to remember that their own attitudes and feelings can also influence patients' receptivity to the information. Nonverbal cues that indicate disapproval or hesitance about a procedure or alternative in question can alter the patient's view of the verbal meaning of the explanation given. The question then remains: Are patients under those circumstances making their own informed consent, or are they being biased by the values and attitudes of the health professional disclosing the information?

Other aspects of the communication process in obtaining informed consent are the timing of the explanation and the amount of time the professional devotes to giving the patient information. As with other patient teaching, if the patient is uncomfortable, distraught, or in some other way preoccupied, information received may not be incorporated by the patient. Although it is not always possible to find an ideal time when the patient is free of pain or concern, it is obvious that some times are better than others. All efforts should be made to give patients explanations when they are most likely to be receptive and when information will have a greater chance of having the most meaning, allowing them to give a truly informed consent.

If at all possible, the patient should be given some time to think about the information and to weigh benefits and risks before making a decision. Giving an explanation and then immediately requesting that the patient make a decision may create undue pressure, resulting in questions about the extent to which the consent was actually informed.

When giving patients explanations, health professionals should not rush the explanation, should give it in an atmosphere as free of distraction as possible, and should allow sufficient time for answering questions and addressing concerns. The professional should be accessible to the patient, both physically and through a behavioral style communicating approachability to answer questions and to discuss concerns. If the patient is intimidated by the health professional's style or if, after the initial explanation, the professional is not available to answer questions that occurred to the patient later, the patient may not have all the information needed to make the consent informed.

FAMILY INVOLVEMENT IN INFORMED CONSENT

Informed consent remains an individual decision. However, most individuals also live in a social or family group on whom their decisions have an impact. When making decisions of whether or not to consent to a procedure, many patients weigh the risks and benefits not only in terms of themselves but also in terms of what their decisions may mean to their families.

The influence of family or social group cannot be discounted in the informed consent process any more than it can be discounted in any other form of patient education. It must also be remembered that the term *family* might be defined broadly to include not only relatives but other persons the patient feels close to or who have special concern for the patient and his or her well-being. The values and attitudes of the individual patient in making decisions may not correspond to those of the health professional. However, patients often make decisions based on how having the procedure or not will affect their own lives and the social groups in which they live.

There are no standard rules that apply to everyone, even when conditions or procedures appear the same. Take, for example, two patients receiving information about treatment for the same type of cancer, both at the same advanced stage. Mrs. He refused further treatment, including chemotherapy, stating that she was concerned about the added burden and strain such treatment would have on her family, since the potential for cure or remission at this stage was slight. Although the prognosis for cure or remission was the same for a second patient, Mrs. Boyd, she consented to additional treatment even though she had a clear understanding of what the procedure would involve. Mrs. Boyd had two small children and felt that even if the treatment extended her life for only a few weeks, the extra time with her children was well worth the discomfort and strain of treatment.

In both instances, the patients' families were major considerations in giving consent. The family can often help provide additional support and encouragement to patients if it is involved in the decision-making process. Health professionals may occasionally feel that involving the family causes too much confusion and that diversity of opinion may actually impede the patient's ability to make a decision. Each patient's situation, of course, is different and at times family involvement may not be advantageous or even desired by the patient.

In many instances, directly involving the family in the information process can enhance communication between the patient and the health professional as well as providing the patient with a sounding board on which to discuss pros and cons. Family members may also help clarify information that the patient may otherwise be hesitant to ask about or that the patient may have difficulty understanding. Including the family in information giving may also facilitate discussion between family members that may be beneficial throughout the course of the patient's illness or treatment. Family members who also have an understanding of the procedure the patient has undergone are in a better position to offer support as well as assisting the patient in follow-up care that may be required.

Although family involvement in helping the patient to make an informed decision about care and treatment can enhance communication between patient and health professional, and may even enhance the patient's course through the condition and treatment, it must also be emphasized that some families provide more hindrance than help. In some situations, the patient may specifically not want family members involved. Except for the special patient problems mentioned earlier, the patient maintains the right to make his or her own informed choice without input from other individuals. The decision of whether or not to involve family members, then, may best be discussed with the patient in advance. Even if the family is insistent on being involved in the decision-making process, it is the responsibility of the health professional to make it clear to the family that, ultimately, it is the patient who has the right to the information that will help yield an informed decision.

REFERENCES

Canterbury v. Spence, 464 F 2d. 772 (C.C. Cir. 1972).

Natanson v. Kline, 186 Kan. 393, 409–10, 350 p. 2Nd 1093, 1106; rehearing denied, 187 Kan. 186, 354p. 2D 670 (1960).

President's Commission for the Study of Ethical Problems in Medicine and Biomedical and Behavioral Research. 1982. Making health care decisions: the ethical and legal implications of informed consent in the patient-practitioner relationship. 1, October. Washington, DC: Superintendent of Documents, US Code Annot US 1982: Title 42, Section 300V.

16

Instructional Aids for Patient Education:

Used or Abused

There has been considerable excitement generated in recent years by the introduction of a number of materials to be used in patient education. Instructional aids can be powerful tools when attempting to convey health information to patients. However, as with any innovative technique, it is important to recognize the potential abuses and misuses of these new innovations as well as their constructive uses.

Use of instructional aids in patient education can be faddish to the point that their use is almost thought to be obligatory in patient teaching without consideration of the quality of the material used. Sometimes health professionals may become so preoccupied with use of instructional aids that they forget about the message the material is intended to convey.

Placing extreme value on instructional aids can lead to dehumanization of the relationship between the patient and health professional, which is so necessary if the patient education interaction is to be effective. Before using instructional aids, health professionals should examine not only the materials, but also their own motivation for their use. In some instances, if health professionals are anxious and inexperienced in patient teaching, they may use instructional aids excessively as a substitute for active presentation of information.

Not only can misuse of instructional aids lead to poor patient education results, sometimes misuse can be traumatic. Some materials that use graphic representation of concepts may be used by health professionals to "shock" the patient into compliance. Such examples would be slides of mutilated bodies in an attempt to coerce patients into using safety belts in cars. Another example may be showing a patient who smokes pictures of diseased or cancerous lungs. There has been little empirical evidence that shows that the shock value of such methods is effective in motivating patients to comply. In fact, in some instances, the shock is so great that it tends to have the paradoxical effect. Use of any instructional aid should be considered in the context of the primary purpose of patient education; to provide the highest quality of patient teaching.

Teaching aids in the form of video- or audiocassettes, movies, pamphlets, books, and fact sheets are available on a wide variety of topics—ranging from prevention and health maintenance to information that is disease-specific or that focuses on certain treatments or procedures.

The abundance of teaching aids, although helpful in providing numerous sources and types of materials from which to choose, can also be overwhelming. Health professionals may have difficultly determining which materials are best, which types of materials are needed, and how materials may be most appropriately used.

Health professionals may have a number of misconceptions about teaching aids, such as: patients learn best when they are exposed to many educational resources; costly or elaborate educational materials are more beneficial than those developed by health professionals themselves; or the "packaging" of the materials is equal to the quality of the information inside.

As with most other procedures or technology, teaching aids can be useful if used appropriately. If not used appropriately, materials can be costly as well as ineffective in patient education. An important part of patient education is the knowledge and skill of the professional in using educational materials in the most effective manner.

USING TEACHING AIDS

The importance of keeping patients informed may be viewed by some health professionals as requiring more time than they have to spend. In other instances, health professionals may feel insecure about their ability to teach patients effectively or may feel they have inadequate patient education skills. They may equate information with education, believing, therefore, that the more information the patient is given, the more educated he or she will be.

Any of these views may lead to misuse of teaching aids. Such misuse can result in needless expenditure of money and less than desired results. Dr. Arnold serves as an example. Dr. Arnold, just out of family practice resident teaching, set up a solo practice in a small rural community near the town where he grew up. He remembered lectures he had heard in medical school about patient education and the importance of keeping patients informed about their condition and treatment. Eager to offer the most up-to-date medical care, he began planning how he could implement a patient education program in his practice. Although he believed patients should be given information, he was also concerned that being in solo practice would require more time than he had available. He was concerned that if he took the time to give patients all the information he thought they needed, the number of patients he could see each day would be severely limited.

In addition, although he had heard some lectures about patient education, there was no actual skill training in how to conduct patient teaching. As a consequence, Dr. Arnold felt somewhat unsure of his ability to relay information to patients effectively.

He had begun to receive numerous brochures describing a variety of educational materials. In addition, at several conferences he had talked with company representatives about materials to implement a comprehensive patient education program.

After reviewing the brochures and talking with the sales representatives. Dr. Arnold bought a video monitor and videotapes on a variety of disease conditions, numerous pamphlets dealing with aspects of prevention, and many other pamphlets dealing with a variety of disease conditions. Dr. Arnold asked his nurse to file the materials in as easily retrievable a way as possible and also asked that pamphlets be distributed to appropriate patients on a routine basis. For instance, all prenatal patients were to receive the pamphlet on preparation for childbirth; all patients requesting birth control were to receive the pamphlet on choosing birth control methods; and all patients with hypertension were to be given the pamphlet on hypertension.

In addition, Dr. Arnold asked that patients with the diagnosis of hypertension or diabetes be shown the videotape about their respective disease. Women having a regular physical examination were expected to view the videotape on breast self-examination.

Feeling confident that he was providing his patients with the best patient education program possible, Dr. Arnold spent very little time talking with his patients about their condition or treatment on a one-to-one basis. The nurse was the only other person in the office and, likewise, had little extra time to spend with patients. Involvement in patient education from the nurse's standpoint became a matter mainly of organizing materials, distributing pamphlets, and starting the videotape machine.

After some time, Dr. Arnold became concerned when the nurse reported that many patients were not viewing the tapes, saying they could not afford the extra time. In addition, many of the pamphlets distributed to patients were found lying in the examining room or waiting room, seemingly untouched. Dr. Arnold became further dismayed that patients seemed no more prone to follow recommendations after receiving the additional materials than before. They actually seemed to have no clearer understanding of what their condition and treatment involved than the patients he had worked with previously who had had no exposure to patient education at all.

Somewhat exasperated by the whole experience, Dr. Arnold discussed the matter with a physician friend in private practice in a nearby town. Dr. Arnold was surprised to hear that his friend, although an advocate of patient education, had actually spent little money on educational materials. His friend had, however, been very selective about the materials that were purchased. In addition, Dr.

Arnold's friend appeared to have more patient cooperation and rapport while still seeing as many patients per day as Dr. Arnold.

Through discussion of the issue with his friend, Dr. Arnold discovered that the educational materials in his friend's office were used to supplement information received from the physician or his nurse, not to act as the sole source of information. Although supplying much information in the form of educational materials, Dr. Arnold supplied little information himself, nor did he encourage his nurse to do so. Patients had begun to interpret Dr. Arnold's lack of personal information giving as cold and impersonal. Also, many of the materials given them were difficult to read or poorly written. The expense and time spent in purchasing and managing the materials were not achieving the results Dr. Arnold had anticipated.

Luckily, rather than viewing patient education as generally not worth the effort, Dr. Arnold realized that he had been equating information and materials with patient education, rather than seeing them as tools to enhance the process of patient education.

Dr. Arnold, although well meaning, had misconceptions not only about the role of educational materials in communicating health information but also about the process of patient education itself. The most important ingredient in patient education is a trusting relationship between patient and health professional. Without this relationship, teaching aids—no matter how elaborate or comprehensive—have little chance of being effective in the total learning process.

Teaching aids are most likely to be effective if patients view them as an extension of the health professional, not as a replacement for contact with them. Patient education materials should be used to supplement information the health professional has given the patient. Patients frequently forget much of the information they have been given. Giving them materials they can take home provides a resource for reinforcement of information and clarification of facts that may have become cloudy for the patient, who is unable to remember exactly what the health professional said. Visual aids can be helpful in illustrating points. The saying, "A picture is worth a thousand words," is quite true in patient education, especially for patients who are unfamiliar with certain concepts or various anatomical terms. The use of models or pictures can be extremely beneficial in helping patients conceptualize various aspects of their condition or treatment. Audiovisual aids in the form of tapes or movies can help supplement information given by the health professional or can provide a mechanism to stimulate discussion.

No matter what type of teaching aid is used in patient education, it will be more useful if health professionals have taken the time to select the material carefully themselves. Information contained within teaching aids should be consistent with that presented by the health professional, reinforcing the professional's teaching, not confusing it. Teaching aids should also be geared to the level of the patient. Therefore, the same teaching aids are not appropriate for all patients. Just as health professionals are responsible for the accuracy of information they give a patient verbally, so are they responsible for the content of the instructional aids they use. Consequently, health professionals should be as careful in choosing types of instructional aids as they are in delivering information to the patient orally. Appropriate use of teaching aids requires skill to ensure that their use facilitates communication between patient and health professional rather than hindering it. The following points should be considered when utilizing instructional aids:

- Use teaching aids to reinforce and illustrate information, not to replace interaction with the health professional.
- Evaluate the content of teaching aids before using them.
- Make sure information contained within teaching aids is consistent with the oral information presented.
- Tailor use of teaching aids to each patient.

After talking with his friend, Dr. Arnold returned to his office. He and the nurse discussed various changes in the strategy of using teaching materials. Together, they carefully read all the written material, discarding the materials that were poorly written or, in some instances, that even contradicted information contained in other sources. Dr. Arnold began to spend more time talking with patients and encouraged the nurse to spend some time with them after giving them materials or showing them a videotape. During this time, the nurse had the opportunity to answer questions or to address patients' concerns.

Implementation of the new plan for patient education materials changed Dr. Arnold's general approach. Now when a woman came to his office for a physical exam, he explained the importance of regular breast self-examination and demonstrated how to do the exam while he was performing it himself. The videotape on breast exams was shown to women while they were waiting, thus causing little inconvenience and requiring little extra time. The videotape in this instance served as preparation for the instructions Dr. Arnold gave them.

When women requested advice on contraception, Dr. Arnold discussed various methods, along with advantages and disadvantages of each. When giving them a brochure on contraception, he would say this:

> This brochure contains much of the information I've discussed with you. Sometimes hearing so much information all at once can be confusing, and it can be difficult to make a decision. I'd like for you to take the brochure home where you'll have time to look it over at your leisure and think about which method you feel might work best for you. When you've decided or if you have questions or would like more information, make another appointment with me.

Using the brochure this way offered a review of the instruction Dr. Arnold had given and helped the patient assess the information at her own pace.

When patients were diagnosed as hypertensive, Dr. Arnold would explain their condition to them briefly and then say the following:

> Hypertension can be controlled, but it requires understanding and coop-eration on your part. Because I feel it's so important for you to understand your condition so you can really work to control it, I'd like for you to view a short videotape about hypertension. After you've seen the tape, we'll talk some more about how we'll treat your condition.

After viewing the tape and engaging in further discussion with the nurse or Dr. Arnold, the patient was given the handout on hypertension. The handout reinforced what the nurse or Dr. Arnold had said and what the patient had seen in the film. Patient learning can be enhanced through repetition of informa-tion and use of different sources of information.

Dr. Arnold's patients who had diabetes were also asked to view the video-tape about their condition and treatment. Viewing the tape was set up as a reg-ular office visit and as part of the patient's comprehensive treatment. After patients viewed the tape, the nurse spent some time talking with them about var-ious aspects of their disease, reinforcing and clarifying points in the tape as well as points in instructions given them by Dr. Arnold. At subsequent visits, the nurse helped patients to assess problems or concerns they might be having about their condition or following the treatment. The nurse supplemented information with pamphlets and brochures as needed.

Dr. Arnold's situation was in the outpatient setting. The same principles regarding use of patient education materials apply, however, regardless of the set-ting in which that education takes place or who is conducting the teaching. Educational materials are valuable only to the extent that they facilitate com-munication between patient and health professional by offering an accurate description of the material discussed at the teaching session at a level the patient can understand. Using educational materials in patient teaching is an impor-tant skill for health professionals to learn. However, skill in assessing and devel-oping materials to be used is just as important.

WRITTEN AIDS

Written teaching aids can increase the effectiveness of patient education if used appropriately. Written aids can have many uses, depending on the teaching sit-uation and the associated goals of patient teaching. For example, written aids can be used to provide preliminary information in preparation for additional patient teaching. A nurse teaching new mothers on the postpartum unit may find that many of the same questions recur frequently. A written brochure or pamphlet addressing common concerns may be distributed to new mothers before the teaching session, possibly providing answers to some routine questions or stim-ulating additional questions in other cases. As a result, more time may be avail-able for the nurse to give in-depth coverage of information or to elaborate on patients' concerns that are still unresolved. Written aids may be given to patients before health professionals give instructions about a procedure or test. The information contained within the teaching aid thus provides the patient with a general outline of what will be covered. Giving the patient teaching aids before the actual teaching session, though at times helpful, can also have certain pitfalls. The technique needs to be carefully undertaken. Some specific disadvantages of this technique are as follows:

- patient misinterpretation of the material contained within the teaching aid, which may then affect receptiveness and understanding of further teaching
- increase in patient anxiety level before teaching takes place
- overreliance by the health professional on the patient's absorption of the material before patient teaching
- reluctance of patients to ask questions because they believe the health professional expected them to pick up most of the information from the teaching aid
- lack of personal interaction and communication on initial contact, thus potentially affecting the degree of rapport developed

Written aids may also be used to reinforce information provided by the health professional or to assist the patient in remembering complex information provided in the teaching session. A pharmacist, for example, may give the patient a written instruction sheet that emphasizes important points about the prescribed medication. After explaining exercises to a patient with low back pain, a physical therapist may give the patient a pamphlet illustrating the exercises.

Another use of written aids is to increase patients' understanding of their condition or treatment by providing more detailed information. A dietitian who has taught a newly diagnosed diabetic about the diet may give the patient a more comprehensive booklet on diabetes and diet that the patient can study in more detail in free time. A nurse who has instructed a patient on ostomy care may give the patient a book called *Life with an Ostotomy*, which can be shared with family members.

Written aids can be used to stimulate thought and ideas or can be directed toward attitude change. Such might be the case of the physician who spends considerable time teaching patients about their condition and treatment but who also feels strongly about prevention. Although the physician may not take additional time with every patient to talk about health risks and prevention in detail, the seed can still be planted by having written materials in the waiting room or examining room or by including such materials with the patient's bill.

It obviously is not practical for most health facilities to have written teaching aids for every condition or situation in which the health professional may be doing patient teaching. In some instances, written aids may be more useful to help patients reach their goals than in others. It is therefore important for health professionals, before ordering, developing, or using written teaching aids, to have a general knowledge of what the aid is expected to accomplish, and in what situations the use of such aids might be most worthwhile.

Written aids are most practical for those conditions or situations that are seen the most frequently. Investing in materials that will seldom be used wastes time and money. For example, even though the health professional identifies an excellent written teaching aid available on pheochromocytoma, if only one patient with that diagnosis has been seen in the health facility in the past, having large quantities of such a written aid is probably not very beneficial. Having written aids available for conditions seen frequently is a better use of resources.

CHOOSING WRITTEN AIDS

A variety of printed teaching aids is commercially available. In some instances, health professionals may find it more beneficial to develop materials themselves. The source of the aid chosen is dependent on the resources available—in terms of money, time, and interest—and on the particular nature of the objectives the teaching aid is to meet. For example, the physician reviewing commercially prepared materials for teaching prenatal patients in the clinic may not find one teaching aid that alone covers all the material he or she feels is important to emphasize. Therefore, the physician may elect to develop his or her own written handout. Thus, the physician is assured that all the information considered important is covered in one comprehensive handout and that the information reflects his or her own personal recommendations.

In other instances, health professionals may find that commercially available sources of written materials cover the information comprehensively and that there is no need to develop further materials. At times, health professionals may not have the time or expertise to develop materials and may feel that commercially available materials can be of the same benefit. A nurse involved in teaching diabetic patients on the inpatient unit, for example, may find that developing written aids to illustrate or emphasize points would be a needless expenditure of time when materials already available have been used with relative success.

Financial resources may also be a determinant of the types of written aids used. Although it may seem that, in the long run, aids developed by the health professional are cheaper, the time invested in developing the aid, printing costs, or photocopying costs also must be considered. Commercially prepared written materials are frequently less expensive if purchased in large quantities. Many excellent written materials may be obtained free of charge from local sources, such as cancer associations or heart associations, or other governmental or private sources. Although the cost of materials must be considered, the extent to which the teaching aid helps health professionals meet their goals for patient teaching is more important. Also to be considered are the materials' accuracy and the likelihood that patients can understand them; how up to date are they? Before incorporating any written material into patient teaching, it should be carefully scrutinized by the health professional.

If health professionals remember that the purpose of the teaching aid is to supplement information they give the patient rather than to supplant it, they

TABLE 16-1	Checklist for Choosing Written Teaching Aids

1. Are information and illustrations accurate?
2. Are information and illustrations up to date?
3. Is information appropriate to breadth and scope?
4. Is information appropriate for the intended audience?
5. Is information organized in a way that is logical and easy for the patient to follow?
6. Does information address issues that are of general concern to most patients with the condition?
7. Is information consistent with the philosophy of the health institution/health professional using the teaching aid?
8. Is the reading level appropriate for the intended audience?
9. Does the teaching aid avoid the use of jargon?
10. Is the technical quality of the material adequate in terms of attractiveness, readability, simplicity?
11. Has the material been developed by a credible source?
12. Is the teaching aid practical in terms of cost, accessibility, and usability?
13. Could the same objective be reached just as well without use of the teaching aid?

may be guided in the types and numbers of teaching aids needed. If health professionals depend too much on written materials to communicate instructions to patients, the effectiveness of the materials may be diluted, and needless time and money may be spent ordering or developing materials that do little to achieve established goals.

Health professionals should remember that not all written aids are of the same quality, nor can written aids used successfully in one health facility necessarily be used with the same effectiveness in another. The type of written aid chosen should be based on the patient population served by the health facility, the conditions that occur most frequently, and goals and objectives patient teaching is to accomplish. The number of written aids possessed by health professionals or health facilities is not nearly as important as the quality and applicability of the aid to the specific population served. Specific criteria for choosing written teaching aids are found in the checklist in Table 16-1.

Assessing Readability

As with patient education in general, to be effective, information contained in written instructions must be read, understood, and remembered. The effectiveness of a printed teaching aid depends to a great extent on how it is written and organized. Information should be structured in a logical way that patients are able to follow. Subheadings separating major content areas are frequently helpful in separating material into "bite-sized" pieces, so that the information can be put into the proper perspective. Subheadings also help patients identify areas they may want to review or clarify.

In general, information contained in written aids should be presented in an appropriate sequence, starting with simple concepts and moving to more complex issues. Basic concepts should be introduced first, as building blocks for more complicated ideas. For example, a handout on diabetes that begins with a description of insulin-producing cells in the pancreas, before giving more basic information about diabetes in general, would probably do more to confuse patients than to increase their understanding of the condition.

Although goals or objectives of the written teaching aid may not be stated explicitly in the material, there should be implicit objectives that are easily inferred from the instruction. For instance, which learning outcomes does the author of the written material expect the patient to achieve? Is the written material geared toward increasing the patient's knowledge of the condition or treatment? Is it directed toward attitude change? Or is it directed toward helping the patient achieve a specific skill? The types of outcomes expected can be inferred from the content of the teaching aid, repetition of important ideas for emphasis, or the general level of detail presented. Are the objectives inferred in the handout congruent with the teaching objectives of the health professional? For example, the health professional may have spent time teaching the patient how to give an insulin injection. At the end of the teaching session, the patient may be given a handout that will review the points discussed and that may give cues for carrying out each of the steps involved in insulin injection. If the handout only addresses the importance of accuracy in administration of insulin, however, or explains how the insulin acts, the teaching aid does little to meet the objectives the health professional had in mind when giving the patient the teaching aid.

Sentence structure, style, and word use are also important considerations when assessing printed teaching aids. The reading level should be appropriate for the audience. Teaching aids chosen by the health professional for an inner-city clinic may be quite different from those chosen by a professional working in a university health service. Although it may be tempting to use written materials that use slang terms appropriate to various cultures or subcultures, it is important to remember that such terms may date otherwise useful materials as well as having the potential to cause resentment if the health professional does not belong to the patient's culture or subculture. In most cases, written materials using these terms should be avoided.

In general, no matter where written materials are to be used, they will be more useful if sentences are short and simple, using common words rather than medical jargon. If one of the health professional's objectives in teaching is to acquaint patients with some medical terms, medical terminology interspersed throughout the handout should be explained in lay terms placed in parentheses after the medical term. It should also be remembered that at times even nonclinical words may cause difficulties. Such words as *predispose* or *incapacitate* may not be clearly understood by patients or may be misinterpreted. In evaluating written materials for use in patient education, especially for situations in which the patient population comes from all walks of life or consists of many different age groups, written materials most likely to be understood by the majority are probably also the most practical and the most likely to be effective.

It is also important that health professionals consider the length of the handout. Although longer written aids may seem more comprehensive, health professionals should remember that they will be of little use if the patient discards the material before reading it because of its length. Generally, the longer and more complicated the written aid, the less likely patients are to read or understand it.

The technical quality of the printed material is also important. Health professionals should assess print size and determine whether it is adequate or whether patients with visual problems will have difficulty reading it. Especially in situations where a majority of patients are geriatric, teaching aids with larger print and more ample spacing may be important. The general appearance of printed material may also be important in attracting patients' attention and motivating them to read the handout.

Illustrations and diagrams may help catch the patient's eye as well as clarify points. Illustrations can be helpful if a patient has difficulty visualizing a procedure or anatomical part. Just as language contained within the aid should be simple, so should illustrations. A detailed, anatomically correct diagram of the heart may not be nearly as effective as a simple line drawing when illustrating to the patient the placement of a pacemaker. Illustrations can make the written material more interesting. Health professionals should also be aware, however, of the messages that pictorial representations may convey that can interfere with the effectiveness of the handout. For example, some illustrations may be offensive to different groups. Other illustrations may be perceived by the patient as treating lightly issues that to them are serious. In these instances, illustrations can defeat the purpose of the written aid itself. Illustrations are most effective when they are done tastefully and are sensitive to patients' concerns. Humor must also be viewed within patients' frame of reference.

In general, the tone of the written teaching aid should be personal and informal and should make patients feel as if the content of the handout is a personal extension of the health professional rather than a mass-produced general handout impersonally supplied to every patient. The more readable the teaching aid is, the more likely the patient is to take the time to read it and incorporate the information it contains.

Assessing Content

Even if patient education materials are well organized and attractive in presentation, the issue of major importance is the quality of information contained within. Health professionals are often swayed by the appearance of the written material rather than by careful evaluation of its content. Since the purpose of using written teaching aids is to communicate information to patients, it is crucial that the information in the aid is what the health professional wants the patient to have.

Health professionals should be familiar with the content of all teaching aids before distributing them to patients. Information and illustrations should be factual and accurate. Health professionals should continue to check written materials used in patient teaching on a regular basis, so that any materials that require updates or that no longer accurately represent current views are identified and changed. Because verbal information given by the health professional may also change over time, periodic checks of handouts help ensure that information in the handouts is still consistent with the verbal explanation and still represents the general view the health professional wants to emphasize.

Information presented in the written aid should also be presented in an objective way, with no major distortions. Although the health professional may be tempted to choose or to develop written aids that present only one side of controversial issues, or that address only positive aspects of a treatment or procedure, it is important to remember that the purpose of the teaching aid is to extend the information given verbally. It is also important to remember that the purpose of patient education is to help patients make informed choices based on facts, not bias. Therefore, if all relevant material is not presented by the teaching aid or if information presented in the material is distorted to give patients biased information, they have not received adequate facts on which to make an informed choice about the degree to which they will comply with the recommendations outlined. In most instances, as with verbal communication, it is important that both sides of issues are presented in an objective fashion so as to give the patient the benefit of factual information.

Written aids can serve as reminders or reinforcers of information given patients by health professionals. If the content of the teaching aid does not accurately reflect the content of the teaching session, however, it is of little value. For example, a nurse may teach a patient about the use of postmenopausal estrogen to help prevent osteoporosis, explaining the advantages and disadvantages as well as potential risks. If the nurse then gives the patient a handout that contains only positive information, however, with none of the potential problems of using estrogen listed, the patient may well forget the information given in the teaching session, depending only on the written materials to make her decision. If the patient later experiences complications because of taking estrogen, even though the nurse verbally discussed the possibility of complications, the patient may feel she was not aware of all the facts before making her decision. Likewise, avoiding negative aspects of a condition or treatment or slanting material in the written aid to one viewpoint can cause health professionals to lose credibility if patients later discover that the information in the written aid was not entirely accurate.

In assessing patient education materials, health professionals should also check to see whether the breadth and scope of the information is sufficient for the purpose intended. They should note whether more or less detail is needed to accomplish the objectives of patient teaching. Sometimes written materials can overinform patients. Patients may not be prepared to deal with all the information presented in the printed aid, especially if it is more detailed than the personal explanation given by the health professional. In this case, the printed aid may do more harm than good. Patients may become confused rather than gaining increased understanding, or may become anxious or overly concerned because they are overwhelmed by the information provided. For example, consider the following case. A pharmacist filling a prescription for a patient was anxious to supplement verbal information given the patient by the physician. The pharmacist made sure the patient was given the drug insert accompanying the medication. The pharmacist warned the patient of key side effects but did not realize that the patient might be affected by the many additional side effects listed on the insert. The patient became so apprehensive about taking the medication after reading the long list of potential side effects that he discontinued the medication of his own volition. If the drug insert was to be useful, the pharmacist should have underlined key side effects, explaining that there was little probability that the others listed would develop.

Health professionals should also be aware of messages that written materials convey that may not be directly related to the accuracy of information but rather to the views of the manufacturers or producers of the materials. Although these views may not be those of the health professional, patients receiving written aids may interpret the information as representative of the attitude of the health professional. For instance, in an effort to be supportive and encouraging, written aids may be written in a "Polyannish" way. This may tell patients that their concerns, fears, and anxiety are negative attributes rather than a natural part of adjustment or adaptation to their condition or treatment. Other pamphlets may portray unrealistic images of situations to which patients may be exposed. For example, a written aid describing breast-feeding may contain factual information but may be presented in such a way that the patient is made to feel inadequate unless she is able to breast-feed. In instances where the mother actually does not want to breast-feed or for some reason is unable to do so, she may experience guilt and may be reluctant to discuss her feelings with the physician or nurse, assuming that the written aid reflects their feelings as well. In assessing written materials, it is important to be alert to value orientations presented in the teaching materials and to determine the extent to which they will hinder the effectiveness of patient teaching.

USE OF AUDIOVISUAL AIDS

In an age of automation and technology, it is not surprising that use of audiovisual aids for patient education has gained increasing popularity. These teaching aids take the form of videotapes, audiotapes, slide tapes, films, or closed-circuit television. As with written materials, the effectiveness of audiovisual aids is dependent to a great extent on how accurate and complete they are as well as how they are used. Before incorporating audiovisual aids into patient teaching, health professionals should review and evaluate their content and presentation. Health professionals also need to review their objectives for patient teaching and determine whether or not using the audiovisual aid is the most effective way of reaching those goals.

Although there has been a proliferation of commercially produced audiovisual aids, there is no evidence that using these aids will drastically increase patient compliance. Use of visual aids can supply an additional means of communication through representing concepts that may be difficult to communicate through words alone. This might be especially true of procedures, such as colostomy irrigation or various types of surgical procedures. Visual aids may be useful in education to increase patient understanding when it is not possible for the patient to observe an actual situation or to observe a demonstration of a particular situation, such as showing prenatal patients a film on childbirth to prepare them for their delivery room experience.

Use of audiovisual aids in patient education definitely has its merits; however, there are also a variety of factors health professionals should consider before incorporating them as a major portion of the educational interaction. First, audiovisual aids can be costly. Films and tapes are usually available either for purchase or for rent, but at considerable expense. Use of audiovisual aids also requires special equipment, such as a movie or slide projector, a slide/tape machine, a tape recorder, or a video monitor. If not already available, the purchase of special equipment can take up all or most of the patient education budget, leaving little money for software that might be needed. Health professionals should also check to see if audiovisual aids, such as videocassettes, can be used with all types of equipment or if purchase of special equipment is also needed.

Commercially prepared materials may not be appropriate for the patient population with whom the health professional is working, or materials may not address specific issues the health professional wants to emphasize. The personal development of films or tapes, while perhaps better suiting the patient population and goals, also requires considerable time and expertise, as well as resources and equipment to produce the aid.

Films or tapes, like written teaching aids, can be outdated quickly. However, because of the expense of purchasing the audiovisual aid, it may not be possible to replace it as easily as written materials. Even if content remains up to date, visual portrayal of people or environments in the film may seem irrelevant to present-day circumstances. Hairstyles, clothing, or specific situations within the film may date it and detract from its credibility despite the accuracy of the material it presents. Patients viewing the film or tape may become more absorbed in noticing the differences in styles than in absorbing the information the aid was meant to confer. In addition, patients may automatically assume that because the visual presentation is dated, the content is also dated and not to be taken seriously. Obviously, audiovisual aids using cartoon characters do not have the same properties of change with regard to time. Cartoon representations may, however, not be the most effective or appropriate way to present information for a variety of conditions, and may in fact insult some patients who feel they are being talked down to or that their condition is being taken less than seriously.

The danger of using any type of instructional aid in patient education lies in substituting the aid for personal contact. The temptation may be even greater with audiovisual aids, which may appear to be more personal and comprehensive than written aids. Effective use of audiovisual aids should be as a supplement to verbal information given by health professionals. Use of such aids will be more cost-effective if they are chosen carefully and if the number of patients with a partic-ular condition is sufficient to warrant purchase of the teaching aid. Effective use of audiovisual aids requires resources in terms of time, money, and equipment as well as effective coordination. The checklist in Table 16-1 can be applied to audiovisual aids as well as printed material. Health professionals should not lose sight of the fact that one of the most important components of effective patient education is the relationship between the patient and the health professional.

PRESENTING TEACHING AIDS

The manner in which a teaching aid is used can be as important, if not more so, than the teaching aid itself. Printed or audiovisual aids alone are not strong moti-vators. Without personal contact with the health professional, teaching aids are of little benefit in patient education. If patients feel that health professionals are using teaching aids to avoid questions or to avoid additional contact, receptivity to the aid and the material it contains will not be nearly as great. Consider the following examples of appropriate and inappropriate presentations of an instruc-tional aid:

> *Patient:* I did have some additional questions about Johnnie's asthma. What can we do at home to minimize his attacks?
>
> *Inappropriate Response:* Here's a pamphlet that will explain it all. Johnnie should make a follow-up appointment for his asthma in a week.
>
> *Appropriate Response:* Why don't you take this pamphlet home with you and read it over at your leisure? It points out a variety of things that might be helpful. When you come back next week for Johnnie's follow-up visit, we'll discuss some of the points covered in it and answer any questions you might have about it.

The health professional in the second example communicated interest in continuing discussion of the material and the patient's questions. In addition, because of how the material was presented, patients may be more motivated to take the time to read the pamphlet and incorporate the information within it.

As with most patient teaching, timing is also important in the presentation of teaching aids. If the patient is anxious or upset, he or she will probably be no more receptive to teaching aids than to any other method of patient teaching at that time. The health professional who gives a teaching aid at this point risks having the patient misinterpret the action as a demonstration of noncaring or aloofness. Consider the following examples:

Patient: (crying) The doctor just told me that I'm going to have to have surgery. Although he says it's a fairly routine procedure, I've always been frightened of the thought of anesthesia and of not being in control.

Inappropriate Response: The procedure is as routine as the doctor says. Here's a pamphlet that explains the procedure in detail, so you'll have a more realistic idea of what to expect.

Appropriate Response: I know you're frightened. Can you tell me a little more about your fears?

In the first example, the health professional communicated a lack of sensitivity and concern. Not only will the information in the pamphlet probably not be read, but the relationship between the patient and the health professional has probably also been weakened. The pamphlet may more appropriately be given to the patient at another time, after initial fears and concerns have been addressed.

Teaching aids should be an extension of interaction with health professionals rather than a replacement. The health professional who is uncomfortable talking with patients about various situations or who uses patient teaching aids to avoid certain situations will probably find that the aid will also not accomplish the desired results. Even though the health professional may feel that exposing patients to the information in the teaching aid is better than giving them no information at all, such a presentation may do more to hinder reaching the objectives of patient teaching than to help it. The following clinic situation illustrates this point:

Dr. Joyner had encouraged her nurse to set up a plan to do patient education with adolescents about sexuality. Being rather shy in nature, the nurse reviewed a variety of pamphlets and audiovisual aids on the subject and selected those that were felt to be the most appropriate for the patients in Dr. Joyner's practice. Dr. Joyner also reviewed the aids and agreed that they conveyed the information she felt was important.

As part of their regular physical exam for school, all adolescents in Dr. Joyner's practice were first referred to the nurse for teaching on sexuality. The nurse placed each teenager in a room that had been established as a patient education resource center, turned on the videocassette machine, and left the room. After the adolescents viewed the tape, the nurse gave them several of the pamphlets on sexuality and took them to the exam room to wait for Dr. Joyner. The patients were given no opportunity to ask the nurse questions, nor did the nurse attempt to engage in discussion or to elaborate on points illustrated in the videocassette or in the pamphlets.

The nurse, in her avoidance of discussion with adolescents, communicated discomfort and embarrassment with the information presented. This in turn caused the adolescents embarrassment. Using audiovisual aids and pamphlets in place of discussion also communicated that perhaps questions and further discussion with the nurse or the physician were to be avoided. Consequently, rarely did the teens bring up questions with the physician during their exams. The physician, assuming that the teens had had their questions answered when they viewed the tape, likewise took little time to ask if they had any questions or to discuss the topic of sexuality further.

The films and pamphlets could have been useful teaching aids had they been used to "break the ice" and to stimulate questions or discussion. By being available for and open to questions or by encouraging the teens to discuss their concerns, both physician and nurse could have increased the effectiveness of patient teaching greatly.

DEVELOPING TEACHING AIDS

Although many excellent teaching aids are available, health professionals may want to develop teaching aids that most closely align with their own philosophy or their own patient population, or in some instances they may want to use a combination of the two. When developing teaching aids, health professionals should first determine which aids are better developed and which are better obtained commercially to best fit the goal of the patient education delivered. Whether health professionals develop their own teaching aids or use those commercially available depends on these factors:

- Is there money available for purchase of commercial aids, and how does the cost compare to developing them in house?
- Are there sufficient time, interest, and resources available for development of patient education materials?

Once the health professional has answered these questions, priorities for purchase or development of materials can be established. When developing patient education materials whether written, audio, or visual, certain preliminary steps should be taken.

First, an individual with interest and expertise should be identified to supervise the project. In some instances, individuals may be interested in developing materials but may not have the technical skills needed. In this case, outside resources may be needed to assist with printing or layout of written materials or taping audiovisual aids. With special computer programs and graphics, professional-looking documents can be prepared by someone with computer expertise (Baker 1991). Slides can be a relatively inexpensive way of visually portraying a concept or outlining steps to be followed in procedures. Likewise, portable video cameras now readily available make it possible for health professionals to produce patient education videotapes of high quality if they are well planned and executed. Whether the project supervisor is directly related in the production aspect is a matter of interest and expertise. Whether directly involved in production or not, the project supervisor should first choose a committee to establish and prioritize materials to be developed. In reaching these conclusions, the committee should first ask these questions:

- What are the most common conditions or information needs in the particular patient population served?
- Are there commercial materials available that would adequately meet those needs and that could be covered in the existing budget?

When the committee has identified those conditions for which no suitable commercial patient education materials are available, and consequently what materials need to be developed, the conditions should be prioritized according to need. After prioritization, the committee should then address which type of material would best convey the information. In some instances, pamphlets or brochures might be best; in others, video- or audiotapes may be needed.

When the conditions for which patient education materials are needed have been prioritized and the type of patient education materials needed for each area determined, the committee then should decide what resources are needed for the development of the materials. For instance, is a computer with appropriate graphics or desktop publishing capabilities available for producing written materials? If so, is there someone available with the time and computer skills needed to produce the materials? Is there a need to allocate money for commercial printing? Is audio or video equipment available, or does production of videocassettes require an outside contract or consultation?

After resources needed for production of materials have been identified, costs associated with those resources should be established and a budget prepared and submitted for review for funding.

Planning Materials

For either written or audiovisual materials to be useful and effective, certain basic steps must first be taken. First, the health professional should determine what specific knowledge, skills, attitudes, or behavior changes the patient education material will be designed to help patients achieve. Specifically listing these behaviors and translating them into objectives before the materials are developed helps maintain focus. Being as specific and behaviorally oriented as possible provides a means for observable, testable outcomes that can assist in the evaluation of the material's effectiveness. For instance, a knowledge objective that reads, "The patient will understand potential complications associated with diabetes" is vague and difficult to measure, whereas an objective that reads, "The patient will be able to list at least five possible complications of diabetes" provides a more concise view of what is to be accomplished and can be measured.

After behaviors have been identified and objectives written, health professionals should decide what information is essential for patients to have to achieve the objective. Listing topics or categories of information relevant to the stated objectives prevents inclusion of superfluous information that could confuse patients. For example, a long description of research leading to the consensus that a particular treatment is now state of the art may not be essential in the patient education material if the main objective is for the patient to be able to carry out the specific treatment.

The next step is to determine how the material is best organized. An outline of the sequence in which the information is to be presented should be developed. The outline will help to clarify thinking, will make sure material appears in a logical sequence, and will prevent extraneous information from being included. A general rule in organizing content is to progress from general to specific, ending with the most important points.

Written Aids

After completing the steps above, health professionals should decide how the material should look visually. It should be attractive, drawing the patient's interest, and it should be easy to use. The extent to which graphics or illustrations are used will depend on the type of information contained, the type of population for which it is designed, and the talent and resources available.

The reading level to which the material is written will depend on the majority of patients for whom the material is designed. (See Chapter 10 for assessment of reading level). Larger print is generally easier for most people to read and is less intimidating. For the most part, to increase ease of reading, fancy type or script should be avoided.

In most instances, technical terms and jargon should be avoided, and short sentences should be used as much as possible. Generally, material should be written in a conversational style. As much as possible, the material is usually best written directly to the patient, such as, "When first getting up in the morning you should . . ." rather than "When a patient gets up in the morning he/she should. . . ." The flow of information should sound natural and clear, and words should be used consistently. For instance, if using the term *high blood pressure* in the handout, it should not be alternated with the term *hypertension* or vice versa. Whichever term is used, it should be used consistently.

As much as possible, each paragraph should contain a single idea. Presenting more than one concept in a paragraph can be confusing and interfere with patient understanding of the main point to be gleaned from the paragraph. Using subtitles can help provide a broad overview for patients regarding specific areas to be covered in the handout as well as provide easy reference for patients if they would like to return to a specific section for review.

If illustrations or graphics are to be used in written materials, health professionals should make sure that they add to the content, not distract from it. Illustrations or graphics can help to reduce the amount of writing or explanation needed. They can be used to illustrate key points, or they can be used to draw patients' interest to the material. When using illustrations, health professionals should determine what they are intending to accomplish and then develop them accordingly. In most instances, simple illustrations are better than more complex ones. Although colored illustrations can be eye-catching, an appealing, often simple black-and-white line illustration can be just as helpful for getting a point across and can be less expensive. The illustration should not have to be studied by patients in order to grasp the concept it is attempting to portray. Each illustration should be in close proximity to the written idea it is to reinforce so patients do not have to search the material in order to find the illustration. It may be helpful if illustrations are accompanied by captions that relate to the text; however, if captions are used, they should be kept brief and to the point. When writing captions, health professionals should concentrate on the exact concept the illustration is designed to convey.

Audiovisual Aids

Audiovisual patient education materials can provide an excellent source of supplemental teaching for patients and can reinforce information as well as prepare patients for information to be given in more detail by the health professional. Examples of audiovisual aids are photographs, slides, slide/tape programs, audiotapes, and videotapes.

Although audiovisual aids can be time-consuming to produce, their advantage is that they are more personal and can be tailored to the views and standards of the health professional or health facility producing them. In addition, they can be tailor-made for the specific type and level of patient population for which they are to be developed.

Regardless of the type of audiovisual aid the health professional produces, the same steps should be taken as for developing written materials. That is, specific objectives that the audiovisual aid is to accomplish must be established; essential information to be contained within the audiovisual aid must be determined; and an orderly, logical sequence for presentation of material must be developed. Likewise, although the message is spoken or visually transmitted in this instance, rather than written, the understandability of the audiovisual material should be established, just as the readability of written material must be determined. If a script is used, such as for audio- or videotapes, the same readability formula used for written materials may be utilized. In the case of slides or photographs, the health professional may want to test the materials and ask the opinion of a sample of patients representative of the population for whom the materials were developed.

Slides and Photographs

Slides and photographs may be used in isolation or in combination with audio- or videotaped patient education presentations. In some instances, health professionals may use photographs arranged in a loose-leaf teaching manual to supplement patient education information the patient is receiving on an individualized basis. In other instances, slides or photographs may be incorporated into a videotape presentation to illustrate or demonstrate specific points. In addition, slides may be incorporated into a slide/tape presentation.

Good slides and photographs can be produced easily and with relatively little effort if time is spent in planning. Again, health professionals should have a good idea of what the visual content contained within the slide or photograph is to convey. Visual content should be kept as simple as possible, with distracting backgrounds and extraneous visual images avoided as much as possible. Health professionals should attempt to avoid introducing too much information in one slide or photograph. As much as possible, each slide or photograph should be used to convey one idea. Color and lighting are crucial as are good focus and clarity of the slide or photograph.

Slide/Tape Programs

Using a combination of slides and audiotapes can be an effective way of communicating patient education information to patients. The availability of individual slide/tape units that advance automatically and a taped soundtrack that corresponds to each slide can be a valuable supplement to reinforce information previously given by the health professional or to prepare the patient for information to be given by the health professional at a later date. Discussion of development of audiotapes follows.

Audio- and Videotapes

Both audio- and videotapes developed for patient education require the same steps discussed previously. The advantage of audio- or videotapes is that patients can use them at their convenience. In some instances, the health professional may make them available to patients on loan so they can review them at home as well. If resources permit, professional actors or speakers can be used; however, the voice or visual image of the health professional adds a personal aspect that may enhance the effectiveness of the tape.

As with written materials, the message should be kept simple. When developing audio- or videotapes, health professionals should avoid using jargon and technical terms and should avoid complex sentences and multisyllabic words. The speaker should speak in a slow, clear, and distinct manner, and avoid speaking in monotone but should also avoid being overly dramatic. Inflections appropriate to the material being presented should be used.

Whether developing audio- or videotape, a specific script should be developed. It is important to keep in mind that patients' attention span is limited. The script should be long enough to convey the message, but not so long that patients lose interest. The goal is to provide patients with essential information in a time that they will be maximally receptive. Therefore, during script development, specific timelines for each section of the tape should be predetermined. This also helps health professionals avoid spending too much time, for example, on the introduction, so that there is insufficient time left for the key points of the message.

In the case of videotapes, cue cards may be used to help the actor/speaker cover the material in an orderly sequence so nothing is left out. If other scenes or illustrations are to be used on a videotape, the health professional should look at the script and outline specifically what scene, action, or illustration would best fit at specific points of the script.

One technique that may be useful when developing audio- or videotapes is the use of dialogue to convey the message. For instance, a teaching tape for acquired immunodeficiency syndrome (AIDS) prevention may use a dialogue between patient and health professional as follows:

Patient: I've been reading a lot about AIDS lately. It's pretty scary, but since I don't use IV drugs, I guess I don't have to worry.

Physician: That's only one way people can get infected with HIV, the organism that causes AIDS. But there are other ways as well.

Patient: You mean it's not just IV drugs? How else could you get it?

Physician: The virus is contained within all body fluids; therefore, although it's in the blood, it's also contained in the semen. Consequently, sexual contact with a person infected with HIV can also lead to infection.

Whether making audio- or videotapes, health professionals should consider using high-quality tapes, which will produce high-quality recordings. In either instance, the sound quality should be tested before making the tape. The actor/speaker should make sure they are speaking directly into the microphone and not turning away from it, which creates fluctuations in sound. Background noises should be avoided.

If videotapes are made, lighting should be considered. If lighting is not adequate, then supplemental lighting may be needed. When developing videotapes, health professionals should consider the use of other visual aids within the tape, rather than merely speaking into the camera for the duration of the message. For instance, introduction of slides, posters, illustrations, or other methods can help to illustrate specific points to be made on the tape as well as maintain patients' attention. For example, a poster prepared with a felt-tip pen may illustrate specific points to be reinforced or illustrations or diagrams, which the camera can focus on at the appropriate time.

If editing of the videotape is possible, different scenes or other outside illustrations may be used as part of the tape. However, editing may not be possible because it requires fairly sophisticated equipment and expertise that are not always available to the health professional.

DEVELOPING A PATIENT EDUCATION NEWSLETTER

Patient education newsletters are a way to communicate general health information to patients who may not come in contact with the health professional on a regular basis (Aukerman 1991). Although perhaps most beneficial in an outpatient setting where there is a specific patient population, many inpatient facilities have also developed newsletters that are distributed to the community at large.

Newsletters can be used to convey information about specific conditions, nutrition, safety, or prevention as well as the availability of specific patient education programs or resources. In addition, newsletters enable health professionals to address specific health issues that currently may be receiving considerable attention in the media, but for which all the facts are not always presented.

Newsletter production also follows many of the same development steps as those discussed earlier for written materials. The layout of the newsletter should be attractive and easy to read. Print should be at least letter quality. Many computer programs now available can produce professional-looking copies. In the event that a computer or expertise to use these programs is not available, professional printing may be considered an option and may be less expensive in bulk than for smaller numbers. The size of the newsletter and format will depend on the resources available.

How the distribution of the newsletter is handled will depend on the facility producing it and the resources available. For example, if there is no money in the budget for mailing, the newsletter may be placed in the waiting room of the health facility, if it is possible to use bulk mailing, newsletters may be mailed to a specific patient population or to the community at large. In some instances, a copy of the newsletter may be included in regular patient mailings, such as with monthly billing statements.

There are a number of advantages to producing a customized newsletter. Not only does it enable health professionals to communicate important health information to patients who may otherwise not receive it, the newsletter may also stimulate patients to contact their health professional with questions they otherwise may not have asked.

COMPUTERS

A variety of patient education software is now available for use in inpatient and outpatient facilities. Programs that offer a number of print-on-demand patient education products can cut down on the need for storing, filing, and reordering patient education brochures, pamphlets, or other information sources. Many of these programs have been tested for readability and acceptability to patients, many of whom use computers at home and are already used to this type of technology (Deye et al. 1997).

Some programs enable health professionals to customize and personalize information presented. Computer programs may also be available in several languages and be able to be adjusted for print size, making it easier for older patients or patients with visual disability to read. Patient education software programs are usually purchased at an initial price, which then includes periodic updates for a minimal fee.

As with other patient education materials, health professionals should assess accuracy, usability, and cost when making decisions about the extent to which patient education software can be used effectively. Evaluation of the content of the educational material as well as whether the range of topics is sufficient for the patient population served are considerations, just as they would be with other types of patient education materials. Health professionals should determine whether material is appropriate for the patient population in terms of acceptability and readability and whether it meets the educational goals the health professional wants to accomplish. Cost-effectiveness may also be an issue. Are there hidden costs to keep the system running or updated? Will additional equipment be needed? Health professionals should make sure that software packages are compatible with their hardware, operating system, and storage capacity and that everyone using the system has the appropriate skills for efficient use.

Computerized patient education materials, if carefully chosen and evaluated, can serve as an excellent reinforcement of patient education information. Most important, however, is recognition by the health professional that nothing can replace the interpersonal interaction between patient and health professional in which the patient's individual needs and concerns are addressed face to face.

USING THE INTERNET

Patients gain health information from many sources. The Internet has become an increasingly important source of health information for patients and can complement or complicate patient education effectiveness. Information sources vary from national health and disease organizations, to pharmaceutical companies, to consumer groups. The type of information available also varies, from information about specific disease and treatment to prevention and alternative health practices.

Health information gained over the Internet can be a major influence in patients' decisions about treatment (Fox and Rainie 2000) and consequently can have a major impact on patient compliance. Although health professionals may not always have control over the type of information patients access from the Internet, it is important to be aware of patients' use of this type of information and to help patients become educated consumers of Internet health-related information.

The appeal of Internet information for patients is the easy and private access to information. Unfortunately, depending on the information source, information may be incomplete, inaccurate, or generally deficient in presenting facts patients may need to make decisions about their health and health care (Beredjiklian et al. 2000).

Quality of information gained by patients on the Internet is dependent upon search engines used and links provided. Web sites differ in quality, depending on whether they are from commercial organizations, government agencies, or nonprofit educational organizations. Some sites, for example, are designed as advertisements to encourage site users to purchase products, use services, or participate in research programs. Others present a viewpoint based on the philosophy of the organization sponsoring the Web site.

Accuracy of information can also vary, as well as the extent to which complete information about a condition, treatment, or adverse of treatment or nontreatment are presented (Soot et al. 1999, Griffiths and Christensen 2000, Jiang 2000, Berland et al. 2001). Patients using information from Web sites as a basis for medical decision making may have deficient information on which to act. Usefulness of information gained from the Internet also depends on readability and how easily the information is understood and interpreted correctly by the user.

Health professionals should ask patients whether they use the Internet as a health information source. Providing guidance to patients who use the Internet can help health professionals ensure that information will be a helpful supplement rather than a barrier to patient education efforts and subsequently to patient compliance. Being open to the information patients find on the Internet as well as being noncritical or judgmental of its use will decrease the likelihood that patients will use the Internet as a substitute for consultation with the health professional. Patients should be encouraged to bring questions or concerns about information they have read on the Internet to the health professional's attention rather than changing treatment on their own.

Patients should be cautioned to check information sources to assure that information is unbiased and not being presented in such a way as to sell a product or idea. Patients should be taught how to assess credibility of agencies or organizations sponsoring the Web site and to check for references and timeliness of information presented.

USING TEACHING AIDS EFFECTIVELY

Teaching aids should not be used without verbal instruction. Patients should be told why they are viewing a tape or film or why they are being given a pamphlet or brochure. They should also be told how they are to use the information contained in it. Does the aid supply additional information? Does it review the information presented verbally? Is the information in the aid to provide cues to patients to help them perform skills discussed? Patients will take the teaching aid more seriously if health professionals take time to point out major areas in the pamphlet that are of particular importance.

Teaching aids, in and of themselves, are useless if not presented within the context of the total process of patient education. Teaching aids should enhance progress toward the general objective of teaching in a particular area. Aids should be appropriate to the patient, the situation, and the particular problem. Most important, teaching aids should enhance communication with health professionals, not replace it.

REFERENCES

Aukerman, G.F. 1991. Developing a patient education newsletter. *Journal of Family Practice* 33(3):304–305.

Baker, G.C. 1991. Writing easily read patient education handouts: a computerized approach. *Seminars in Dermatology*, 10(2):102–106.

Beredjiklian, P.K., Bozentka, D.J., Steinberg, D.R., Bernstein, J. 2000. Evaluating the source and content of orthopedic information on the Internet: the case of carpal tunnel syndrome. *Journal of Bone and Joint Surgery* 82:1540–1543.

Berland, G.K., Elliott, M.N., Morales, L.S., Agazy, J.I., Kravitz, R.L., Broder, M.S., Kanouse, D.E., Munoz, J.A., Puyol, J.A., Lara, M., Watkins, K.E., Yang, H., McGlynn, E.A. 2001. Health information on the Internet: accessibility, quality, and readability in English and Spanish. *Journal of the American Medical Association* 285(20):2612–2621.

Deye, D.L., Kahn, G., Jimison, H.B., Renner, J.H., Wenner, A.R. 1997. How computers enrich patient education. *Patient Care* Feb 15:88–113.

Fox, S., Rainie, L. 2000. The online health care revolution: how the Web helps Americans take better care of themselves. Washington, DC: Pew Charitable Trusts.

Griffiths, K.M., Christensen, H. 2000. Quality of web based information on treatment of depression: cross sectional survey. *British Medical Journal* 321:1511–1515.

Jiang, Y.L. 2000. Quality evaluation of orthodontic information on the World Wide Web. *American Journal of Orthodontics and Dentofacial Orthopedics* 118:4–9.

Soot, L.C., Moneta, G.L., Edwards, J.M. 1999. Vascular surgery and the Internet: a poor source of patient oriented information. *Journal of Vascular Surgery* 30:84–91.

17

Issues in Research and Evaluation in Patient Education and Patient Compliance

IMPORTANCE OF RESEARCH AND EVALUATION

Few would argue the importance of patient education in patient care. Until recently, conducting patient education was based on common sense, experience, and trial and error. As patient education has evolved, however, there has been increasing emphasis on accountability. Does patient education bring about positive health outcomes? Are some approaches to patient education more effective than others? Do the benefits of patient education outweigh the cost in terms of time and resources? Research and evaluation as a way of testing and validating effectiveness of patient education interventions has, consequently, grown in importance.

To strengthen and enhance the quality of patient education, research and evaluation are essential. Results from well-designed studies can help health professionals make rational choices between alternative patient education approaches and materials, validate various patient education interventions, and build a stable foundation of effective patient education practice. Well-planned and well-executed research provides the basis from which conclusions regarding patient education can be drawn. Sound research acts as a safeguard against proliferation of patient education practices that may be fashionable or faddish, but ineffective.

Well-designed research and evaluation are necessary not only to enhance the quality of patient education but to increase its credibility and, in some instances, its potential for survival. Although lip service is given to the importance of patient education in the provision of quality health care, the extent of support, both financial and otherwise, is often contingent on evidence of cost-effectiveness. There has been a recent upswing by the patient education industry of development of new materials, equipment, and other innovations that are marketed as tools to increase quality of patient education and to increase patient education effectiveness. Decisions regarding which, if any, of these products should be purchased or implemented should be based on research that has demonstrated effectiveness. Too often, health professionals caught up in enthusiasm and who are influenced by the popularity of products and overwhelmed by the availability of patient education materials rush out to purchase products and implement use without first ascertaining their effectiveness. If benefit of product use has not been shown to justify the cost, when budgetary decisions are made, and especially when financial cutbacks are necessary, patient education may be viewed as a luxury rather than a necessity. As a result, resources for patient education may be the first targeted for reduction or, in some cases, elimination.

There is a dearth of well-controlled, randomized research that attempts to evaluate patient education methods and their impact on patient compliance. Likewise, do patient education activities designed to increase patient compliance actually improve patients' health status? Controversy also exists regarding the extent to which compliance should be a goal of patient education. Should a major goal of patient education be increasing patient compliance, or should the goal be increasing patients' ability to make their own informed choices about the extent to which they will follow recommendations?

Research and evaluation are essential for strengthening and enhancing patient education and for contributing to increased understanding of the phenomenon of patient compliance. Although much valuable information already exists as the result of patient education and patient compliance research, much research has been conducted by researchers in academic or industrial settings. These individuals may have an interest in patient education and patient compliance and may have expertise in research and evaluation methodology, but they may have little direct involvement with patient education and patient compliance issues in practice. Research and evaluation of various materials, methods, and programs are most relevant when built upon the experiences and perceptions of those individuals most involved with patient education on a day-to-day basis. These health professionals are in the best position to identify specific patient education problems, recognize patient compliance issues, help establish research priorities, set goals, collect and analyze data, and assist in interpreting conclusions. Many health professionals, however, have not been trained in research and may be intimidated by the concept. Not all research has to be complicated to be valuable. The most elegant research and the most important findings can come from simple projects that have been well designed, planned, and executed.

It is important for health professionals to remember that the quality of research findings is directly related to the quality of research design, attention directed to implementation of research protocol, objective analysis of data, and careful interpretation of data. This is true whether health professionals are conducting research or evaluation as single investigators or in collaboration with experts in research methods; whether conducting research to test a hypothesis or theory or merely evaluating a specific method or material; whether conducting a study within their own setting or cooperating with a variety of individuals within other settings; or whether merely being a consumer of findings from other researchers. The importance of good research and evaluation techniques cannot be overemphasized. Planning is essential to both good research and evaluation.

DEFINING RESEARCH AND EVALUATION

Research and evaluation are often used synonymously. Although both may use many of the same procedures, they are two separate processes, with different purposes. Research, purely defined, is oriented toward the development of theory, with its purpose being to search for new knowledge or to establish facts or principles. Evaluation, on the other hand, is directed toward appraising or judging worth, or judging the degree to which a program, process, or material has met its predetermined goal. Inherent in evaluation is judgment of value, or degree to which it can be judged as good or bad. Research remains objective, reporting facts, but making no value judgment related to the facts. Research frequently involves manipulation of variables, whereas evaluation does not.

As an illustration, consider the following problem. A rural health clinic had identified a low rate of screening mammography utilization by women over the age of 50. The nurse, Ms. Dunn, designed a research project to study the problem. Ms. Dunn hypothesized that the low usage was related to lack of physician encouragement and patient education related to mammography. In reviewing other research that had been conducted, she noted that findings from previous studies appeared to indicate that more active physician involvement in giving recommendations was correlated with the likelihood that the patient would follow through with the recommendations provided. She therefore hypothesized that patients who received more encouragement and patient education about mammography from their physicians would have greater likelihood of obtaining mammography than patients who did not. To study the problem, she divided patients into two groups. One group would be given specific information about mammography from the physician according to a specific protocol, and the second group would not. After collecting and analyzing the data, she found that her hypothesis had been correct. Those women who had received the information from their physicians were twice as likely to have obtained a mammogram as those who did not.

Now consider the same problem, but with an evaluation focus developed by a nurse, Ms. Janesky. In this situation, Ms. Janesky designed a specific program, the goal of which was to increase women's use of screening mammography. The program consisted of developing a brochure that explained the importance of mammography after the age of 50 and addressed common concerns women may have about mammography. She also developed a videotape that demonstrated the procedure of mammography and that women were to view while waiting to see their physician. After implementing the program for a specified time,

Ms. Janesky evaluated women's perceptions of the brochure and videotape, evaluated their attitudes about mammography before and after receiving the brochure and viewing the videotape, and evaluated the number of women who had received a mammogram after being exposed to the patient education program. She found that although women evaluated both the brochure and videotape positively, the number of women who actually had a mammography after participating in the program had not increased. She concluded that the program was not effective, and the program was discontinued.

In the first case, Ms. Dunn conducted research. She formulated a hypothesis based on findings of other research; manipulated the amount of patient education groups of women would receive; made a comparison of the two groups; and after analyzing the data, reported findings objectively, making no judgment regarding the merit of the innovation.

Ms. Janesky, on the other hand, had developed a program with specific goals. She evaluated data related to the effectiveness of the program in meeting the stated goals, using the outcome as a basis for deciding whether or not the program should still exist. In this situation, when looking at other ways to increase usage of mammography, she may consider Ms. Dunn's findings when designing a patient education innovation, but her evaluation will always revolve around how successful the program was in meeting its predetermined goals.

Whether conducting research or evaluation, an organized, systematic approach should be used. For both research and evaluation, a specific problem must first be identified. In the case above, the problem was the same—low mammography usage in women over the age of 50. Ms. Dunn developed her hypothesis based on the problem and developed research protocol to study it. Ms. Janesky developed a patient education intervention with specific goals of what it was to accomplish. It is these goals on which the evaluation is based. In both instances, Ms. Dunn and Ms. Janesky had a period of implementation in which, in Ms. Dunn's case, the study was carried out, and in Ms. Janesky's case, the program was implemented. At the end of a specified time, both analyzed the data and reached conclusions based on their analysis.

Both research and evaluation are needed in patient education. Both require careful planning and a clear-cut statement of exactly what is to be examined or evaluated. A brief description of the steps within the process of research and evaluation is discussed below.

STEPS IN PROGRAM EVALUATION

Before evaluation can be conducted, a program, a course of study, or materials must first be developed and implemented. Although it is not the purpose of this chapter to discuss program development, program planning and evaluation should always be integrated functions. Thorough program planning leads to logically linked, expected outcomes. The term *evaluation* implies systematically planning and implementing activities carried out as part of the program and measuring the effects or outcomes resulting from those activities. Evaluation, then, is a way of determining the degree to which previously determined goals or objectives of the program were reached.

The first step in program planning, and essential to comprehensive evaluation, is to conduct a needs assessment. The needs assessment should identify the major needs the program is to address. Too often there is little relationship between needs being measured and activities being carried out as a part of a specific program. Unless there is a link between needs, activities carried out as part of the program, and expected outcomes, it is impossible to evaluate effectively whether or not a program was successful in meeting a specific need. A need can be defined as the difference between what is and what should be. It is from needs that program goals and, consequently, measurable objectives are developed. It should be noted that evaluation is dependent on the clarity and observable, measurable goals and objectives that the program is designed to accomplish. The more clear, observable, and measurable the goals and objectives, the easier the task of evaluation.

Assessing individual patient needs was discussed in previous chapters. Although some of the steps and principles are the same, assessing needs on which to build a specific patient education program is somewhat different. Needs assessment at a program level requires input from more people in the planning process.

Determining needs at the program level can be best illustrated by example. Ms. Janes was a nurse practitioner working with three physicians in a satellite clinic outside a large city. Although all practitioners at the clinic provided one-to-one patient education to their individual patients, Ms. Janes had begun to feel that patients could also benefit from a more formalized and structured patient education program. She arranged a meeting for the medical staff and asked them to list what they perceived to be the greatest patient needs in their particular patient population with regard to patient education. It is important to note that Ms. Janes focused on patient-oriented needs rather than on preferences of individual health care providers. After a list of needs had been established, Ms. Janes asked the staff to rank order the needs as high, moderate, or low importance. This was important because it was unlikely that equal resources could or would be given to ease all identified needs at once.

Ms. Janes and the staff decided to begin with only the area that was designated as the highest priority. The staff then determined goals for the program and from the goals developed measurable objectives. Then they needed to design the program itself based on the stated goals and objectives. Key issues involved questions such as:

- What is needed to reach the stated objectives?
- Who will be responsible for carrying out or facilitating various parts of the program?
- What financial and other resources are available?

- What type of budget needs to be established in order to implement and maintain the program?
- What criteria will be used to judge program effectiveness?

It should be noted that the most effective program is based on and responsive to patients' actual needs. When formulating programs, ideally, having patient input as well is important to achieve a more realistic view. Health professionals' perceptions of patient need are not always the same as patients' perceptions. In Ms. Janes's case, in addition to assessing and prioritizing needs as identified by the clinic staff, she may also have polled a selected sample of patients to assess their needs and priorities. (Sample selection is addressed later in the chapter.)

The second step important to planning and subsequent evaluation is development of goals and objectives. Program goals and objectives should be based on the identified needs and should be stated in terms of desired outcomes. As stated previously, specifically stated goals and objectives that are measurable are crucial to evaluation. When developing goals and objectives, there should be a logical relationship between goals, objectives, resources, and activities by which the goals and objectives are to be accomplished.

Although goals can be somewhat idealistic, serving as an ideal to strive for, objectives should be more reasonable, realistic, and attainable. For example, if Dr. Farris develops a patient education program for hypertension, an idealistic goal may be, "All complications of hypertension will be prevented in the patient population." However, since the likelihood of reaching this goal is remote, objectives should reflect a more realistic view of what the program is to accomplish. In writing program objectives, Dr. Farris should make sure that the true mission of the program is reflected. In other words, although he may list as an objective, "Patients will list the complications of hypertension," Dr. Farris's real objective in implementing the program is probably not limited to patients regurgitating facts but rather incorporating the facts into their lives so that their hypertension may be better controlled, thus striving for the goal of reducing complications. Consequently, an objective of the patient education program in hypertension may be, "To maintain blood pressure below 140/ 90." In the same vein, the objectives should be clear and readily measurable. An objective that states, "The patient will understand the potential complications of hypertension" lacks both clarity and measurability. If an objective relating to patients' knowledge of complications is to be written, a more precise, measurable objective might be, "The patient will be able to list five complications associated with hypertension."

It should be noted that program evaluation may have several different focuses. Using the program described previously as an example:

- Did the program make a difference? For instance, did patients participating in the program develop few complications? Did patients attending the program show greater compliance with recommendations, such as engaging in a regular exercise program, lowering blood cholesterol, losing weight, adhering to medication instructions?

- Was the program cost-effective? Did resources expended result in desirable outcomes? Was the benefit worth the cost? Cost/benefit can be measured either in actual program costs (e.g., materials, personnel time) or in terms of more global cost vs. outcomes (e.g., cost of hospitalizations, days lost from work).

- Are there changes that need to be made to make the program more effective? For example, if the program was planned for six sessions, but patients stopped coming after two, what might be done to encourage fuller participation?

Program evaluation can be conducted in two phases. These two phases are called formative and summative evaluation. The first phase, formative evaluation, is a means of obtaining feedback about the program and how well it is making progress toward its stated objective. This type of evaluation takes place during program implementation, enabling midcourse corrections or refinements to be made if necessary to better achieve the stated objectives or to keep the program in line with its original design. This type of evaluation focuses not only on the results of the program activity, but on the activities themselves. For example, in Dr. Farris's hypertension program, he may find that didactic sessions and video sessions are equally effective in relaying information, but that patients prefer the personal interaction of the lecture and are more likely to continue participation in the program if this format is used.

The summative evaluation takes place at the end of the program or after its full implementation to determine the extent to which objectives were achieved. From summative evaluation information gathered may help health professionals make decisions about whether or not the program should be continued and about modifications to improve or maintain the program in the future. In this case, evaluation focuses not only on whether the objectives were met, but whether the objectives were appropriate. All objectives of the program might have been met, but the objectives themselves may have been meaningless. For instance, if Dr. Farris's only objective was patient participation in the hypertension program, but patients gained no new knowledge or behavior change that increased the likelihood of their well-being, although the stated objective was met, it would be hard to judge the program as effective.

There are many models of program evaluation. The type chosen depends on the needs of the specific individual or facility implementing the program and the general purpose of the evaluation. For example, in some instances, the major objective and thus focus of evaluation may be patient outcomes. In other instances, evaluation may focus on the effectiveness of various materials or other patient education innovations.

Accountability in patient education assigns responsibility to those doing patient teaching for monitoring and assessing measurable outcomes. The validity of the evaluation results will, in a large part, also be determined by the accuracy of measurement used in the evaluation process. Different processes for evaluation are used for different evaluative purposes.

Measurement of effectiveness of individual patient education programs is important for maintenance of program quality and for program accountability. In a broader context, the importance to the field of patient education is study of the extent to which a successful program can be implemented in different settings with similar results. Development of effective patient education strategies that can be demonstrated to have positive effects on patient outcomes have the greatest utility if the program is effective in other settings as well. In addition, it is important to make sure that positive outcomes are a direct result of the patient education program being evaluated and not other confounding factors. For example, if the major determining factors in achievement of the objectives of Dr. Farris's program are patient loyalty and respect for Dr. Farris and not the program itself, evaluation results could be misleading. It might be difficult to determine whether the increased attention to compliance with recommendations is a function of the patient education program itself, Dr. Farris's individual personality, or both. These two factors are confounded, and the effects of each cannot be determined.

Many of the same procedures are used for program evaluation as for evaluation of individual teaching effectiveness. A key consideration in program development, implementation, and evaluation is that none of these elements exists in a vacuum. The social context of patient education programs includes a wide variety of people, from administration, to staff, to the initiator of the project, to patients. To blindly proceed without considering all these levels is foolhardy and limits the potential for program effectiveness. This is especially true in evaluation, and specifically when evaluation of program effectiveness may be a determining factor regarding whether or not the program will still be in existence.

Program evaluations must be conducted with an awareness and sensitivity to the political atmosphere of the program's setting. Persons directly and indirectly related to the program probably represent different levels of power, influence, and authority and have their own values and priorities regarding specific goals. Program evaluation is based on scientific principles and procedures for collecting and analyzing data. Because any program operates within a social and political context, to obtain a meaningful evaluation, the relationship between these various factors must be considered.

STEPS IN RESEARCH

As with evaluation, central to good research is careful planning. The first step to conducting research is identifying a problem to be studied. The more clearly stated the specific problem to be studied, the easier it is to develop a sound research plan, which will result in valid conclusions. An ambiguous or general research question such as "Does patient education make a difference in health care costs?" is so general that interpretation of findings that result would be extremely difficult.

The problem selected for study should be of interest to the health professional conducting the research and should be based on a conceptual framework grounded in research findings reported in the current professional literature. A comprehensive literature review provides the researcher with deeper insights into the research topic by acquainting him or her with current thinking in the area of interest as supported by research findings from other studies. Literature review also provides insights into various methods used by other researchers studying similar research problems and can stimulate new ideas for additional research.

Depending on the research question being investigated, the literature review may include classic studies from the past as well as studies most recently published. Research on the specific topic of interest as well as studies in related research areas may be included.

Several sources may be used to search the literature. Professional journal indexes compile listings of articles by year and generally categorize articles by topical area. Computer searches are also convenient sources for identification of articles related to specific research topics. A number of computer search engines dedicated to health related studies are available for quick and easy identification of related topics. Bibliographies from articles obtained are also good sources for identifying additional articles related to the topic being studied.

When conducting a literature review, health professionals should keep their own research topic in mind, looking for literature that relates specifically to it. Without maintaining this focus, it is easy to become overwhelmed by volumes of articles which may have minimum relevance to the research problem being investigated.

The second step in the research process is to develop a clear and precise research question. Refining and narrowly defining the research question is the beginning of good research design and protocol. The best stated research question is simple, brief, and unambiguous. The research design and methods are based on the research question. Consequently, the more clearly and precisely the question can be stated, the more clearly the research design and methods can be outlined.

A common mistake made by beginning researchers is to collect data before a clear research question has been formulated, hoping that some sense can be made of the data at a later time. Another common error is taking data that already exist and attempting to develop a research problem to fit them. Although retrospective studies may also have their place in research on patient education and patient compliance, if existing data are used, health professionals must still have a clear idea of what the specific project is designed to study and a specific plan to achieve that goal. Too often existing data are used merely because they are convenient and too little thought has been put into the real purpose of analyzing the data. Again, unless there is a precise research question, a sound plan for analyzing data cannot be developed.

When the research question is clearly established, other issues regarding the feasibility of the project must be considered. Such issues relate to whether the researcher has the skills, resources, or time to carry out the research. This includes access to subjects, ability to obtain a sufficient number of subjects, administrative support, financial support, and access to programs for data analysis. Although study design is important and should be appropriate to the research question being asked, health professionals must also consider the realities of the research situation. Listing resources needed for completion of the study and assessing their availability can help health professionals assess the feasibility of the study realistically as well as help identify potential resources.

The quality of findings of research is directly related to the study design and methods used to carry out the study. Research in patient education and patient compliance is applied research. Many methodological issues may not be present in research conducted under more controlled conditions, as is the case for research conducted in laboratory settings. Consequently, health professionals must also consider the setting in which research is to be conducted. Different settings present their own particular problems in conducting research. Conducting research in a clinic setting may present different issues than conducting research in a hospital setting. Issues of staff cooperation, patient recruitment and availability as study subjects, and political considerations may be factors that have different ramifications in different settings. Being aware of potential problems and identifying them early can save health professionals both time and money in the long run, as well as help them to develop and maintain a sound research protocol.

Many different research designs can be used when conducting research. The research design merely refers to the plan or strategy used to study the research question. It specifically addresses selection of research subjects, measures, and procedures used. The design of a research project is dependent on the purpose of the study, the nature of the problem to be studied, the setting in which the research is to be conducted, and the resources available for the investigation. The importance of good research design cannot be overemphasized. If a study is conducted and the research design is flawed, the data will be meaningless, and no amount of statistical manipulation can repair the damage.

One of the goals of good research design is to eliminate confounding effects. Without doing this, it is difficult to determine how much of the findings are due to the variables of interest in the study and how much are due to something else. For example, Dr. Lewis conducted a research study in which he investigated the effect of his prenatal classes on infant mortality and morbidity in infants of mothers who attended the classes. The classes consisted of four different sessions. He conducted the classes for three years. At the end of the three-year period, he collected follow-up information regarding outcome for infants born to women attending the classes. He compared this figure with infants born to other patients in his practice who had not attended the prenatal classes. His findings demonstrated that the rate of morbidity and mortality in infants born to parents who had attended the classes was significantly less than that in infants whose parents had not. He concluded that his prenatal classes had a significant effect on reducing infant morbidity and mortality. Dr. Lewis's conclusions were invalid, however, because he had not considered all the other factors that could also affect infant morbidity and mortality. In his particular situation, those attending the classes were, in general, well-educated, upper-middle-class individuals living in two-parent homes. A large number of the remaining prenatal patients in Dr. Lewis's practice were unwed teenagers from lower socioeconomic backgrounds. Given the difference in the two groups, it is unlikely that the prenatal classes themselves had an effect on infant mortality, but rather that age, general health, and socioeconomic status of the mothers had more of an effect.

Using another example with a different research question, suppose that Mr. Roseman, a nurse, was interested in studying whether or not exposure to a videotape on how human immunodeficiency virus (HIV) is transmitted increased patients' knowledge about how HIV infection could be prevented. He showed the videotape to a group of patients selected to participate in the research, and after having them watch the tape, administered a questionnaire he had developed to assess the patients' knowledge. This study has major flaws. First, since Mr. Roseman had not assessed the patients' knowledge level of HIV transmission or prevention prior to the videotape, he had no way of knowing whether or not scores on the questionnaire were a reflection of knowledge gained because of the intervention. To observe changes, baseline information must be gathered against which comparisons can be made. Second, since he had developed the questionnaire but had not tested it to see how accurate and sensitive it was as an actual measurement of patient knowledge, he had no way of determining that the scores on the questionnaire were a valid measurement of patient knowledge of HIV. Last, there was no provision for comparison. In other words, how did the knowledge level of those individuals who had not viewed the videotape compare with those who had?

For sound research design, precautions should be taken. Certain types of studies require a control group by which comparisons can be made. Factors other than the particular intervention being studied may also contribute to any differences found. Consequently, a group that does not receive the intervention provides a means for "controlling" for confounding factors so that a comparison can be made. Otherwise, there is nothing against which to compare effectiveness of the specific procedure. In the example used above, Mr. Roseman had no basis for comparison since he did not use a control group.

Sampling

Another precaution that must be taken when conducting research relates to choosing study participants. This process is called *sampling*. Sampling procedures are critical to a good study, and to the usefulness of results. One of the objectives of conducting research in patient education is to gain information that can be applied to other settings. If, for instance, a patient education technique used in a certain setting has been found to be effective in reducing patient noncompliance, findings are of little value unless the same techniques are found to be effective in other settings as well. The extent to which research findings in one setting can be applied to other settings is called *generalizability*. This is accomplished in part through proper sampling techniques. Two issues are important in sampling: (1) representativeness and (2) sample size.

Although larger sample sizes tend to increase the probability of obtaining statistically significant results, perhaps even more important is the degree to which the sample is representative of the group to which generalizations can be made. In order to increase the possibility of generalization as much as possible the sample studied should be representative of the type of patient to which conclusions regarding the study could be drawn. For example, in a study of the effect of a specific patient education intervention on patients' compliance with treatment recommendations for rheumatoid arthritis, before reaching a valid conclusion the health professional would have to make sure that the study sample included individuals representative of those with rheumatoid arthritis. Only including Caucasian women in the sample, for example, would not allow any conclusions to be drawn, except perhaps as results applied to Caucasian women.

Sample size is often an issue. In the case above, although it would be ideal to study the entire population of patients with rheumatoid arthritis, this would not be feasible. Therefore, a sample of the total group is used. Health professionals need to identify the minimum sample size needed so that if significant differences between groups in the study exist, those differences can be determined. When considering sample size, precision is important, but so is cost. Larger samples are more costly in time and effort as well as financially, but results are more reliable and representative. Even if resources are available for a larger sample, the number of individuals in a certain area or situation who are available to participate as subjects in a research study may be limited. When it is not possible to use a large sample, smaller samples may be used. One way of determining sample size is through the use of a power table. These are available in a number of research texts. The goal is to make the power as large as possible given the practical limitations on the sample size.

An additional problem related to sample size is the fact that some patients may drop out of the study or fail to follow through with the research protocol. At times, patients drop out of the study because of excessive demands of time or effort required in study participation. When planning the study, health professionals should consider demands on study participants and adjust the sample size to accommodate the anticipated number of patient drop-outs. One way to test the effectiveness of the research plan as well as to assess the potential for drop-outs is to conduct a pilot study with a small number of patients before beginning the study. This enables health professionals to test the feasibility of the research and to identify and correct any problems in the study before additional resources are used. Patients participating in the pilot study should, of course, be eliminated from selection for the major study.

Another important concept in sampling is randomization. Randomization in sampling diminishes the potential of selection bias, helping to ensure that groups are similar with respect to characteristics that may be important. Random samples are obtained in a way that ensures that every member of the population to be studied has an equal chance of being chosen for the study and that selection of each person for the study has no effect on the selection of another person in the population. For example, if the health professional were comparing the effects of computerized instruction on levels of compliance for patients in their practice with gout, first all patients in the practice with gout would need to be identified. Unless the total number of patients in the practice with gout was very small, the health professional would probably decide to choose a random sample of the total group. Choosing every seventh patient from the list of patients with gout is not a random sample. Most commonly, random selection may be accomplished by using a random number table. Random number tables and their method of use can be found in a variety of research texts.

In addition to random selection of study participants, random assignment of individuals into different treatment groups is also important. In the example used above, from the random sample selected, the health professional would then assign patients to one of the different groups using a random selection process. This type of randomization helps to avoid the possibility that there was bias from one particular treatment group or the other. Again, a random table could be used.

In patient education settings, randomization can be difficult. Whereas in laboratory settings, animals easily may be randomly assigned to different study groups, in conducting research with patients, the task is not always as easy. Patient rights must be considered. Patients must be informed of benefits as well as risks that might be involved through their participation in the study. In addition, patients have the right to refuse participation. They cannot be coerced to participate as subjects or to be placed in a specific treatment group. In patient education situations, random assignment and control groups may not always be possible and may also not be feasible for ethical reasons. For instance, if the health professional were interested in studying the effectiveness of two different methods of patient education for new diabetics, ideally patients would be randomly assigned to three different groups. Each of two groups would receive patient education by two different methods, and the third group would receive some intervention, but unrelated to diabetes. Obviously, in this example, it is not feasible or ethical to withhold patient education from a group of diabetic patients. In other situations, in addition to issues of confidentiality, it may not be possible to identify all patients within a setting who have a specific condition. Consequently, a true random sample could not be drawn.

Researcher and Subject Bias

Another issue to be considered when designing research concerns diminishing researcher and subject bias as much as possible. The degree to which this precaution is followed varies and avoiding bias is not always possible. Ideally, neither the researcher nor the subjects should know which treatment group is which. Less ideal is when the researcher knows, but the subjects do not. Although bias on the part of the researcher or the patient may not be intentional, it can subconsciously affect interpretation of the data by the researcher and behavior of the research subject. Patients who know they are being assigned to a specific group may feel and/or act differently compared to patients not in the group. This is even more problematic if the patient knows what the group is intended to demonstrate. For instance, take a study being conducted to see whether patients who receive detailed instructions about their treatment are more compliant than those who do not. If patients are told "We're conducting a study to see if receiving instructions about your medication will make it more likely that you will take it as prescribed," it is possible that any increased compliance of the group may be more related to the fact that patients know they are in a study group than from the special instructions they received. In the case of researchers, there may be an unconscious tendency to project into the study or into the interpretation of the data what they expected or hoped to find so that the data are subtly shaped to meet the expected outcomes. The fact that all patients participating in research must be volunteers, rather than blind participants, also introduces some bias.

MEASUREMENT IN RESEARCH AND EVALUATION

When a research study is conducted, observations of some type take place. In order to be meaningful, these observations must be measured. Again, the validity of research or evaluation results will depend on the clarity of the definition of what is to be observed or measured and the exactness of the tool used to measure it.

If, for example, the health professional is interested in assessing differences in patient learning about colostomy irrigation when either of two patient education methods are used, learning must first be defined and a way of measuring it established. Learning is not directly observable. Consequently, the health professional must define precisely what will be considered as learning for purposes of the study. For example, learning could be defined in terms of a score on a test, or it could be defined by direct observation of behavior, such as being able to irrigate the colostomy. In order to avoid ambiguity, these definitions should be even more precise, such as providing a cut-off score on the test, below which scores would not be considered indicative of learning, or carefully defining each step of colostomy irrigation so that learning may be defined as performance of the procedure with some percentage of accuracy. A third level of defining learning would be the extent to which the patient continues to follow the protocol accurately and consistently at home when not under the watchful eye of the health professional.

Definitions should be constructed carefully to avoid obtaining results that lead to misleading conclusions from the research or evaluation. For example, consider evaluation of a specific intervention, such as determining the effect of a computerized patient education program on patient compliance with a prescribed antihypertensive medication regimen. The health professional has defined what will be measured (medication compliance). In interpreting results, however, whether or not the procedure is concluded to be effective will depend on how the health professional defined compliance. If, for example, compliance was defined as taking the medication 10 percent of the time, the program may be more likely concluded to be highly effective than if the standards were set at a higher level, such as 70 percent or 80 percent.

The type of measurement depends on the research question being asked. In all instances, no matter what type of measure is used, it is crucial that the measure be as accurate and as valid as possible. Two key issues in measurement are validity and reliability. Validity refers to how accurately the instrument actually measures what it is intended to measure. Reliability refers to how consistently the instrument measures. Before an instrument or observational technique is used, some attempt should be made to assess validity and reliability. Methods for doing this also may be found in a variety of research texts. When feasible, it is desirable to find an existing instrument that has had tests of reliability and validity already performed.

Some research questions are such that measurement can be done with direct observation. For example, if the outcome variable of interest were appointment keeping, measurement could be done by simply observing whether or not patients kept their appointments. When the simultaneous observation of two observers is required, attempts should be made to assess the degree of reliability of the two separate ratings.

The least accurate means of measurement may be patients' self-reports. Although accuracy can be increased if the health professional approaches the patient in a nonthreatening way, for the most part, this type of measure has low credibility.

QUALITATIVE METHODS IN RESEARCH

Most health professionals, if exposed to research, have been exposed to empirical, experimental, or quantitative research described above. This type of research begins with a theoretically based hypothesis and emphasizes objectivity, prediction, and control, striving to separate the researcher and the subject so that specific values or bias of the research is eliminated as much as possible when gathering data and interpreting results. The hypothesis in quantitative research is confirmed or rejected through systematic investigation, manipulation, and analysis of some body of empirical data.

There are a number of instances, however, when experimental control is not possible and when strict experimental research design is not appropriate to study the particular question at hand. For example, Dr. Dean, who conducted patient education for patients undergoing chemotherapy, wanted to gain more understanding into patients' feelings and fears about chemotherapy, so he could gain more insight that could then be used to improve the patient education program. Although he could give patients a structured questionnaire, with questions developed from a variety of validated theories gleaned from the professional literature, the information would not provide him with the same depth of information regarding patients' feelings as if he talked with them directly and elicited their spontaneous remarks. In this case, use of more subjective, qualitative methods may be more appropriate.

To obtain this type of information, many behavioral and social sciences utilize an approach called *qualitative research* or *naturalistic inquiry* to study special areas of interest. Until recently, the credibility of qualitative research when applied to research issues in health care has been widely disputed. The usefulness, appropriateness, and applicability of qualitative methodology in research related to patient education and patient compliance is becoming more widely accepted.

Qualitative research differs from quantitative or experimental research not only in method but also in philosophy. Qualitative research is based on the premise that the nature of a variety of social phenomena is markedly complex, and only by in-depth investigation and integration of information can an accurate description of the phenomena result. Rather than beginning with a theory or hypothesis as in quantitative research, theoretical categories in qualitative research are developed from the data. Rather than beginning with a specific research question, the individual using qualitative research methods formulates the research questions as the study progresses. The premise is that all human behavior must be studied within the context of the social situation and the meaning of the behavior to the individual being studied. Consequently, qualitative research is nonmanipulative and descriptive, providing vivid details rather than fitting data into predetermined, standardized categories.

Qualitative research emphasizes a more subjective approach, is more intuitive, and is based on direct and vicarious experience. Qualitative research necessitates more direct interaction between the researcher and subject so that insight can be gained subjectively without necessarily separating facts and values.

In qualitative research, most data are drawn from direct communication with or observation of subjects. One of the most used devices for obtaining information is the interview, which can be used to identify relevant dimensions of the research questions of interest. Interviews can be structured so that the researcher predetermines questions or has an initial outline of the interview, or the interview can be informal, relying on the natural flow of conversation to elicit spontaneous information of relevance to the research question.

Data gathered by qualitative means are usually presented in more informal, narrative form. The researcher may present information through the use of case reports in which the opinions or responses of the subjects are described, rather than placing a numerical value on whether the majority of individuals felt strongly one way or the other.

COLLABORATION IN RESEARCH AND EVALUATION

If the health professional has limited training or experience in conducting research, using a consultant or working in collaboration with another individual with research skills and experience is desirable. The benefits of collaboration to both parties, and consequently to the field, are obvious.

If using consultants, it is usually important to involve them in the early stages of designing the study rather than waiting until all data are collected. In some instances, consultants may request a fee. In other instances, they may be willing to work as a coinvestigator and coauthor on any manuscripts resulting from the study. In either case, it is wise at the onset of the relationship to establish the role each person will play and to outline specific responsibilities each person will have. In order to benefit most from consultants, however, health professionals should have a clear idea of what they want to accomplish with the project.

MANAGING A RESEARCH PROJECT

Even a well-designed and well-planned research project does not run itself. Almost all research or evaluation, no matter how simple, requires some coordination. Depending on the nature of the project, other staff may be used for implementation of protocol, recruitment of subjects, or collection of data. Enlisting the cooperation of these individuals is crucial to a successful study. For example, Ms. Segel, a nurse, had developed a well-designed patient education study in which recruitment of subjects was to be done by the receptionist when the patient checked in for a physician visit. She told the receptionist what to do and assumed the protocol was being carried out. After a month, however, Ms. Segel grew concerned that the number of patients recruited for the project was so low. When she checked with the receptionist to see why she thought more patients were not agreeing to participate, Ms. Segel found that the receptionist had failed to follow the recruitment protocol in most instances, resenting what she considered extra work on her part and a disruption of patient flow.

To be successful, there must be a mechanism for quality control. Data must be recorded accurately and uniformly. If a number of different people are involved in data collection or data coding, the chance for error is great. Consequently, the health professional should make certain that people assisting understand the importance of accuracy. The accuracy of data collected and accuracy of coding should be randomly checked so that any systematic errors or errors of precision can be identified and corrected.

When attempting to gain cooperation from others, it is important to approach them with respect and sensitivity. No one likes to be ordered or threatened into participation. Health professionals should take time to explain the project and its purpose to all involved and clearly outline what is expected. Health professionals should be open to questions and suggestions and demonstrate appreciation for assistance received. There should be regular communication with all individuals involved with the project and updates of the study's progress.

SPECIFIC ISSUES IN PATIENT EDUCATION RESEARCH AND EVALUATION

Research and evaluation in patient education are means to determine the most effective way to provide patients with information about their condition, treatment, or ways to prevent disease or complications from disease. Research and evaluation in patient education also helps health professionals test and expand new ideas, test new theories, and determine the extent to which current patient education practices meet stated goals.

Research and evaluation are means by which patient education credibility and accountability can be established. Several issues are problematic, however, in research, evaluation, and interpretation of data in studies related to patient education. The first issue relates to the variation in definition of patient education in various studies. Patient education can be described in a variety of ways. It can be formal or informal; conducted in a group setting or on a one-to-one basis; or consist of passive patient participation such as use of audiovisual aids or written aids, or active patient participation such as use of self-directed learning through computerized patient education programs or return demonstrations. Although each of these interventions are patient education, techniques for each are different, each may be used separately or in combination, and each has different factors that may produce different results. Because there is no consistent definition of what constitutes patient education, there is no definitive way of interpreting results. For example, if Dr. Gephart were interested in determining whether patient education made a positive difference in blood pressure control of patients with hypertension, she may first survey the literature and evaluate the results. She would probably find a number of studies that used patient education about hypertension as a means of effecting blood pressure control but might also find it difficult to reach a conclusion. Some studies may consist of patient education about hypertension in a group setting, whereas others use an individualized approach. Others may test patient education materials or computer simulations about hypertension as a means of helping patients understand consequences of not following recommendations. Some studies may use a combination of patient education approaches. Comparisons between such different approaches cannot be made categorically. Each intervention has different variables that could influence results. For instance, the dynamic of a group setting is different from that of a health professional and patient on a one-to-one basis. Passive approaches, such as giving patients written materials to read, have a different impact than more active patient participation, which would occur in computer simulations. Consequently, although Dr. Gephart may find evidence in the literature that indicates that one form of patient education has been shown to be more effective than another, she would have difficulty finding definite proof that patient education per se made a positive difference in blood pressure control.

Another issue involves the wide variation of topics addressed by patient education. Patient education can be directed toward primary prevention such as immunization or secondary prevention such as reduction of risk of heart disease through helping patients learn about lowering cholesterol. Although both are topics addressing prevention, variables contained in each topic present different issues that could affect patient education effectiveness. Patient education may also be directed toward tertiary goals, such as controlling progress, symptoms or complications of disease.

Another problem regarding interpretation of results of research and evaluation in patient education relates to defining outcome. Generally, education may be said to be effective if learning has taken place; however, learning in patient education may also be defined broadly. Learning may be defined as knowledge acquisition or as expressed changes in attitudes. In other instances, learning may be defined as skill acquisition or ultimately as readily observable behavioral change. In some instances, outcome is defined as the degree of patient compliance. In each of these cases, patient education effectiveness is determined by specific outcomes as defined by the health professional. However, might an acceptable patient education outcome also be patients choosing not to follow recommendations when based on their own values and informed choice?

A third problem in interpreting results from research and evaluation in patient education relates to the inconsistency of methods used to assess patient education effectiveness. In some instances, effectiveness has been assessed through patients' written or oral responses to questions developed by the health professional or some other source. In other instances, direct observation of patient skill in performing a task or of other behavior has been used as a method of assessment. In each of these instances, there may be inconsistent definitions of what constituted a "successful" or "effective" intervention. For example, must the patient score 100 percent of items on a questionnaire correctly in order for the intervention to be considered effective, or is the difference in the score prior to the intervention and after the intervention the method of measurement used? If the method of assessment is patient compliance, how is the compliance measured? Is the health professional able to observe the patient's behavior directly, such as in appointment keeping, or in other instances must the health professional rely on patients' self-reports? Can the patient's health status be used as a reliable assessment of the success or effectiveness of a patient education intervention?

Not only are methods of assessing patient education effectiveness often inconsistent, there are also problems related to timing of measurements. Although a specific patient education intervention may be found to be effective in the immediate period following the intervention, would the same benefits be present if measured longitudinally? Another problem relates to the practicality of patient education programs or interventions that are tested and/or evaluated. Even if a specific patient education intervention is shown to be effective in a particular setting, if its complexity and cost would preclude its subsequent implementation in a wider number of settings, then the findings are of little benefit.

In research and evaluation, the patient education intervention, as well as outcomes to be measured, must be defined with precision so that results can be more accurately interpreted. Detailed explanation of research or evaluation methods used is also important so that those who wish to replicate the study or apply the intervention to their own practice may do so.

SPECIFIC ISSUES IN PATIENT COMPLIANCE RESEARCH

Although considerable time and effort have been and continue to be spent studying patient compliance and variables that affect it, there is still little definitive information that would enable the health professional to ensure patient compliance in all areas for all patients. Major questions remain unanswered and warrant further research. First, although compliance is influenced by a variety of psychological and socioeconomic variables, little is known about how these variables may be changed by treatment management. Second, even interventions that have been shown to have a positive influence over compliance in the short term may not be as effective over time. Longitudinal research should be conducted for increasing understanding of compliance to long-term treatment regimens for chronic conditions. Likewise, little is known about change in compliance rates for the same individual as a result of progressing to different life stages. Longitudinal studies of individuals could identify potential barriers to patient compliance that may be shared by a number of individuals at different stages of life.

Most emphasis has been placed on studying interventions to increase compliance; however, much might also be learned from ineffective interventions by examining them closely to establish why they did not work. In addition, although there appear to be no specific demographic variables that can be used to predict compliance behavior, it may be valuable to study in more detail issues related to noncompliance in an effort to increase understanding of the concept, thereby guiding efforts to improve it.

A number of issues are also problematic in patient compliance research. As in the case of patient education, the definition of patient compliance must also be precise and unambiguous as well as appropriate to the research setting. Inconsistency of findings in patient compliance research relates to a great extent to the inconsistency in definition of the term. There are many forms and levels of compliance. If, for example, the researcher is interested in compliance with appointments, does this mean those initiated by the patient, follow-up appointments initiated by the health professional, or both? Variables that impact on patient compliance are different for each. Health professionals conducting patient compliance research must be aware of the importance of defining terms clearly so that others who wish to replicate the work or use the results in practical application will be able to do so without difficulty.

Difficulty in interpretation of research results may be related to measurement of compliance both in degree and at different levels. For example, to be considered compliant, does the patient need to follow recommendations 100% of the time or is the standard for compliance set at a lower percentage level? What percentage of time must the patient follow recommendations to be considered compliant or noncompliant? Is the patient considered compliant if they follow some of the recommendations but not all of them? For how long must the patient continue to follow treatment recommendations? Are they considered compliant if they follow all the recommendations but do so incorrectly? Will follow-up of compliance be conducted? How long does the patient need to follow recommendations to be considered compliant? For instance, an intervention to increase compliance may have different results if applied to patients with acute conditions rather than chronic conditions.

Another issue in compliance research is how compliance is measured. Compliance measures must be appropriate to the research question being investigated as well as appropriate to the recommendations and the setting. Indirect measures of patient compliance, such as self-report, are probably the least costly but are also the least accurate. More direct measures, such as direct observation or results of laboratory tests, are more accurate but more costly and difficult to accomplish. For example, research on patient compliance with taking a pre-scribed medication may use the direct measure of blood samples to assess com-pliance, however such a measure cannot be obtained for research purposes without the knowledge and permission of the patient. If the patient knows that their compliance is being monitored, how much does this knowledge alone impact on the degree to which they follow recommendations?

Consideration of ethical issues should be inherent in any research. In patient compliance research, there are two relatively unique problems that must be con-fronted. First, if patients as research subjects are fully informed about the purpose of the study, there is a potential for biasing results. Is it ever appropriate to not fully disclose to patients the purpose of the study in order to gain more accurate information about compliance? Second, are strategies that are designed to alter patient compliance in and of themselves ethical to apply? Is investigation of strate-gies that are designed to manipulate patients into behavior appropriate, or should strategies be directed to finding the most appropriate means to help patients make informed and rational choices based on their own goals and values?

How to determine the most effective way to increase compliance causes con-cern for many health professionals. Given research from the past 25 years, how-ever, it appears that one of the most effective ways to increase compliance might also be in keeping with the goals of patient education—that of formation of a partnership between patient and health professional to facilitate communica-tion and decide upon a plan that can help them both attain their goal, that of improved health status.

FUTURE DIRECTIONS FOR RESEARCH

The proliferation of patient education materials and expansion of patient edu-cation programs attest to the belief that information about prevention, as well as about diseases and treatments used to cure and control them, is important to the provision of good health care. In this proliferation of materials and efforts to educate the patient, an underlying perception that patients, given factual information designed to help them, will incorporate the information into their lives. This, of course, is not always the case. The fallacy that merely providing patients with comprehensive information is sufficient to bring about significant educational impact can be best alleviated through well-designed and well-con-trolled research that investigates the effectiveness of a variety of different patient education interventions for different medical conditions. The impact patient education has on patient outcomes both in terms of prevention and control of disease as well as patients' health status and perceived well-being must be care-fully studied and evaluated. In addition, the role patient education has in reducing health care cost as well as human cost related to illness and disability warrants further intensive investigation.

As the field of patient education grows and more technologies and methods for delivering effective patient education are developed, it behooves both practitioners and academicians to continue to search for ways to improve and maintain the quality and accountability of practices used. This is best accomplished by sound research and evaluation, the results of which are directed toward not only maintaining credibility regarding the usefulness of patient education, but also ensuring that patient education interventions continue to be sound and feasible means that contribute to higher-quality health care.

INDEX